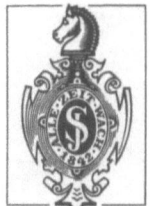

Y. Yoshida
T. Yamaguchi C.G. Caro S. Glagov R.M. Nerem (Eds.)

Role of Blood Flow in Atherogenesis

Proceedings of the International Symposium,
Hyogo, October 1987

With 169 Figures and 10 Tables

Springer-Verlag
Tokyo Berlin Heidelberg New York London Paris

Prof. Dr. YOJI YOSHIDA
Department of Pathology, Yamanashi Medical College
Tamaho, 409-38 Japan

Dr. TAKAMI YAMAGUCHI
Department of Vascular Physiology
National Cardiovascular Center Research Institute
Suita, 565 Japan

Prof. Dr. COLIN G. CARO
Physiological Flow Studies Unit, Imperial College
London, SW7 2AZ, England

Prof. Dr. SEYMOUR GLAGOV
Department of Pathology, University of Chicago
Chicago, IL 60637, USA

Prof. Dr. ROBERT M. NEREM
Biomechanics Laboratory and School of Mechanical Engineering
Georgia Institute of Technology
Atlanta, GA 30332-0405, USA

ISBN-13: 978-4-431-68401-5   e-ISBN-13: 978-4-431-68399-5
DOI: 10.1007/978-4-431-68399-5

Organization

Host

The Organizing Committee of the International Symposium on the Role of Blood Flow in Atherogenesis and the Japan Heart Foundation

Sponsors

Japan Atherosclerosis Society, Japanese College of Angiology, Japanese Society of Biorheology, and the British Council

Organizing Committee

Honorary President

H. Manabe, National Cardiovascular Center, Osaka, Japan

Advisory Board

C.G. Caro, Imperial College, London, England

S. Glagov, University of Chicago, Chicago, USA

R.M. Nerem, Georgia Institute of Technology, Atlanta, USA

T. Azuma, Juntendo University, Tokyo, Japan

Y. Nimura, National Cardiovascular Center, Osaka, Japan

T. Omae, National Cardiovascular Center, Osaka, Japan

G. Ooneda, Gunma University, Maebashi, Japan

T. Takeuchi, Yamanashi Medical College, Yamanashi, Japan

K. Tanaka, Kyushu University, Fukuoka, Japan

Conference Committee

Chairman: Y. Yoshida (Yamanashi Medical College, Yamanashi)

Members of Committee: T. Fukushima (Shinshu University, Matsumoto); F. Kajiya (Kawasaki Medical School, Okayama); A. Kamiya (Hokkaido University, Sapporo); A. Kitabatake (Osaka University, Osaka); H. Masuda (Akita University, Akita); M. Mitsumata (Yamanashi Medical College, Yamanashi); S. Murota (Tokyo Medical and Dental University, Tokyo); N. Sakata (Fukuoka University, Fukuoka); M. Sato (Tsukuba University, Ibaraki); K. Sueishi (Kyushu University, Fukuoka); T. Takano (Teikyo University, Kanagawa); H. Ueda (National Cardiovascular Center, Osaka); T. Yamaguchi (National Cardiovascular Center, Osaka); C. Yutani (National Cardiovascular Center, Osaka)

Scientific Secretaries: General, T. Yamaguchi (National Cardiovascular Center, Osaka); S. Hanai (National Cardiovascular Center, Osaka); M. Mitsumata (Yamanashi Medical College, Yamanashi)

Foreword

As the honorary president of the organizing committee, it is my great pleasure and honor to be able to contribute to the Proceedings of the International Symposium on the Role of Blood Flow in Atherogenesis.

Diseases related to atherosclerosis, particularly coronary heart diseases, have long been the leading cause of death in most westernized societies. Those diseases have recently become one of the leading cause of death in Japan, too. It is almost certain that changes in the environment and life-style which have occurred in the past 20-30 years are responsible for this phenomenon in Japan. This is why the National Cardiovascular Center, over which I preside, and the Ministry of Health and Welfare are very keen to support collaborative studies in the fields of atherosclerosis and related cardiovascular diseases.

One such collaborative study group, chaired by Prof. Yoji Yoshida, represents the core of the organizing committee of this symposium. This is a unique group composed of scientists selected from many different fields, including pathology, physiology, chemistry, and engineering. This group has carried out excellent research on the mechanisms of the initiation, development, and localization of atherosclerosis with respect to the fluid mechanics of blood flow.

I am delighted to see such a fruitful symposium being held at the end of the 3-year collaborative study program with the participation of leading scientists in this interdisciplinary field. I was truly impressed by the active discussions held in the sessions involving scientists from all over the world. I have the greatest belief that our understanding about the disease will progress considerably as a result of this symposium and these proceedings will be of immense help to those who could not attend.

HISAO MANABE
Honorary President
Organizing Committee

Preface

It has long been recognized that atherosclerosis tends to develop in particular areas of the artery. Thus, blood flow is considered to play an important role in such development. The direct mechanism of the influence of blood flow on atherosclerosis is, however, controversial. A number of studies in this field have been carried out in Japan in the past few years, the most recent being a team project organized by the Cardiovascular Center in 1985 under the sponsorship of the Japan Ministry of Health and Welfare. In this the final year of the project, members of the project team, in collaboration with active investigators in the field, invited top scientists from around the world to a symposium in Japan to discuss "The Role of Blood Flow in Atherogenesis." It is to be hoped that the discussions held during the symposium as well as the actual results of the studies presented will provide new insights into our understanding of atherosclerosis.

I would like to thank once again the people who made the symposium possible, particularly Profs. C.G. Caro, S. Glagov, and R.M. Nerem of the International Advisory Board, the Organizing Committee presided over by Dr. Hisao Manabe, all speakers, chairmen, and participants. I would also like to extend my sincere gratitude to all the sponsoring organizations, including the pharmaceutical and other companies, who made generous contributions to help meet the financial obligations of the symposium held at Green Pia Miki in Hyogo, Japan.

YOJI YOSHIDA
Chairman
Organizing Committee

Acknowledgments

The Organizing Committee gratefully acknowledges the support of the following:

Banyu Pharmaceutical Co., Ltd.; Bayer Yakuhin, Ltd.; Beecham Yakuhin K.K.; Carl Zeiss Co., Ltd.; Chugai Pharmaceutical Co., Ltd.; Ciba-Geigy (Japan) Limited; Daiichi Seiyaku Co., Ltd.; Dainippon Pharmaceutical Co., Ltd.; Eisai Co., Ltd.; Farmitalia Carlo Erba K.K.; Fuji Chemical Industry Co., Ltd.; Fujisawa Pharmaceutical Co., Ltd.; Fukujin Co., Ltd.; Funai Pharmaceutical Co., Ltd.; Fuso Pharmaceutical Industries, Ltd.; Grelan Pharmaceutical Co., Ltd.; Hoei Pharmaceutical Co., Ltd.; Iwaki Seiyaku Co., Ltd.; Japan Upjohn Ltd.; Kaken Pharmaceutical Co., Ltd.; Kanebo Ltd.; Kanebo Pharmaceuticals, Ltd.; Kirin Brewery Co., Ltd.; Kissei Pharmaceuticals Co., Ltd.; Kowa Company, Ltd.; Kowa Shinyaku Co., Ltd.; Kuraya Pharmaceutical Co., Ltd.; Kyorin Pharmaceutical Co., Ltd.; Kyowa Hakko Kogyo Co., Ltd.; Maruho Co., Ltd.; Maruishi Pharmaceutical Co., Ltd.; Meiji Seika Kaisha, Ltd.; Mochida Pharmaceutical Co., Ltd.; Mohan Medicine Research Institute; Morisita Pharmaceutical Co., Ltd.; Nagai Co., Ltd.; Nihon Pharmaceutical Co., Ltd.; Nihon Schering K.K.; Nikken Chemicals Co., Ltd.; Nippon Boehringer Ingelheim Co., Ltd.; Nippon Chemiphar Co., Ltd.; Nippon Glaxo Co., Ltd.; Nippon Kayaku Co.,.Ltd.; Nippon Sherwood Medical Industries Ltd.; Nippon Shinyaku Co., Ltd.; Omori Yakuhin Co., Ltd.; Ono Pharmaceutical Co., Ltd.; Osaka Pharmaceutical Manufacturers Association; Otsuka Pharmaceutical Co., Ltd.; Otsuka Pharmaceutical Factory, Inc.; Pfizer Taito Co., Ltd.; Sandoz Pharmaceuticals, Ltd.; Sankyo Co., Ltd.; Santen Pharmaceutical Co., Ltd.; Sanwa Kagaku Kenkyusho Co., Ltd.; Sato Pharmaceutical Co., Ltd.; Sawai Pharmaceutical Co., Ltd.; Searle Yakuhin K.K.; Shin Osaka Shokai Co., Ltd.; Shionogi & Co., Ltd; Shiraimatsu & Co., Ltd.; Showayakuhinkako Co., Ltd.; Squibb Japan Inc.; SS Pharmaceutical Co., Ltd.; Sumitomo Pharmaceutical Co., Ltd.; Taiho Pharmaceutical Co., Ltd.; Taisyo Pharmaceutical Co., Ltd.; Takeda Chemical Industries, Ltd.; Tanabe Seiyaku Co., Ltd.; TEAC Corporation; Teikoku Hormone MFG. Co., Ltd.; Teysan Pharmaceuticals Co., Ltd.; The Green Cross Corporation; The Life Insurance Association of Japan; The Pharmaceutical Manufacturers Association of Tokyo; Tobishi Pharmaceutical Co., Ltd.; Tokyo Garasu Kikai Co., Ltd.; Tokyo Tanabe Co., Ltd.; Torii & Co., Ltd.; Toyama Chemical Co., Ltd.; Toyo Jozo Co., Ltd.; Toyota Motor Corporation; Tsumura Juntendo, Inc.; Wakamoto Pharmaceutical Co., Ltd.; Warner-Lambert K.K.; Yakult Central Institute for Microbiological Research; Yamanouchi Pharmaceutical Co.. Ltd.; Yoshitomi Pharmaceutical Industries, Ltd.; Yufu Itonaga Co., Ltd.; Zeria Pharmaceutical Co., Ltd.

Contents

Chapter 1
Fundamental Observations on Human and Animal Atherosclerosis

Chapter 2
Fluid Mechanics of Blood Flow in Atherogenesis

Chapter 3
Cellular or Tissue Reactions to Blood Flow

Chapter 4
Transport Phenomena and Underlying Mechanism of Atherogenesis

List of Contributors

The page numbers given below refer to the page on which contribution begins.

ANDO, J., Hokkaido University, Japan 195

ASAI, M., Keio University, Japan 139

ASAKURA, T., Montreal General Hospital, Canada 67

CARO, C.G., Imperial College, England 215

CERVÓS-NAVARRO, J., Freie Universität Berlin, Germany 19

CHIEN, S., Columbia University Medical School, USA 253

DAVIES, P.F., Harvard University Medical School, USA 201

DEWEY, Jr., C.F., Massachusetts Institute of Technology, USA 201

DUTTA, A., The Pennsylvania State University, USA 103

ERIKSON, U., Uppsala University, Sweden 123

FRIEDMAN, M.H., The Johns Hopkins University, USA 41

FUCHS, L., The Royal Institute of Technology, Sweden 123

FUJII, K., Osaka University, Japan 179

FUJIWARA, T., Kawasaki Medical School, Japan 117

FUKUSHIMA, T., Shinshu University, Japan 11, 81

FUKUZAKI, H., Kobe University, Japan 245

GIDDENS, D.P., Georgia Institute of Technology, USA 3, 63, 73, 185

GIMBRONE, Jr., M.A., Harvard University Medical School, USA 201

GLAGOV, S., University of Chicago, USA 3, 63, 73, 185

GOTLIEB, A.I., University of Toronto, Canada 157

HAMADA, M., Wakayama Medical College, Japan 217

HANAI, S., National Cardiovascular Center, Japan 109

HARAKAWA, K., Shinshu University, Japan 81

HASHIDA, R., Teikyo University, Japan 231

HATANI, M., Kobe University, Japan 245

HOMMA, T., Shinshu University, Japan 11, 81

HORI, M., Osaka University, Japan 179

IMAKITA, M., National Cardiovascular Center, Japan 25

ISHIBASHI-UEDA, H., National Cardiovascular Center, Japan 25

ISHIHARA, K., Osaka University, Japan 179

ISHIKAWA, C., Hokkaido University, Japan 195

ISHIKAWA, Y., Kobe University, Japan 245

ITO, H., Osaka University, Japan 179

KAJIYA, F., Kawasaki Medical School, Japan 117

KAMADA, T., Osaka University, Japan 179

KAMIYA, A., Hokkaido University, Japan 195

KANAZAWA, S., Kawasaki Medical School, Japan 117

KARINO, T., Montreal General Hospital, Canada 67

KASHIHARA, M., Taoka Hospital, Japan 19, 205

KATO, K., Tokyo Medical and Dental University, Japan 223

KAWAI, H., Kanegafuchi Chemical Industry Co., Ltd., Japan 131

KAWAMURA, K., Akita University, Japan 163, 171

KIM, D.W., University of Toronto, Canada 157

KITABATAKE, A., Osaka University, Japan 179

KLANCHAR, M., The Pennsylvania State University, USA 103

KOMATSUDA, T., Hokkaido University, Japan 195

KU, D.N., Georgia Institute of Technology, USA 3, 63, 73

KUSUYAMA, Y., Wakayama Medical College, Japan 217

LANGILLE, B.L., University of Toronto, Canada 157

LEVER, M.J., Imperial College, England 237

LEVESQUE, M.J., Georgia Institute of Technology, USA 189

LIEPSCH, D., The Eisenhower Medical Center, USA 91

MABUCHI, S., Montreal General Hospital, Canada 67

MASUDA, H., Akita University, Japan 163, 171

MASUYAMA, Y., Wakayama Medical College, Japan 217

MATSUMOTO, K., The University of Tokushima, Japan 19, 205

MATSUOKA, S., Kawasaki Medical School, Japan 117

MINEO, C., Teikyo University, Japan 231

MITSUMATA, M., Yamanashi Medical College, Japan 33

MIYAZAKI, N., Kobe University, Japan 245

MORAVEC, S., Fachhochschule München, Germany 91

MORITA, I., Tokyo Medical and Dental University, Japan 223

MUKODANI, J., Kobe University, Japan 245

MUROTA, S., Tokyo Medical and Dental University, Japan 223

NAKAGAMI, K., Teikyo University, Japan 231

NAKAZATO, K., Keio University, Japan 139

NARUSE, T., Keio University, Japan 139

NEREM, R.M., Georgia Institute of Technology, USA 153, 189

NEWMAN, D.L., Royal Melbourne Institute of Technology, Australia 209

NISHIO, I., Wakayama Medical College, Japan 217

NISHIYAMA, A., The Jikei Univesity School of Medicine, Japan 55

OGASAWARA, Y., Kawasaki Medical School, Japan 117

OHBA, K., Kansai University, Japan 145

OHKUMA, S., Teikyo University, Japan 231

OHYAMA, N., The Jikei University School of Medicine, Japan 55

OKAMOTO, R., Kobe University, Japan 245

OKAMURA, T., The Jikei University School of Medicine, Japan 55

OONEDA, G., Geriatrics Research Institute and Hospital, Japan 33

OYAMA, T., Yamanashi Medical College, Japan 33

PEDLEY, T.J., University of Cambridge, England 97

PFEFFER, R., The City University of New York, USA 253

POLL, A., Eisenhower Medical Center, USA 91

RALPH, M.E., University of Cambridge, England 97

SAKAGUCHI, S., Kansai University, Japan 145

SAKATA, N., Fukuoka University, Japan 11

SATO, MAKOTO, Kansai University, Japan 145

SATO, MASAAKI, University of Tsukuba, Japan 189

SAWADA, T., Keio University, Japan 131

SHOZAWA, T., Akita University, Japan 163, 171

SKALAK, R., Columbia University, USA 261

SMEDBY, O., Uppsala University, Sweden 123

STEHBENS, W.E., Wellington School of Medicine, New Zealand 47

TAKAICHI, S., National Cardiovascular Center, Japan 25

TAKANO, S., Kobe University, Japan 245

TAKANO, T., Teikyo University, Japan 231

TAKEBAYASHI, S., Fukuoka University, Japan 11

TANAHASHI, T., Keio University, Japan 131

TANIGUCHI, T., Kobe University, Japan 245

TANISHITA, K., Keio University, Japan 139

TANOUCHI, J., Osaka University, Japan 179

TARBELL, J.M., The Pennsylvania State University, USA 103

TOHDA, K., Akita University, Japan 163, 171

TOMINAGA, N., Osaka University, Japan 179

TSUJIOKA, K., Kawasaki Medical School, Japan 117

TSUKITANI, M., Kobe Univesity, Japan 245

TSUNEMITSU, M., Kobe University, Japan 245

TUTTY, O.R., University of Southampton, England 97

UEDA, S. The University of Tokushima, Japan 205

UEMATSU, M., Osaka University, Japan 179

URA, M., Wakayama Medical College, Japan 217

WANG, S., Yamanashi Medical College, Japan 33

WATANABE, N., Kobe University, Japan 245

WEINBAUM, S., The City University of New York, USA 253

WENN, C.M., Royal Melbourne Institute of Technology, Australia 209

YAGYU-MIZUNO, Y., Teikyo University, Japan 231

YAMAGUCHI, T., National Cardiovascular Center, Japan 33, 109

YAMAMOTO, A., National Cardiovascular Center, Japan 25

YAMANE, T., Yamanashi Medical College, Japan 33

YOSHIDA, Yoji, Yamanashi Medical College, Japan 33

YOSHIDA, YUTAKA, Osaka University, Japan 179

YOSHIKAWA, H., Wakayama Medical College, Japan 217

YOSHIMURA, H., Nippon Zoki Pharmaceutical Co., Ltd., Japan 179

YUTANI, C., National Cardiovascular Center, Japan 25

ZARINS, C.K., University of Chicago, USA 3, 63, 73, 185

Chapter 1
Fundamental Observations on Human and Animal Atherosclerosis

Establishing the Hemodynamic Determinants of Human Plaque Configuration, Composition and Complication

S. Glagov[1], C.K. Zarins[2], D.P. Giddens[3], and D.N. Ku[3]

[1]Department of Pathology, University of Chicago, Chicago, IL 60637, USA
[2]Department of Surgery, University of Chicago, Chicago, IL 60637, USA
[3]The School of Mechanical Engineering, Georgia Institute of Technology, Atlanta, GA 30332-0405, USA

ABSTRACT

We now have sound information concerning the distribution of intimal thickenings and atherosclerotic plaques at clinically important sites in humans. Low and/or oscillatory wall shear stress are the associated hemodynamic conditions at these locations. It is also evident that artery walls may compensate for hemodynamic changes and for the development of atherosclerotic disease and maintain lumen diameters and configurations consistent with adequate flow. Obstruction occurs when the adaptive processes do not keep pace with plaque enlargement or when plaques are disrupted. Future investigations must therefore include studies of plaque growth and composition in relation to variations in geometric configuration, pulse rate and flow velocity. Until the disease can be prevented it is necessary to identify those features of plaque composition and configuration which underlie susceptibility to instability and to characterize the hemodynamic and other mechanical circumstances which may induce plaque disruption and those which favor the maintenance of an adequate and stable channel. Such studies place renewed emphasis on the fact that the artery wall and the atherosclerotic plaque are living tissues, capable of healing and adaptive restructuring as well as degeneration and disruption.

INTRODUCTION

The papers presented at the opening session of the International Symposium on the Role of Blood Flow in Atherogenesis had as a common theme the distribution of human intimal thickenings and atherosclerotic plaques in relation to position in the arterial tree and about specific geometric configurations where flow field characteristics may be determined and correlated with precise plaque localization. Flow patterns in specific human vessels and in relation to configurational features associated with lesions were described also in Session II. On the basis of image analysis techniques, topographical studies of adequately prepared human material, and measurements in models of human vessels, conclusions have been drawn concerning the hemodynamic conditions which may either favor or inhibit plaque formation or the development of predisposing or precursor intimal changes. In general, departures from unidirectional, laminar and symmetrical flow profiles are considered to induce or at least to potentiate the induction of plaques. In particular, the data from adult human carotid and aortic studies indicate that atherosclerotic plaques tend to occur in regions of low and/or oscillating wall shear stress, while relatively high shear rates and unidirectional, laminar flow patterns such as those which occur at or near flow dividers tend to be associated with sparing [1-3]. The special propensity of coronary arteries to become atherosclerotic has been associated with features of flow variation in these vessels during the cardiac cycle. The coronary arteries are exposed to greater fluctuations in flow direction and amplitude during systole than are other systemic arteries and increases in heart rate result in decreased diastolic time while systolic time remains nearly constant. Individual differences in the relative involvement of the coronary arteries compared to other vessels in the same arterial tree have therefore been attributed to differences in heart rate. Both experimental [4] and clinical [5] studies tend to indicate that elevated heart rate is a risk factor for coronary artery disease.

ADAPTIVE REACTIVITY OF ARTERIES

It does not however follow from these considerations that intimal thickening, per se, in regions of departure from laminar flow, or where flow velocity and/or direction are altered, is necessarily evidence of vessel injury, incipient atherogenesis or inevitable progression to stenosis. Intimal reactions such as advanced atherosclerosis and obstructive intimal hyperplasia underlie clinically significant interferences with flow, but well organized focal and diffuse fibrocellular intimal thickenings occur frequently without occlusion or lipid accumulation (Fig. 1A). These changes appear to be related to hemodynamic stimuli, suggesting that they represent adaptive reactions, regulated in such a manner as to maintain levels of mechanical stress consistent with normal function. Increased flow velocity has been shown to result in artery enlargement until baseline shear stress levels of about 15 dynes/cm^2 are restored [6,7]. Artery enlargement could result in intimal thickening in order to reestablish normal levels of tensile stress. Conversely, reduced flow velocity could stimulate intimal thickening to reduce effective diameter and increase wall shear stress to more normal levels. Such intimal reactions are most often self-

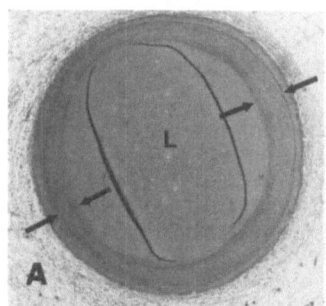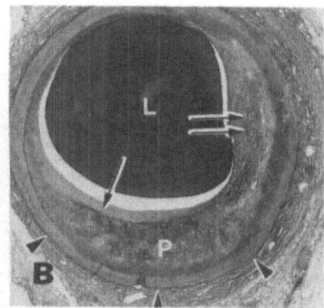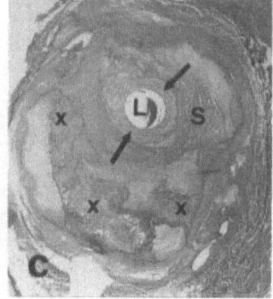

Figure 1. Sections of human coronary arteries. A-Diffuse circumferential fibrocellular intimal thickening (arrows). This is not an atherosclerotic plaque and is not necessarily the site of future plaque formation or stenosis. The lumen (L) contains a gelatin mass introduced during controlled pressure-fixation. B-Characteristic eccentric atherosclerotic plaque (P) with evidence of compensatory artery enlargement as well as sequestration of the plaque by outward bulging of the media beneath the plaque (arrowheads) and a well formed fibrous cap (arrow) of about the same thickness as the media. A zone of dense intimal sclerosis (double arrow) is also noted. The lumen (L) remains nearly circular. C-Advanced, complex plaque which almost totally occludes the still circular lumen (L) and contains zones of sclerosis (S) and calcification (X) as well as a circumferential fibrocellular zone (arrows) about the lumen.

limiting in venous or arterial bypass grafts, at anastomoses between vessels or between vessels and prosthetic grafts, and about geometric modifications associated with radial and/or axial artery enlargement and tortuosity. Changes in pressure or outflow resistance are also associated with intimal thickening.

Even advanced and extensive atherosclerotic disease may be associated with artery enlargement, widely patent artery lumens and persistence of adequate flow (Fig. 1B). Recent studies reveal that, on the average, coronary arteries tend to enlarge with increasing plaque cross-sectional area [8]. Not until about 40% or more of the potential lumen area is occupied by plaque does there seem to be a transition to progressive lumen narrowing. In addition, despite the formation of complex, eccentric plaques, lumen shape nearly always remains circular (Fig. 1B) or slightly oval [9]. The impression that uncomplicated plaques bulge into the lumen on cross-section is nearly always based on artefacts of preparation. Modelling of the plaque, incorporation and organization of mural thrombi (Fig. 2B), and development of a circumferentially structured fibrous cap are also suggestive of adaptive reactions designed to restore and maintain optimal conditions for adequate, laminar flow for as long as possible. Plaque disruption or ulceration is a major critical complication for it may result in the exposure of plaque components to the circulation (Fig. 2A), thereby engendering occlusive and/or embolizing thrombi and may also be associated with sudden obstructions due to plaque hemorrhage even when plaques are not markedly stenotic. Even marked disruptions may undergo remodelling leaving defects suggesting healed or restructured walls (Fig. 2C). Thus, eventual critical lumen narrowing (Fig. 1C) and/or plaque complication (Fig. 2A) at one or a few critically located lesions are the significant determinants of clinically manifest ischemia rather than plaque size per se. Despite the apparent capability of arteries to compensate for hemodynamic deviations both focal and regional in order to maintain mural integrity and stability, arteries do become obstructed and in some cases aneurysmal and fragile. The nature and limits of arterial adaptability therefore need to be defined, particularly in relation to hemodynamic and other mechanical forces.

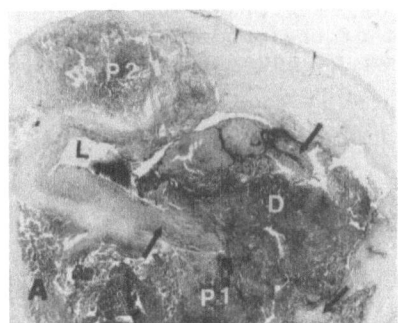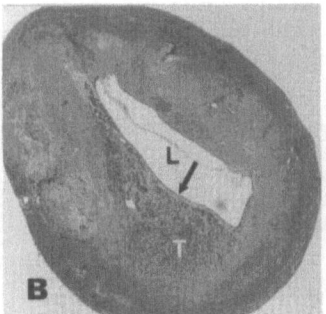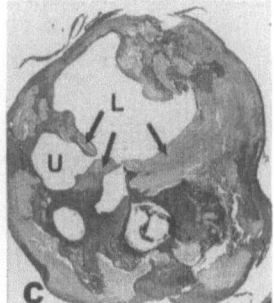

Figure 2. Endarterectomy specimens. A-Proximal internal carotid artery. Disruption (ulceration) of a plaque (P1) results in extrusion of plaque debris (D) into the lumen (L) across the breached remnants of the fibrous cap (arrows). Another plaque (P2) has also eroded its fibrous cap. B-Thrombus (T) organized and incorporated into the wall of a coronary artery. A thin fibrous cap (arrow) has formed between the thrombus and the lumen (L). C-Internal carotid artery. Defects (U) within the complex plaque connect with the lumen (L). They are in all likelihood healed disruptions or ulcerations. Remnants of the fibrous cap (arrow) remain.

MECHANISMS OF PLAQUE TRANSITION

In consideration of the evidence a) that the initial fatty streak may be reversible, b) that the complex, fibrous plaque is the potentially harmful lesion, c) that little is known regarding the pathogenetic relationship between fatty streak and fibrous plaque or between diffuse intimal thickening and eccentric plaque formation, and d) that complex plaques differ in composition and architecture and probably in rate of development in different locations (Figs. 1 and 2), evaluation of the relationship between hemodynamic factors and atherogenesis must extend beyond considerations of plaque localization and initiation alone. If we are to approach the mechanisms which underlie the focal and regional propensities for plaque formation and particularly for plaque occlusion and complication in human arteries, we will need to understand how specific mechanical forces associated with blood circulation influence not only the form and function of artery cells and the occurrence of intimal thickening but also how these forces influence the architecture, composition and evolution of plaques. Suggestions have been forthcoming from investigations conducted in cell culture, utilizing systems designed to subject cells to measureable degrees of mechanical stress. These studies provide data of interest with respect to cell biology and may furnish clues to the manner in which mechanical forces modify the function of artery cells and could affect the architecture and composition of blood vessel walls and plaques [10]. These data should however direct us to devise corresponding studies in arteries designed to probe the mechanisms by which human arteries adapt to alterations in flow and pressure and cope with the occurrence and enlargement of atherosclerotic lesions. Application of current techniques to the study of the natural history of plaques should permit us to delineate the degree to which mechanical factors influence plaque composition and growth and determine whether plaques stabilize or disrupt or whether stenoses or aneurysms develop.

QUANTIFYABLE FEATURES OF ATHEROSCLEROSIS

In order to proceed with such studies, it follows that we need to distinguish among the relevant features of atherosclerosis which are subject to quantitation when we describe changes which may be related to hemodynamic conditions [9]. The extent of the process may be defined as the degree of involvement of a given expanse of lumen surface.

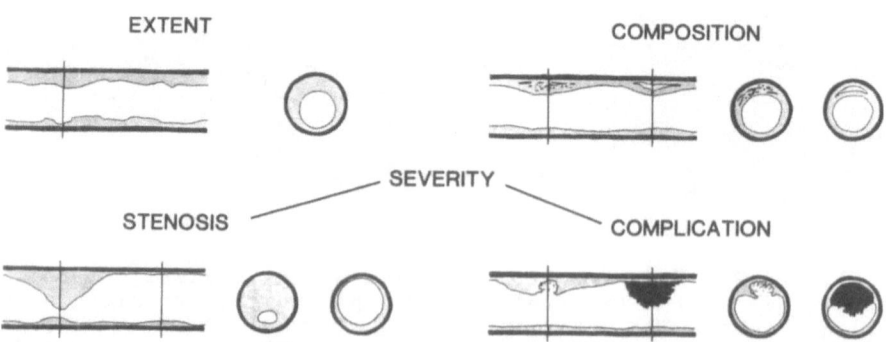

Figure 3. Diagrammatic representation of plaque features which require detailed quantitative study in order to identify those hemodynamic and other mechanical variables which determine lesion stability and those which favor stenosis and complication. "Intimal thickening" may not per se provide information which implies an actual or ultimate disease state.

and/or as the number of arteries in a particular vascular region involved by plaques (Fig. 3). Severity is a term with direct clinical implications and is determined by the actual or potential interference with flow. Thus, regardless of the extent of involvement, critical lumen narrowing and plaque complication are the significant determinants of clinical severity rather than percent stenosis (Fig. 3). Percent stenosis is usually evaluated from angiograms by comparing the diameter of a narrowed lumen segment on axial projection with a presumably uninvolved or less involved adjacent region. Although the absolute diameter at the narrowing is likely to be the best index of the degree of actual or potential obstruction to flow, it is not a reliable indicator of the extent of the disease process. The presumably uninvolved segment is often the site of advanced disease, despite an apparently adequate lumen. Widely patent lumens may actually be associated with larger plaques than are present in the immediately adjacent narrowed segment [11]. Nor is there adequate information on angiograms concerning the composition of plaques, either in the narrowed or relatively wide segment. Newer means of in vivo visualization promise to provide sufficient resolution and discrimination to establish plaque and wall thickness, cross-sectional area and density, and should permit better clinical studies of plaque growth rate and plaque composition. Histological preparations of artery cross-sections do provide reliable information on artery size, as well as on plaque area, composition and the distribution of plaque components, provided that the vessels are prepared with sufficient attention to fixation under conditions of distention by suitable levels of intraluminal pressure. In such material per cent stenosis is defined as the extent to which the area encompassed by the internal elastic lamina is occupied by plaque, assuming that the internal elastica area represents the potential lumen area. Since these data are available only for the particular plane of section, three dimensional reconstructions from sequential sections will be required in order to provide new knowledge concerning plaque organization and the precise location of areas vulnerable to disruption. These features should then be related in to geometry and to presumed or measured flow field characteristics. Although the topography of lesion components and the nature of lesion complication are difficult to delineate with reasonable degrees of confidence from angiograms, more precise visualization methods and methods for simultaneous flow measurements are in the offing.

HEMODYNAMICS AND PLAQUE STABILITY

Susceptibility to disruption, fracture or fissuring of a plaque is likely to be associated with plaque structure, composition and consistency. Thus, plaques may be relatively soft and pliable, friable or cohesive, densely sclerotic or calcific and brittle. Some have well formed fibrous caps, similar in architecture and thickness to a normal artery wall, thereby effectively sequestering the plaque and its contents from the lumen [9], while others are separated from the lumen by a narrow zone of connective tissue or by endothelium alone. Advanced plaques with intact, well organized fibrous caps would be expected to present smooth and regular lumen surfaces to the bloodstream, but abnormal levels of wall shear stress and departures from laminar, unidirectional flow may favor local accumulation, adhesion and deposition of thrombocytes, monocytes and fibrin. These are likely to occur distal to stenoses, at foci of endothelial surface irregularity or extrinsic mechanical trauma and in regions of softened plaque consistency. Local mechanical stresses resulting from sudden changes in pressure, flow or pulse rate, or from torsion and bending in relation to organ movements may precipitate disruption of friable or brittle plaques.

Conversely, changes in vessel configuration associated with plaque progression and stenosis may create conditions favoring the development of complex flow instabilities and vibrations. Although vessel segments distal to tight stenoses tend to be spared, degrees of stenosis not tight enough to prevent distal plaque formation may nevertheless engender unstable flow conditions which could modify plaque composition and configuration. Plaques in experimental animals which are located immediately distal to a region of moderate narrowing have been shown to be more complex in structure and composition than those which occur in the same region in the absence of a proximal stenosis [12]. The likelihood of turbulence is also enhanced as vessels enlarge and become tortuous with age or when multiple plaques occur in the same vessel in close axial proximity. Since regions of high flow velocity tend to be spared, increasing flow velocity at progressive narrowings could also conceivably be associated with local slowing of the atherogenic process. Decreased flow velocity due to distal obstruction, decreased pressure or increased peripheral resistance would have the opposite effect.

RELATED MECHANICAL FACTORS

Although we are occupied at this conference with the effects of blood flow at the blood-vessel wall interface in relation to atherogenesis, there are associated mechanical factors related to flow and pressure which must eventually receive close attention. The physical properties and composition of the media and the modifications of its structural components in response to short and long-term alterations in flow and pressure are also factors both in plaque initiation and in the consequences of plaque formation. Motion of the artery wall in relation to pulsatile flow has been shown to be related to plaque localization in an experimental animal model and to artery wall metabolism [13]. In addition, the transport of circulating substances through the wall from the lumen is necessarily related to the density and composition of the media [14] and to the width of a diffusely thickened intimal [15]. Thus, whatever blood-vessel wall interface conditions favor increased diffusion through the endothelium or uptake of circulatory elements by the wall, accumulation in the intima is likely to be a function also of those mechanical factors which govern wall and intimal composition and therefore affect transmural transport. Accelerated frequency of tensile stress variation due to increased pulse rate, acute and chronic elevations of mean tensile stress associated with blood pressure and with changes in artery diameter in response to changes in flow as well as wall vibrations related to turbulence distal to stenoses are all physical factors likely to affect wall composition and therefore transport. Changes in smooth muscle tone in response to vasoactive substances [16] would also be expected to influence medial microarchitecture and transport. Flow velocity as well as early plaque formation have been suggested as factors which may determine the elaboration, release or sensitivity of the cells of the media to the endothelial derived relaxation factor [17-19] and thereby affect the state of media.

DIRECT INTERVENTIONS

Operative procedures, including placement of biologic and prosthetic grafts, operative endarterectomy, transluminal angioplasty including placement of luminal stents, removal of plaque tissue by laser beam searing, excision by atherotome, and fragmentation by drilling cather modify flow fields and therefore hemodynamic conditions at the blood-vessel wall interface in diseased arteries. In addition, tissue reactions are induced in the plaque and wall by these direct mechanical disruptions as well as by the sudden imposition of markedly altered hemodynamic conditions. Both the effectiveness and the consequences of these interventions will depend on the composition of the plaque which has been traumatized and the state of the associated artery wall. Our ability to understand the basis for success or failure of these procedures will depend on our knowledge of the nature of the interaction of various types of injury with hemodynamics and with arterial tissue responses. Parallel research is therefore also needed to establish the nature and degree of individual differences in arterial tissue response to flow, pressure and tensile stress in relation to age, gender, and nutritional and metabolic status.

CONCLUSIONS

It is apparent from the papers in this first session that we now have sound information about where plaques are likely to form at clinically important sites in humans and about the probable associated hemodynamic conditions at these locations. We know little however about the mechanisms by which flow conditions initiate or potentiate plaque formation and we have barely begun to address the relationship between hemodynamic variables and the evorution of human atheroscleotic plaques toward stability or toward symptomatic disease. Correlative phenomenological research has advanced to a point which should now permit us to compare lesion-prone and lesion-resistant regions with respect to possible hemodynamic determinants of plaque composition and consistency and of the rate of plaque enlargement. In particular, investigations of the type covered this morning should direct us to develop detailed quantitative studies of plaque growth and composition in relation to variations in geometric configuration, pulse rate and flow velocity. We will then need to identify the features of plaque composition and configuration which underlie susceptibility to plaque instability and to characterize the hemodynamic and other mechanical circumstances which may predispose to plaque disruption, as well as those which favor the maintenance or reestablishment of an adequate and stable lumen channel. Such studies should place renewed emphasis on the fact that the artery wall and the atherosclerotic plaque are living tissues, capable of healing and restructuring as well as undergoing necrosis, degeneration and disruption. Until the disease can be entirely prevented, enhancement of the adaptive and restitutive processes remains an important goal.

REFERENCES

[1] Zarins CK, Giddens DP, Bharadvaj BK, Sottiurai VS, Mabon RF, Glagov S (1983) Circ Res 53:502-514
[2] Ku DN, Zarins CK, Giddens DP, Glagov S (1985) Arteriosclerosis 5, 292-302
[3] Friedman MH, Deters OJ, Bargeron CB, Hutchins GM, Mark FF (1986) Atherosclerosis 60:161-171
[4] Beere PA, Glagov S, Zarins CK (1984) Science 226:180-182
[5] Kannel WB, Kannel C, Paffenbarger RS Jr., Cupples PH, Cupples LA (1987) Am Heart J 113:1489-1494
[6] Kamiya A, Togawa T (1980) Am J Physiol 239:H14-H21.
[7] Zarins CK, Zatina MA, Giddens DP, Ku DN, Glagov S (1987) J Vasc Surg 5:413-420.
[8] Glagov S, Weisenberg E, Zarins CK, Stankunavicius R, Kolettis G (1987) N Eng J Med 316:1371-1375.

[9] Glagov S, Zarins CK (1983) Quantitating atherosclerosis: Problems of Definition, Chapter 2 In: Clinical Diagnosis of Atherosclerosis; Quantitative Methods of Evaluation, Bond MG, Insull W, Glagov S, Chandler AB, Cornhill F (eds) Springer-Verlag, New York pp 11-35

[10] Leung DYM, Glagov S, Mathews MB (1977) Exp Cell Res 109:285-298

[11] Zarins CK, Zatina MA, Glagov S (1983) Correlation of post-mortem angiography with pathologic anatomy: Quantitation of atherosclerotic lesions. Chapter 13 In: Clinical Diagnosis of Atherosclerosis; Quantitative Methods of Evaluation, Bond MG, Insull W, Glagov S, Chandler AB, Cornhill F (eds), Springer-Verlag, New York

[12] Bomberger RA, Zarins CK, Glagov S (1981) J Surg Res 30:205-212.

[13] Lyon RT, Hass A, Davis HR, Glagov S, Zarins CK (1987) J Vasc Surg 5:59-67

[14] Fry DL (1987) Arteriosclerosis 7:88-100

[15] Tracy RE, Kissling GE (1987) Arch Path Lab Med 109:651-658

[16] Lever MJ (1985) Int J Microcirc 4:294

[17] Jayakody L, Senaratne M, Thomson A, Kappagoda T (1987) Circ Res 60:251-264

[18] Freiman PC, Mitchell GG, Heistad DD, Armstrong M, Harrison DG (1986) Circ Res 58:783-789

[19] Smiesko V, Kozik J, Dolezel S (1985) Blood Vessels 22:247-251

Distribution and Endothelial Morphology of Atherosclerotic Lesions at Bifurcations and Curves of Human Cerebral Arteries

N. Sakata[1], T. Fukushima[2], S. Takebayashi[1], and T. Homma[2]

[1] Second Department of Pathology, School of Medicine, Fukuoka University, Fukuoka, 814-01 Japan
[2] Institute of Cardiovascular Diseases, School of Medicine, Shinshu University, Matsumoto, 390 Japan

ABSTRACT

The present study was an attempt to clarify mechanisms related to the development of atherosclerotic lesions at branches and curves in the human arterial tree. The distribution of atherosclerotic lesions, including cloudy thickenings, fatty streaks, fibrous plaques and complicated lesions, was investigated at bifurcations and curves of cerebral branches of the internal carotid artery. Morphological changes of the endothelium over fibrous plaques at bifurcations was also assessed, by means of scanning electron microscopy. Early atherosclerotic lesions occurred predominantly at the outer walls of bifurcations and distal to the center of the inner curvature at curves, where wall shear stress is considered to be low. In contrast, the flow divider of bifurcations and the outer curvature of the bends, presumably high-shear regions, were free of early lesions. Endothelial cells over fibrous plaques without sudanophilia(FP) and with sudanophilia(SP) were significantly less elongated than those in lesion-free areas. In addition, endothelial cells over the FP and SP showed significantly more microvillous projections than did those in lesion-free areas. These results suggest that focal hemodynamic forces are implicated in the development of the atherosclerotic lesions.

Introduction

Since early atherosclerotic plaques tend to be localized at branches and curvatures[1], focal hemodynamic forces are considered to play an important role in atherogenesis. However, little is known of the mechanisms determining localization. Endothelial morphology may be related to focal hemodynamic forces and to atherogenesis[2]. We investigated the topographical distribution and endothelial morphology of atherosclerotic plaques at bifurcations and curves of the cerebral arterial branches of the internal carotid artery, with the objective of elucidating the role of blood flow in the development of atherosclerotic plaques.

Methods

1) Topographical distribution of atherosclerotic lesions was determined at bifurcations of the cerebral artery and at curves of the internal carotid artery.

Randomly collected cerebral arteries, from 107 humans aged 0 to 87 years, were examined. Specimens included 173 bifurcutions of the internal carotid - anterior cerebral- middle cerebral artery (IC-AC-MC bifurcation), and 162 bifurcations of the middle cerebral artery- temporal branch (MCA bifurcation). Each bifurcation was opened lengthwise, stained with Sudan IV, and photographed in stereoscopic microscopy. A parent and two daughter vessels and the central bifurcation area were separated into 16 compartments. The presence or absence of atherosclerotic lesions including the fatty streaks, fibrous plaques and complicated lesions, was established for each compartment. The atherosclerotic index, surface involvement by atherosclerotic lesions and frequency distribution of fibrous plaques in the IC-AC-MC and MCA bifurcations were determined.

The internal carotid arteries of 50 humans aged 1 to 88 years, were examined. After the internal carotid arteries, consisting of the carotid canal and carotid siphon portions, had been perfusion- fixed with 10% neutral buffered formalin, they were dissected free of surrounding tissue. Angles, outer curvatures and vessel diameters were measured. Samples were then cut and divided into the carotid siphon portion (part I) and carotid canal portion (part II). Each was opened longitudinally and stained with Sudan IV. Two separate drawings were made according of the macroscopic apperance. One to outline fibrous plaques and the other to outline a cloudy thickening without the fibrous plaque, which showed the non-fibrotic, raised lesion with pallor and translucency. Complicated lesions were excluded from this study. The proportion of the area of parts I and II occupied by lesions was calculated. The frequency distribution of lesions was examined at the middle of each curve, and at 45-degrees distal and proximal to this site on the inner(I), outer(O) and lateral (L1 and L2) walls.

2) Endothelial morphology of atherosclerotic plaques at the cerebral arterial bifurcation.

Cerebral arteries, obtained from 4 subjects autopsied within 3 hours after death and aged 46, 51, 82 and 86, were used. At autopsy, cerebral arteries were perfused with saline followed by 2.5% glutaraldehyde in 0.1M phosphate buffer(pH 7.4) under a pressure of 120 mmHg. 24 bifurcations were dissected, opened lengthwise and stained with Sudan IV. After stereoscopic observation, the samples were pinned on a board, dehydrated through a graded series of ethanol concentrations, critical-point dried from CO_2, and coated with platinum. The endothelal cells over lesion-free areas(LF), fibrous plaques without sudanophilia(FP) and with sudanophilia(SP) were examined by a scanning electron microscopy. The following parameters were analyzed by means of a semi-automatic image analyzer and point counting method. The surface area(μm^2), width/length ratio and surface density of crateriform hollows (/mm^2) of endothelial cells were obtained by using micrographs of final magnification of X1250. The surface density of microvillous projections(/cm) of endothelial cells was determined on micrographs of final magnification of X5000.

Results

1) Topographical distribution of atherosclerotic lesions at the bifurcations of the cerebral artery and the curvatures of the internal carotid artery.

Both the atherosclerotic index and the surface involvement by lesions in the cerebral arterial bifurcations increased with age, augmenting rapidly in persons over 40. Fatty streaks occurred after the age

13

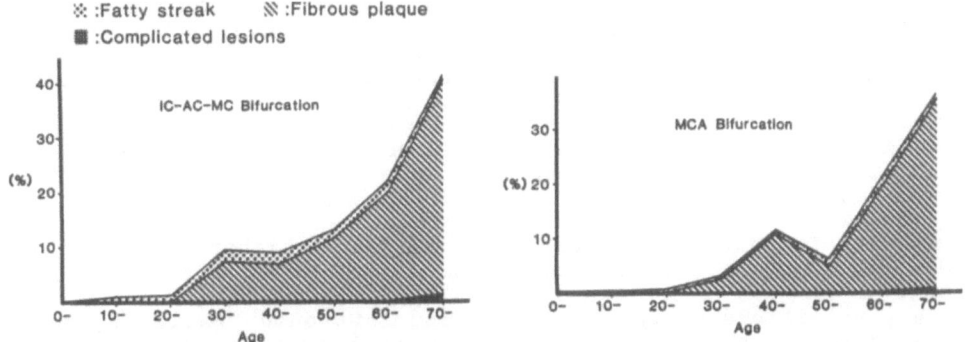

Fig. 1. Changes of surface involvement by lesions with increasing age. Results are mean values for each decade.

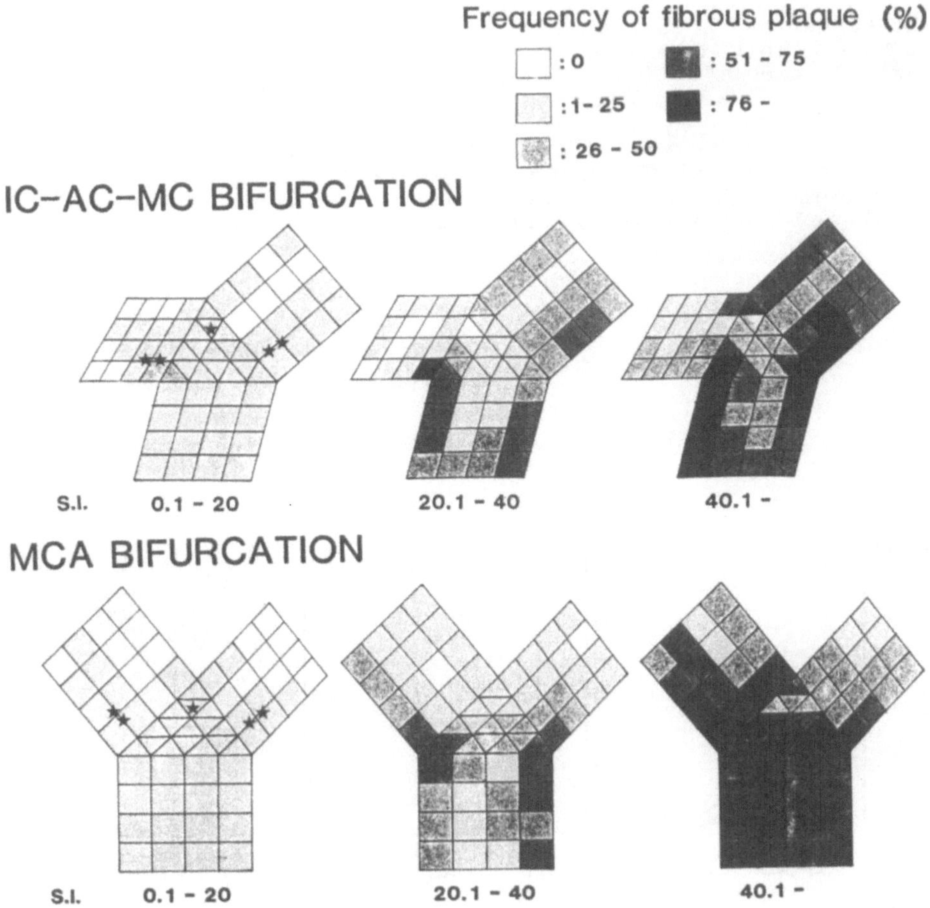

Frequency of fibrous plaque (%)

☐ : 0   ■ : 51 - 75

☐ : 1- 25   ■ : 76 -

▨ : 26 - 50

IC–AC–MC BIFURCATION

S.I.   0.1 - 20   20.1 - 40   40.1 -

MCA BIFURCATION

S.I.   0.1 - 20   20.1 - 40   40.1 -

Fig. 2. Topographical representation of frequency of occurrence of fibrous plaques in IC-AC-MC and MCA bifurcations. An asterisk denotes the apex of the bifurcation, two asterisks the outer wall of the bifurcation.   S.I.: Surface involvement by fibrous plaques.

of 10. Surface involvement by fatty streaks did not increase with age. In contrast, fibrous plaques first appeared after age 30, and surface involvement by fibrous plaques increased with age. Complicated lesions were present only after 70 years(Fig.1). Fig.2 shows a topographical representation of the IC-AC-MC and MCA bifurcations. Fibrous plaques occurred in a distinct pattern with a high incidence on the outer walls of the daughter vessels of the IC-AC-MC and MCA bifurcations. In addition, fibrous plaques were also found predominantly in the middle of the MCA bifurcation. In the IC-AC-MC bifurcation of samples with less than 40 percent involvement, the incidence of fibrous plaques on the outer wall of the anterior cerebral artery was higher than that of the middle cerebral artery, and the former originated from the internal carotid artery at a more acute angle than the latter. There was, however, no difference between right and left outer walls of the daughter vessels of the MCA bifurcation. In both IC-AC-MC and MCA bifurcations, the flow divider was free of atherosclerotic lesions.

Curving site of the internal carotid artery were non-planar and showed three-dimentional complexity. The carotid siphon and canal portions were composed of two curves, termed C-1,2 and C-3,4, respectively. The former had a shorter outer radius of curvature, (mean values of 6.29 ±1.19mm(C-1) and 6.91 ± 1.87mm(C-2)) than the latter,(10.32 ±1.87mm(C-3) and 9.56 ± 2.00mm(C-4)). Vessel diameters (18 samples) had mean values of 5.25 ±0.64mm, 5.51 ± 0.52mm, 5.17 ±0.89mm and 5.22 ±0.76mm(SD),(C-1, C-2, C-3 and C-4 respectively).

In part I, localized cloudy thickening was more frequent in the younger subjects, at the mean age of 22.8 ± 23.2years(SD), than the fibrous plaque, 63.3 ±11.1 years(SD). Fibrous plaques appeared after the age of 40 and increased progressively with age in both part I and part

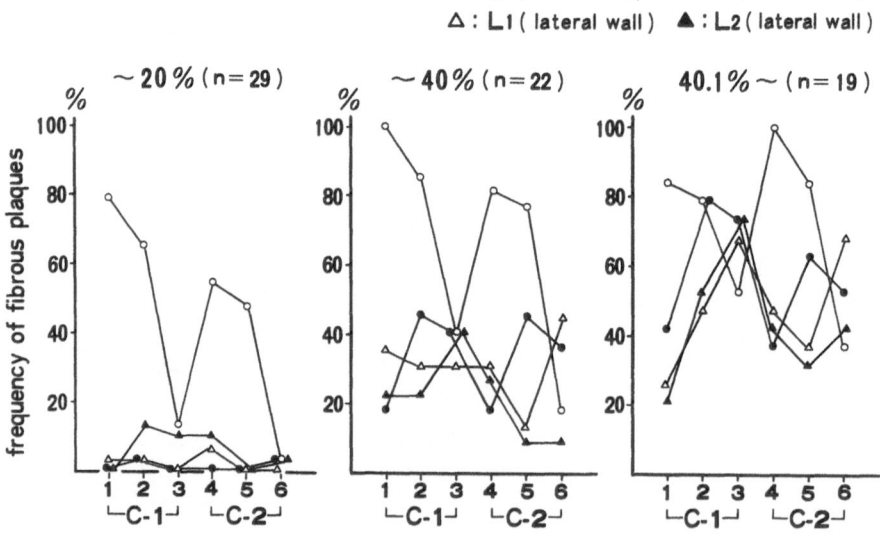

Fig. 3. Frequency of fibrous plaques in carotid siphon portion(part I) composed of curve-1 and 2. 1,4: 45-degree distal point from the middle of curve 2,5: the middle point of curve 3,6: 45-degree proximal point to the middle of curve

II. The mean value of the extent of involvement with the fibrous plaque was greater in part I (26.9%) than in part II (7.85%). Cloudy thickenings and fibrous plaques had the same distribution within each curve, that is, both were located in the distal region from the middle of the inner curvature within each curve. Fig. 3 shows the frequency distribution of the fibrous plaque in the carotid siphon portion including two curves (C-1 and 2). Fibrous plaques were most frequently seen only at the middle and 45-degree distal points (2, 5 and 1, 4, respectively) on the inner walls of C-1 and C-2 in the samples with under 20 percent involvement by fibrous plaques. In 20.1-40 percent involved samples, fibrous plaques were present in some sites as well and became confluent in samples with over a 40 percent involvement. Fig.4 shows a topographical representation. In subjects aged 40 or younger, localized cloudy thickenings were present in regions distal to the middle of inner curvature. In subjects over 40, fibrous plaques occurred at similar sites, and subsequent lesions tended to develop more distally and circumferentially.

2)   Endothelial morphology of atherosclerotic plaques in cerebral arterial bifurcations.
     Endothelial cells over lesion-free areas(LF) were elongated and lay with their long axis parallel to the direction of blood flow. A few microvillous prejections and crateriform hollows with a 0.5-1 micron in diameter were present on the surface. Over fibrous plaques without sudanophilia(FP) or with sudanophilia(SP), endothelial cells were fusiform or round, and showed a loss of streamline orientation. There was no increase in the number of crateriform hollows of endothelial cells over FP and SP, but the microvillous projections were increased (Fig.5). Denudation of the endothelium was not evident at any site. Table 1 shows the results of the morphometric analysis. Surface area of endothelial cells was significantly smaller in FP than in LF and SP, and there was a significant difference between the width/length ratio of endothelial cells in LF, FP and SP. The mean value was highest in SP, followed by FP and LF. Surface density of the microvillous projections of the endothelial cells also showed significant differences.

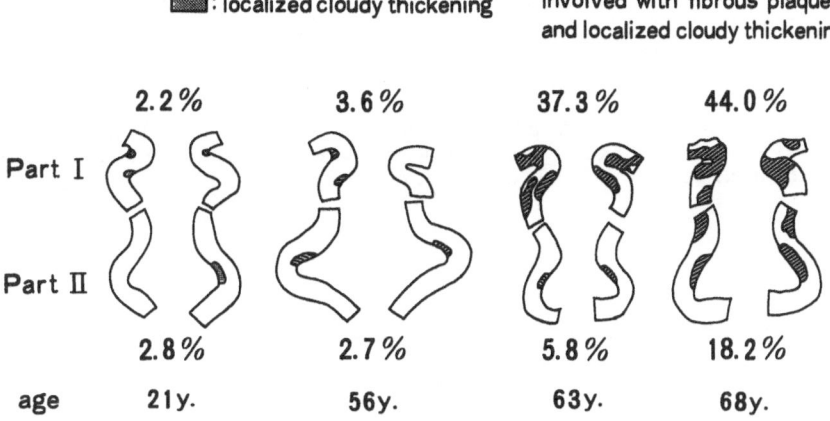

Fig. 4. Topographical representation of localized cloudy thickening and fibrous plaque in carotid siphon and canal portions of internal carotid artery.

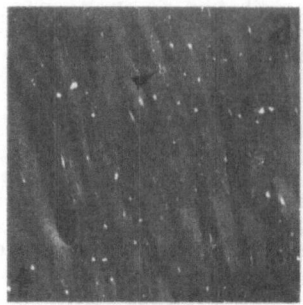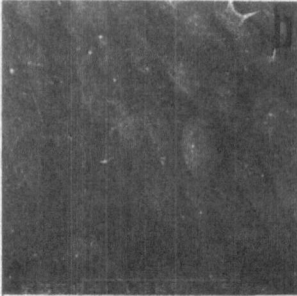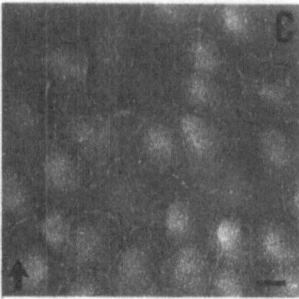

Fig. 5. Scanning electron micrographs showing typical fields of endothelial cells in lesion-free areas(a), over fibrous plaques without
sudanophilia(b) and with sudanophilia(c). An arrow indicates the direction of blood flow. An arrowhead shows a crateriform hollow of endothelial cell. Bar denotes 10 microns.

Table 1. MORPHOMETRIC COMPARISON OF ENDOTHELIAL CELLS.
Results are expressed as the mean ± S.D.. Statistical analysis was made
using two-tailed unpaired t-test.

Examined region	Area (μ m^2)	Width/length ratio*	Surface density of microvillous projections(/cm)*	Surface density of crateriform hollows(/mm^2)
LF	313±160(244)	0.23±0.14(244)	0.12±0.06[22]	4.8±0.5[22]
FP	288±146(610)**	0.35±0.21(610)	0.18±0.06[21]	4.4±0.4[20]
SP	325±147(280)	0.43±0.23(280)	0.34±0.10[11]	2.8±1.2[8]

( ): Total number of endothelial cells examined
[ ]: Total number of areas examined
  * Significant difference between examined regions(p<0.01)
 ** Significantly less compared to LF and SP(p<0.05)

The magnitude was greatest over SP, followed by FP and LF. In contrast, there was no difference between the surface density of crateriform hollows of endothelial cells over LF, FP and SP.

Discussion

     As to the role of wall shear stress in atherogenesis, there are at
least two conflicting hypotheses concerning the hemodynamic mechanisms
involved and concerning the localization of lesions.   One is the
proposal by Fry [3]that high shear stress damages the endothelial
cells, and the other is Caro's hypothesis[4] that the early lesions
occur in regions with a lower shear stress. The present study showed
that the spatial distribution of the early atherosclerotic lesions had
a distinct pattern in the bifurcations of the cerebral artery and the
curves of the internal carotid artery.   The early lesion was
frequently found on the outer wall of the daughter vessels in the IC-

AC-MC and MCA bifurcations of the cerebral artery; in the latter it occurred frequently in the middle of the bifurcation. The early lesion was located only at the distal region from the middle of the inner curvature in the curved sites of the internal carotid artery. Recent studies showed the generation of secondary flows in branching and curving tubes. In the MCA bifurcation, the localization of the early lesion coincided with the region where the secondary flow "horseshoe vortex"[5] was generated. Trapped vortical motions were observed at the inner dowstream region of the curved tube[6]. The present study suggests that these secondary flows may be related to the development of atherosclerotic lesions.

At the IC-AC-MC bifurcation, the incidence of fibrous plaques on the outer wall of anterior cerebral artery was higher than that in the middle cerebral artery. The anterior cerebral artery diverges from the internal carotid artery at a more acute angle than the middle cerebral artery. In contrast, there was no difference between the incidence of fibrous plaques on both outer walls of the daughter vessels in the symmetric MCA bifurcation. In the curving site of the internal carotid artery, the magnitude of surface involvement by fibrous plaques was significantly greater at the carotid siphon portion than in the carotid canal portion. The radii of the former were smaller than in the latter. These findings suggest that development of atherosclerotic lesions may be related to the geometric features of the branching and curving sites of the artery.

There are reports that hemodynamic forces influence endothelial morphology and function. According to Reidy and Bowyer[7], endothelial damage with denudation is consistently found in the high-shear region. On the other hand, there are irregular alignments and shape of the endothelial cells in the low-shear area[8]. The present study showed that 1) the endothelial cells over atherosclerotic lesions were rounder, and had more microvillous projections than did the lesion-free area 2) there was no denudation of the endothelial cells at any site 3) early atherosclerotic lesions developed predominantly in the regions suspected of low shear stress. These results suggest that the non-denuded morphological changes of endothelial cells in the low-shear region may be related to development of human atherosclerotic lesions. The rounder endothelial cells are considered to be more highly metabolic and permeable and occur in areas of high cell turnover[9,10]. In addition, the presence of microvilli may be associated with slower flow of the plasma along the endothelial surface and to facilitate the exchange of metabolites between the arterial blood and the vessel wall[11]. The present study revealed that endothelial cells over the fibrous plaque with sudanophilia, an area where there was an accumulation of sudanophilic materials derived from the plasma, were roundest in shape and had most numerous microvillous projections. Thus endothelial morphlogy may reflect functional changes in endothelial cells.

In conclusion, the present study indicates that atherosclerotic lesions occur predominantly in regions where wall shear stress is considered to be low at the bifurcations and curves of human arteries. Vascular geometry may be an important factor in the development of lesions and endothelial morphology may relate to atherogenesis.

Acknowledgment: This work was supported by a Research Grant for Cardiovascular Disease (60C-2) from the Ministry of the Health and Welfare.

REFERENCES

[1]Sakata N, Joshita T, Ooneda G (1985) Heart and Vessels 1:70-73
[2]Nerem RM, Levensque MJ (1983) The case for fluid dynamic as a localizing factor for atherogenesis. In: Schettler G, Nerem RM, Schmid-
Schonbein H, Morl H, Diehm C (eds) Fluid dynamics as a localizing factor for atherosclerosis. Springer-Verlag, Berlin, pp 26-34
[3]Fry DL (1968) Circ Res 22:165-197
[4]Caro CG, Fitz-Gerald JM, Schroter RC (1971) Proc Roy Soc Lond B
177:109-159
[5]Fukushima T, Azuma T (1982) Biorheology 19:143-154
[6]Chandran KB, Yearwood TL (1981) J Fluid Mech 111:59-85
[7]Reidy MA, Bowyer DE (1977) Atherosclerosis 26:181-194
[8]Woolf N (1982) Pathology of Athrosclerosis. Butterworth Scientific,
London, pp 25-46
[9]Repin YS, Dolgov VV, Zaikina OE, Novikov ID (1984) Atherosclerosis
50:35-52
[10]Caplan BR, Schwartz CJ (1973) Atherosclerosis 17:401-417
[11]Smith U, Ryan JW, Michie DD, Smith DS (1971) Science 173:925-927

Observations on Carotid Bifurcation Atherosclerosis in Human Cadavers

M. Kashihara[1], K. Matsumoto[2], and J. Cervós-Navarro[3]

[1]Taoka Hospital, Tokushima, 770 Japan
[2]Department of Neurological Surgery, School of Medicine, The University of Tokushima, Tokushima, 770 Japan
[3]Institut für Neuropathologie, Klinikum Steglitz, Freie Universität Berlin, D-1000 Berlin, Federal Republic of Germany

ABSTRACT

The atherosclerotic changes in the carotid bifurcation were examined in 70 Japanese and 73 German cadavers. Initially, a fatty streak or dot appeared in the carotid sinus and/or on the anterior side of the common carotid artery. Further progression occurred predominantly in the carotid sinus, resulting in a localized atheromatous plaque. Finally an atheromatous plaque was formed all around the bifurcation. The following speculation was made from observations of many carotid bifurcations; the accumulation of fatty streaks on the anterior surface of the common carotid artery results in an atheromatous plaque in the carotid sinus analogous to accumulation of sand on a sandbank in a river. This concept may be useful in understanding the progression of atheromatous plaques.

INTRUDUCTION

Many regions of the human arterial system are highly susceptible to atherosclerosis. One is the carotid bifurcation in the neck, where the common carotid artery(CCA) branches into the internal carotid(IC) and the external carotid(EC) arteries. A large atheromatous plaque often occurs at the lateral wall of the carotid sinus, i.e., at the junction of CCA and IC. There have been many reports on the pathogenesis of atheromatous plaques in this position, mainly from the hemodynamic point of view. The most widely accepted concept is that plaques in this position are related to shearing stress at the branching site. However, most pathologists and surgeons believe that the distribution of atheromatous plaques is too complex to be explained on the basis of two-dimensional schematic drawing of rheological forces. Moreover, although fatty streaks or dots appear in numerous places in the initial stage of atherogenesis, not all streaks develop into atheromatous plaques. Rheological conditions in the branching vessel are probably very complex and analysis of CCA could be helpful in understanding atherogenesis in this region.

MATERIALS AND METHODS

Carotid arteries were obtained by courtesy of German and Japanese pathologists. In all, 70 Japanese specimens were obtained during 1983 and 1984 in Tokushima, and 73 German specimens during 1985 in Berlin. The aortic arch and both carotid arteries including the carotid bifurcation were excised in block and immersed in 10% buffered formalin for more than a month before examination. After measurement of the length of the CCA, the artery wall was opened

axially on the anterior side, and the inner diameter of each region
of the artery was measured. The regions measured included the IC just
distal to the carotid sinus, the widest part of the carotid sinus,
the origin and distal end of the CCA, and the proximal and distal
regions of the aortic arch. The location and characteristics of
atherosclerotic changes were recorded and mapped on a chart.
Atherosclerotic changes were classified in six grades: grade 1, no
macroscopic change; grade 2, fatty streak or dot; grade 3, localized
thin atheromatous plaque; grade 4, thick localized atheromatous
plaque or diffuse fatty streak; grade 5, plaque with ulceration or
pathological stenosis; grade 6, advanced stage with diffuse
ulcerations.

RESULTS

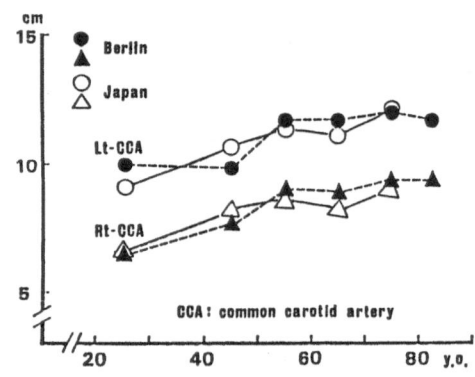

        The length of the common
carotid artery increased with
age(Fig 1). The inner diameter,
especially that of the carotid
sinus, also enlarged with age (Fig
2). With age, the inner diameter of
the distal CCA became slightly
greater than that of the proximal
side in the Japanese group. The
carotid sinus is reported to be the

Fig.1 Length of common carotid artery. The length of the common
carotid artery increaseed with age. The increase was not linear, but
most rapid in subjects in their forties, and only slight in those
over sixty.

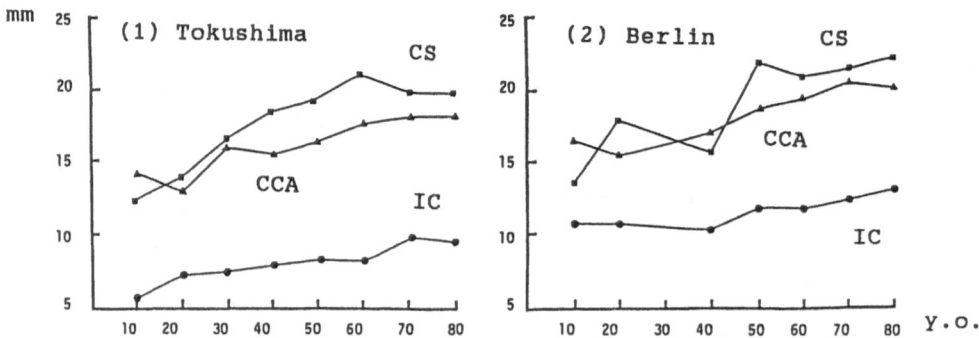

Fig.2   Inner diameter of the carotid artery. The carotid sinus
diameter increased most with age. The artery was smaller in Japanese
than in Germans. CS,carotid sinus; CCA,common carotid artery;
IC,internal carotid artery

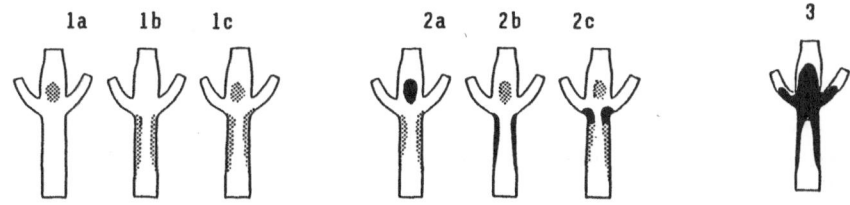

1a 1b 1c 2a 2b 2c 3

Fig.3 Stages in development of carotid bifurcation atherosclerosis. Dotted regions indicate fatty dots or streaks, black regions indicate atheromatous plaques.

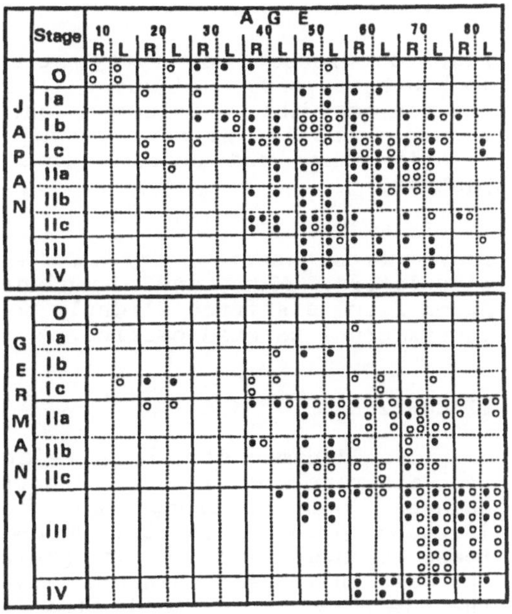

Fig.4 Age and sex distributions of stages in Japanese and Germans. ●:Male, ○:Female.

Stage	10 R	10 L	20 R	20 L	30 R	30 L	40 R	40 L	50 R	50 L	60 R	60 L	70 R	70 L	80 R	80 L
JAPAN																
O	○○	○○		○	○		●	●	●		○					
Ia			○		○		●		●○●○	●○			●	●○		
Ib							●	●○●○	●○●○	○	●○●○	●○	●○●○			
Ic			○	○	○		○		●○●○	●○	●○●○		●○○	●○		
IIa					○			●	●○		●	●○	●○○	●		
IIb								●	●○●	●○	●○	●	●			
IIc							●○	●	●○●○	●○	●○●		○	●○		
III									●	●	●○	●	●			○
IV									●							
GERMANY																
O	○						○		●	●		○				
Ia											○					
Ib									○	●	●		○	○		
Ic			○		●	●			●	●○	○		●○	○		
IIa					○	○			●	●○ ●○	●○●○	○	●○●○	○ ○	○	○
IIb							● ○	●	●	● ○	○	●	●○●			
IIc									●	●○ ●○	●○	○	● ○	● ○●		
III									●	●○ ●○	●○ ●○	● ○	●○●○ ○○○○ ○○ ○	●○● ○○○ ○○	●○ ○	●○ ○
IV										●	● ●	●○ ●	●○ ●	●○ ●		

most common site for atherosclerotic change, and this was confirmed by our study. But we also found that the incidence of atheromatous change was high in the CCA near the EC. Progression of atherosclerosis in the carotid bifurcation followed the following pattern(Fig.3). The initial stage is a fatty streak or dot appearing mainly in the carotid sinus, or in the anterior region of the CCA, or in both regions. Atheromatous plaques enlarged and thickened in the sinus, in the common carotid artery and in the orifice of the external carotid artery. During further progress, these plaques joined to form a larger plaque around the carotid bifurcation. In some cases, the whole carotid artery was covered with atheromatous plaques.

The age and sex distribution of the various stages in Japanese and German cases are presented in Fig.4. Involvement increased with age, and was more rapid in the German group. Progress was also greater in males than in females, especially in older individuals. In most cases, progress was similar in the right and left carotid artery. Of subgroups of stage 1, 1-c was the most common, but 1-b was also frequently noted in the Japanese group. In stage 2, fatty streaks were always noticed in the CCA, and atheromatous plaques were also often found in the carotid sinus. There were also many instances of 2-b and 2-c in the Japanese group. Progress of atherosclerosis to stages 3 and 4 was observed in subjects over 50 years old. Many German specimens from individuals older 70 had severe atherosclerosis.

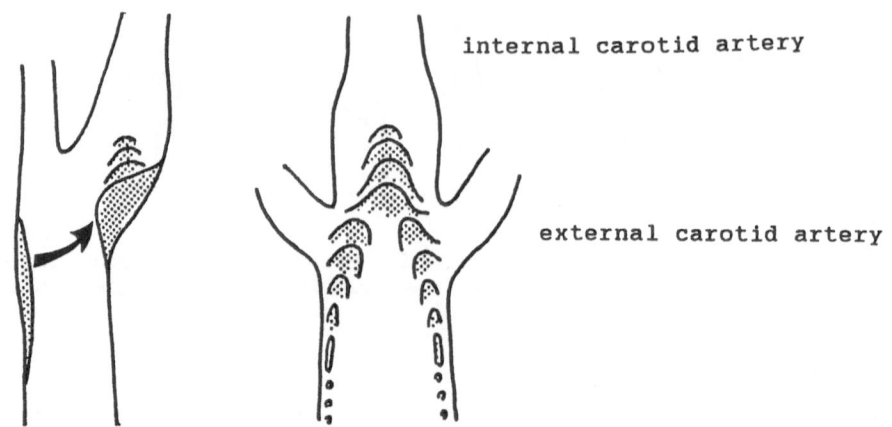

internal carotid artery

external carotid artery

Fig.5 Progression of fatty streaks and dots to atheromatous plaques. Fatty streaks located on the anterior surface of the common carotid artery extend toward the carotid sinus and develop into atheromatous plaques.

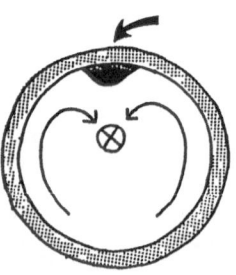

Fig.6 Cross section of a vessel showing circulatory flow and hemodynamic stress. Axial flow is shifted slightly to the side of the external carotid orifice.

DISCUSSION

Hemodynamic stress is related to the initiation and progression of atherosclerosis(1). Atherosclerosis results in morphologic changes, such as elongation of the common carotid arteries and an increase in their diameter. However, the present study indicated that these changes occur most rapidly in subjects in their forties. Increase in vessel diameter was most marked in the carotid sinus, and the distal side of CCA became larger than the proximal side. Little change in vascular size was seen in subjects of over sixty.
Our main interest was in the location of atherosclerotic plaques. The dynamics of formation of an atheromatous plaque appears to be analogous to that of accumulation of sand on a sandbank of a river(Fig.5). The fatty streak or dot originates in the mid- or distal-third of the CCA and progresses toward the distal side. The fatty dot or streak is almost always located in the anterior region of the CCA, i.e., the side of the EC, giving a 1-b type fatty streak. Sometimes a fatty streak appears sumultaneously in the carotid sinus, as in type 1-c, or separately as in type 1-a. The fatty streak in the CCA progresses to the orifice of the EC, where it becomes a plaque, of type 2-c. In other cases, an atheromatous plaque is formed in the carotid sinus or in the anterior part of the CCA, as in type 2-a or 2-b. An advanced, stage 3 athromatous plaque has three extensions, one proximal process on the anterior surface of the common carotid artery and the others on the internal and external carotid arteries. The reason the initial fatty streak appears in the anterior part of

the CCA is unknown, but its formation may result from the turbulent flow in the CCA as shown in Fig.6. If the axial flow is slightly shifted to the external carotid artery side, the circulatory flow and flow separation or turbulent flow could be expected on the anterior surface of the CCA.

CONCLUSION

The accumulation of fatty streaks resulting in formation of an atheromatous plaque may be analogous to that of accumulation of sand on a sandbank of a river.

Acknowledgments: We are very grateful to Prof. Dr. U.Gross and Prof. Dr. H.Stein for allowing us to examine German carotid arteries, and to Prof. K.Hizawa and Prof. H.Ohtsuka for providing Japanese carotid arteries.

REFERENCE

(1)Giddens DP, Zarins CK, Glagov S, Bharadvaj BK and Ku DN (1983) Flow and atherogenesis in the human carotid bifurcation. In: Schettler G, Nerem RM, Schmid-Schönbein H, Mörl H, Diehm C(eds) Fluid Dynamics as a Localizing Factor for Atherosclerosis. Springer-Verlag, Berlin Heidelberg New York Tokyo, pp 38-45

Localization of Lipids and Cell Population in Atheromatous Lesions in Aorta and Its Main Arterial Branches in Patients with Hypercholesterolemia

C. Yutani[1], M. Imakita[1], H. Ishibashi-Ueda[1], A. Yamamoto[2], and S. Takaichi[2]

[1]Division of Pathology, National Cardiovascular Center Hospital, Suita, Osaka, 565 Japan
[2]Department of Etiology and Pathogenesis, National Cardiovascular Center Research Institute, Suita, 565 Japan

ABSTRACT

To find clues to the mechanism of regression of atherosclerosis, we investigated the localization of lipids and cell populations in atheromatous lesions at arterial branches in patients with hypercholesterolemia. Intimal thickening and lipid deposits were found in the proximal areas (low shear areas) to the orifice more markedly than in the distal areas (high shear areas), while the apex (flow divider) was composed of dense fibrous and elastic cushion lesions. Lipid storage was found more frequently and more extensively in smooth muscle cells rather than in macrophages in the deeper areas of the thickened intimas. These observations suggest that smooth muscle cells play an important role in lipid deposition and contribute to atherosclerotic lesions at the sites of arterial branches. This finding may be related to the delay in regression of atherosclerotic lesions in spite of intensive antihypercholesterolemic treatment.

INTRODUCTION

Recent development of anticholesterolemic therapy including oral drugs and plasmapheresis enabled us to reduce serum cholesterol near or into the optimum range(1), leading to the prevention of ischemic heart disease. It has also been shown that xanthomas in skin and tendons and lesions of the aortic valve can regress relatively easily in response to such an intensive treatment(2). However, the regression of athromatous lesions in the arterial wall may not take place so easily, especially at or near branching sites of the aorta and the major arteries.

A variety of physical and physico-chemical factors have been suggested to account for the localization, and initiation of atherosclerosis. The wall shear stress has been suspected to play an important role in this process, because of its inherent non-uniformity (3,4).

Recent human studies(5,6) indicated that the earliest atherosclerotic change occurs preferentially at regions where average wall shear stress is expected to be low.

The purpose of this investiation was twofold: first, to evaluate so called "low shear theory" and, second, to investigate the basis for the wide variation in the ease with which regression of atherosclerosis is achieved. We investigated the localization of lipids in relation to cell populations in atheromatous lesions of the artery wall.

MATERIALS AND METHODS

The aterials which formed the basis for this study were selected from the autopsy files of the National Cardiovascular Center. The patients(mean age 60.7±15.3 years) had a history of hyperlipidemia with serum cholesterol level greater than 220 mg/dl. Among twenty four patients, there were two cases of homozygous familial hyper-cholesterolemia and one heterozygote. Secondary hypercholesterolemia with hypertension and diabetes mellitus were also included in this study. The patients were divided into five groups(Table 1).

Samples were taken from the coronary, carotid, intercostal, celiac, superior mesenteric, and renal arteries. Each section was stained by H.E., elastica van Gieson, Masson's trichrome and Oil red O.

In order to compare the intimal thickening for the various sampling sites, the intima was divided into four areas by longitudinal section; (A) proximal (B) distal (C) upper part (D) lower part(Fig. 1). The first centimeter from the origin of each branch was studied by using a computer system(Cosmozone; Nikon).

The severity of foam cell infiltrate was graded by scoring from 0 to 3 in each area.

To determine the origin of foam cells, either derived from monocytes or smooth muscle cells, the foam cells in the intima were identified by enzyme immuno-histochemical methods with lysozyme(Dako, U.S.A.) and myosin(generously provided by Dr. Fujiwara) and by electron microscopy.

Table 1 Groups of patients with hyperlipidemia and risk factors.

Group	Risk Factors		Age	Sex
I	Familiar Hypercholesterolemia	1	21	F (Homozygote)
		2	30	M (Homozygote)
		3	48	M (Heterozygote)
II	Secondary Hyperlipidemia (HL)[1]	1	38	M
		2	54	F
		3	50	M
		4	47	M
III	HL + HT[2]	1	70	F
		2	66	F
IV	HL + DM[3]	1	67	M
		2	67	M
		3	74	F
V	HL + DM + HT	1	73	F
		2	56	F
		3	73	M
		4	65	M
		5	83	F
		6	78	F
		7	61	M
		8	66	M
		9	67	F
		10	75	M
		11	59	M
		12	69	F

[1] More than total cholesterol 220 mg/dl
[2] Hypertension [3] Diabetes mellitus

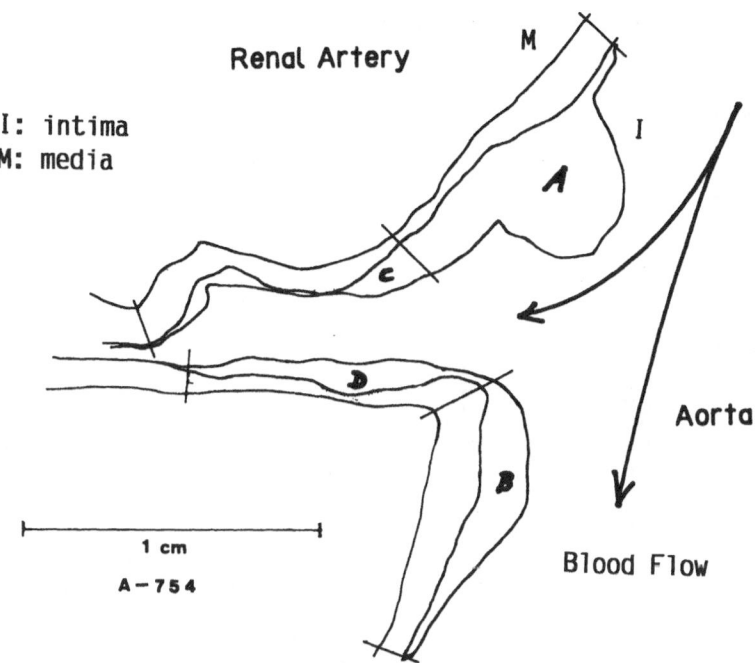

Fig. 1 Schema of the longitudinal section made along blood flow
       showing area A, B, C and D.

RESULTS

   Mean area of the intimal thickening(Fig. 2) as well as the grading
scores of the foam cell infiltrate(Fig. 3) in the proximal part (area
A) was larger than in the distal part (area B) ($P < 0.01$).
   Among the patients with familial hypercholesterolemia, hypertension, diabetes mellitus, or the combination of two or three of
these follows, there was no significant difference with respect to
intimal thickening in proximal portions (area A) (Fig. 4).   Intimal
thickening in patients with hypertension and/or diabetes mellitus
resembled that of patients with familial hypercholesterolemia(7).
   On electron microscopic study, a larger proportion of the foam
cells in area A was composed of smooth muscle cells than that in area
B ($P < 0.01$) (Fig. 5,6).   In area A, there were many synthetic phase
smooth muscle cells accompanied by accumulations of glycosaminoglycans
, while in the area B, collagen fibers were increased and contractile
smooth muscle cells were present (Fig. 6).
   Immunohistochemical examination revealed that lipid storage was
found more frequently and more extensively in smooth muscle cells
which were positive on stains for myosin antigen rather than in
macrophages (lysozyme positive) in the deeper areas of the thickened
intimas.

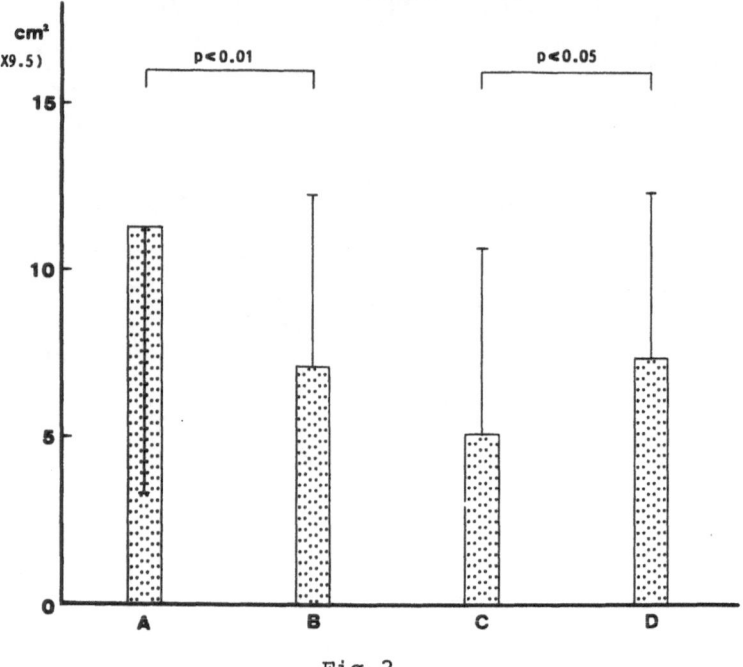

Fig.2

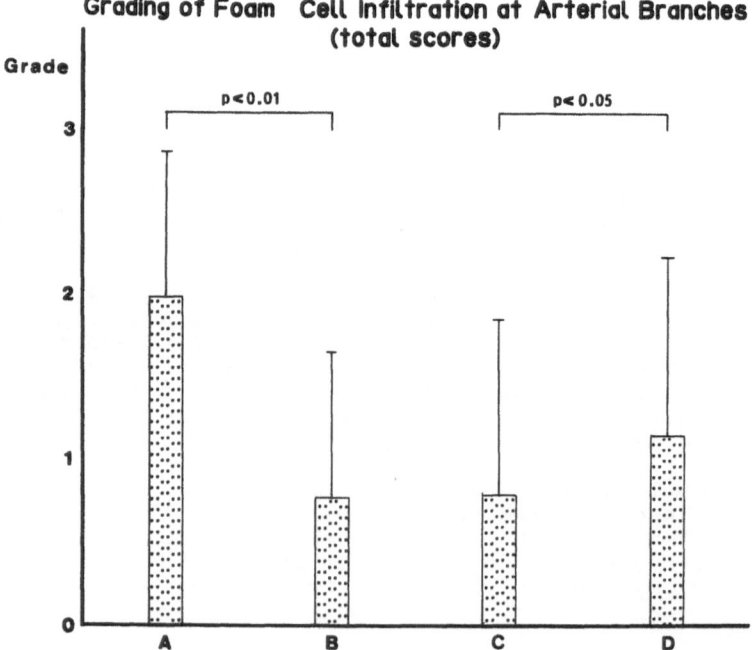

Fig.3

Areas of Intimal Thickening of Each Group

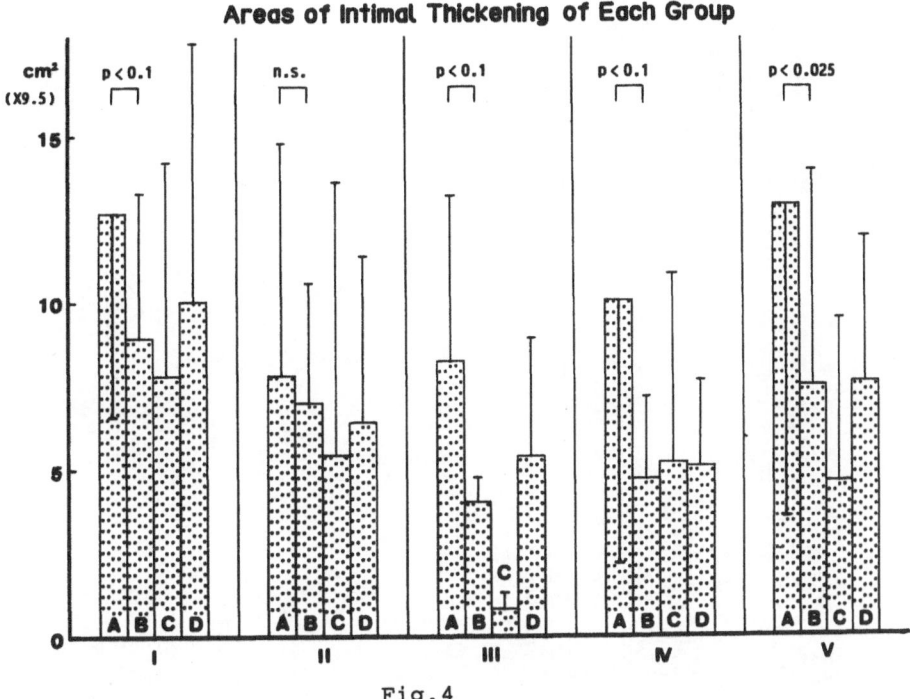

Fig.4

Comparison of SMC-foam cells with macrophage-foam cells
(Branches of intercostal artery)

Electron microscopic examination

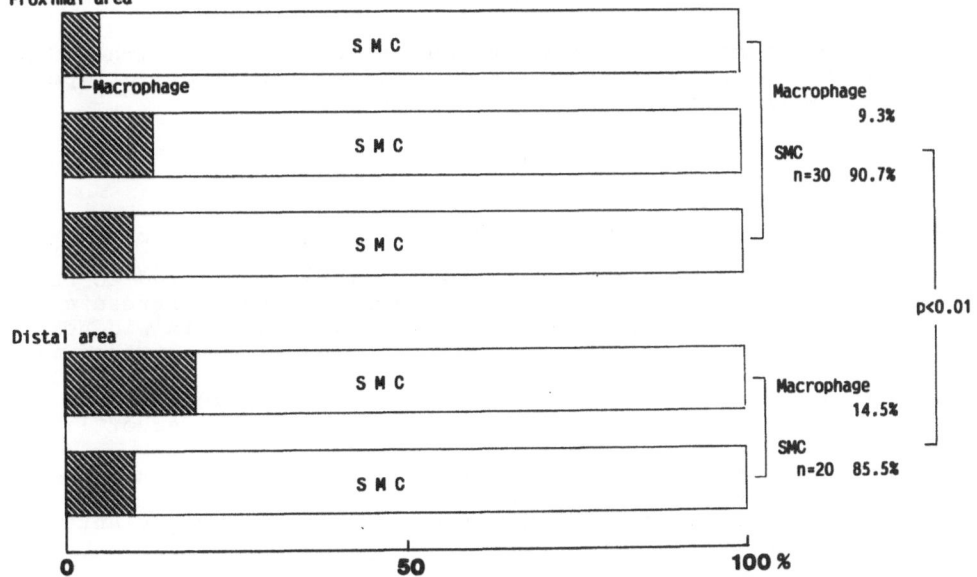

Fig.5

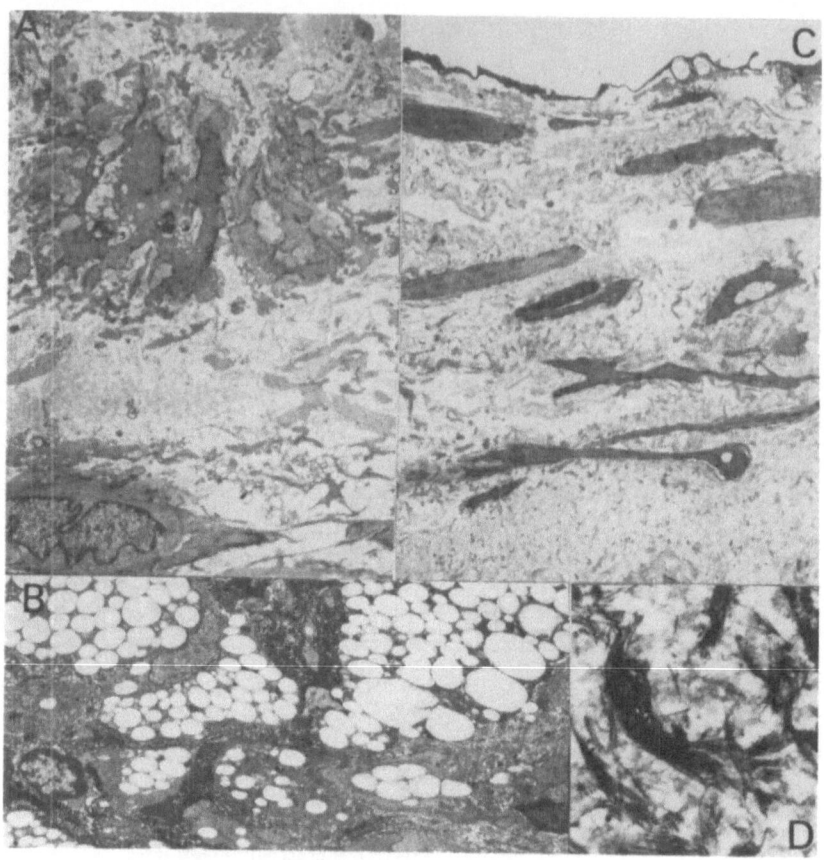

Fig. 6 Electron micrograph showing synthetic mode SMCs with GAG(A) and
       foam cells(B) in the proximal area and contractile type SMCs
       (C) with collagen fibers(D) in the distal area.

DISCUSSION

     In the setting of our study, area A may be considered to be a low
fluid shear stress area, and area B a highfluid shear stress area.
     Intimal thickening in area A was not only larger in wideness width
, but also had foam cell infiltrates to a greater extent than area B.
The results support a hypothesis that an exposure of the vascular
endothelium to low fluid shear stress leads to the formation of
atherosclerosis by adversely affecting the mass transfer of lipoprotein particles across the arterial wall(3).
     Moreover, the foam cells in area A were composed of a larger
population of smooth muscle cells than in area B. It is known that
foam cells derived from macrophages are easily removed by anticholesterolemic theraphy(8).

In most of the experimental animal models, either hereditary or
nutritional, atheromatous vascular lesions are consist mainly of
macrophages and are easy to regress by lowering plasma cholesterol
levels (2). In contrast, a longterm experiment at a moderate
cholesterol level in rabbits showed that smooth muscle cells mainly
constitute the vascular lesion and regression is not easy(9).
It is suggested that the smooth muscle cells play an important role
in lipid deposition and contribute to atherosclerotic lesions at the
sites of arterial branches and that the sitvation may be related to
the delayed regression of atherosclerotic lesions in humans in spite
of intensive antihypercholesterolemic treatment.
     Intimal thickening in patients with hypertension and/or diabetes
mellitus resembled that of patients with familial hypercholesterolemia
who lack functional low density lipoprotein receptors, this finding
indicated that the absence of functional low density lipoprotein
receptors in familial hypercholesterolemia does not appear to alter
the intimal thickening responces at arterial branches in chronic
hypercholesterolemia(7). Hence, risk factors, namely hypercholesterolemia, hypertension, and diabetes mellitus, may play an essential
role for the establishment of atherosclerotic lesions.

Acknowledgment: This work was partly supported by a Research Grant for
Cardiovascular Diseases(60C-2) from the Ministry of the Health and
Welfare.

REFERENCES

(1) Yokoyama S, Hayashi R, Satani M, Yamamoto A (1985) Arterio-
     sclerosis 5:613-622
(2) Fowler S, Shio H, Haley NJ (1979) Lab Invest 41:372-384
(3) Caro CG, Fitz-Gerald JM, Schroter RC (1971) Proc Roy Soc Lond B
     177:109-159
(4) Fry DL (1972) Localizing factors in arteriosclerosis. In: Likoff
     W, Segal BL, Insull W Jr(eds) Atherosclerosis and coronary Heart
     Disease. Grune and Stratton, New York, pp 85-104
(5) Kjaernes M, Svindland A, Walloe L, Wille O (1981) Acta Path
     Microbiol Scand Sect. A. 89:35-40
(6) Zarins CK, Giddens DP, Bharadvaj BK, Sottiurai VS, Mabon RF,
     Glagovs (1983) Circ Res 53:502-514
(7) Rosenfeld ME, Tsukada T, Chait A, Bierman EL, Gown AM, Ross R,
     (1987) Arteriosclerosis 1:24-34
(8) Yamamoto A, Matsuzawa Y, Yokoyama S, Funahashi T, Yamamura T,
     Kishino B (1986) Am J Cardiol 57:29H-35H
(9) Wilson RB, Miller RA, Middleton CC, Kinden D (1982) Arterio-
     sclerosis 2:228-241

Underlying Morphological Changes in the Arterial Wall at Bifurcations for Atherogenesis

Y. Yoshida[1], T. Oyama[1], S. Wang[1], T. Yamane[1], M. Mitsumata[1], T. Yamaguchi[2], and G. Ooneda[3]

[1]Department of Pathology, Yamanashi Medical College, Tamaho, 409-38 Japan
[2]Department of Vascular Physiology, National Cardiovascular Center Research Institute, Suita, 565 Japan
[3]Geriatrics Research Institute and Hospital, Maebashi, 371 Japan

ABSTRACT

Apical and outer wall intimas at branchings of inferior mesenteric arteries from aortas of human autopsy cases were investigated.
The outer wall intima, a low shear stress region, was thicker than the apical intima, a high shear stress region, except in cases younger than one month. Deposit of ß-lipoproteins in the outer wall intima increased with age, but not that in the apical intima. Electron microscopic studies revealed that collagen fibers increased markedly in the apical intima in the third decade. Among the dense collagen fibers, intimal smooth muscle cells(SMC) exhibited contractile phenotype. The outer wall possessed mucinous intima accompanied with synthetic SMC. Atherosclerotic rabbit intimal SMC cultivated on type 1 collagen gel increased cAMP production to change phenotype from synthetic to contractile and to suppress DNA synthesis. Early lipid deposition of rabbits placed on an atherogenic diet within three weeks occurred in special linear areas of flow dividers. As a result, blood flow dynamics may induce cellular and microarchitectural changes in vessel walls which are favorable or resistant to atherogenesis.

INTRODUCTION

Even if one assumes that the distribution of atherosclerosis is, in fact, a direct result of or at least mediated by the detailed characteristics of blood flow[1,2], there are still questions as to mechanisms through which fluid mechanics act. In human arteries the flow dividers at branchings, where relatively high wall shear stress is expected, are generally spared from the disease. The outer walls of branchings, where the blood flow must reduce shear rate, have preference for atherosclerosis[3]. Given precise topographical data relating to the distribution of atherosclerotic lesions of human arteries, it looks very hard to issue interpretations on the mechanisms of atherogenesis. Therefore, we have studied morphological changes in 2 regions expected to have low and high shear stress respectively, to clarify underlying vascular structures which must be altered by blood flow mechanics and, subsequently, have strong influence on atherogenesis. We have also mapped lipid deposition and studied arterial structural changes preceding the deposition in dietary induced hyperlipidemic rabbits.

MATERIALS AND METHODS

1. Human aortas were obtained from 81 autopsy cases ranging from infants to 75 year old persons. Both the flow divider (apex) and the outer wall of inferior mesenteric artery (IMA) branchings from abdominal aortas were investigated histometrically, immunohistochemically, and electron microscopically to study structural changes related to shear forces, and the relation between these forces and atherogenesis.

Histometrical study: On longitudinal paraffin sections through the center of 50 branchings, intimal thickness at 2 regions, the apex and the outer wall; the volume ratio of muscular cellular elements to matrices were measured on specimens stained with Weigert's elastic stain by a micrometer and with Azan's stain by point counting method respectively under a light microscope.

Immunohistochemical study: Histological specimens were prepared from 36 materials fixed in Zamboni's solution to stain with antisera against types 1 and 3 collagen, and ß-lipoproteins.

Electron microscopic (EM) study: Aortas obtained from 25 autopsy cases and fixed with a perfusion of fixatives (2.5% glutaraldehyde in buffers with or without ruthenium red) at 100 mm Hg within 2 hours after death. Small tissue blocks from both the apexes and the outer walls of IMA were postfixed in 1% OsO_4 to process for EM specimens.
Observation on the subendothelial structures under a scanning electron microscope was done on 20 materials which had been fixed in formalin and immersed in 88% formic acid (at 45°C) to dissolve cellular elements.

2. Effects of type 1 collagen on SMC morphology and functions were investigated in vitro in order to clarify the effects of collagen fibers increased in the apical intima of the human artery. Atherosclerotic intimal SMC which had been obtained from plaques of rabbit thoracic aortas were plated on type 1 collagen gel (protein concentration; 1 mg/ml) and incubated in DME with 10% fetal bovine serum. The cells were harvested after pulse labelings with ^{3}H-thymidine for 24 hours at the 1st, 3rd, 5th, and 7th days of the experiment to assay the number of cells and DNA synthetic activities. Amounts of cAMP and fine structures of SMC were also investigated.

3. Branchings in aortic arches and bifurcations of carotid arteries of 30 male rabbits weighing approximately 2 kg and had been on either a stock or an atherogenic diet containing 1% cholesterol and 5% lard for 1-3 weeks, were fixed by perfusion of the glutaraldehyde and then postfixed by the OsO_4 for electron microscopic studies. The earliest changes of atherosclerotic lesions and underlying structural changes in segments of artery, which have become susceptible to atherosclerosis, were investigated. Immunohistochemical studies were performed on specimens fixed with Zamboni's solution with antibodies against rabbit Apo B and E (generously provided by Dr. Tomikawa, Daiichi Pharmaceutical Co., Central Research Institute).

RESULTS

1. Studies on morphological changes in the apical and outer wall intima at bifurcation of IMA from the human aorta

Histometrical and immunohistochemical findings: Humans within 1 month after birth had thick apical intimas, consisting of 3-4 layers, compared to the intimas of outer walls, with only 1 or no layer of SMC. Consequently, the ratio of intimal thicknesses in apical to outer walls (A/O) was at most infinity. In that case, the apical intima

was 15μ thick while the outer wall intima had no thickness (Fig.1).
After one month, thickness in the outer wall intima increased rapidly,
so that the A/O ratio became close to 1. Intimal thickenings developed
more in the outer wall than in the apex of branchings in all ages
after childhood (Fig.2), and the ratio of cellular elements of SMC
to intimal areas had a tendency of decrease, as increased intimal
thickness. Collagen fibers including types 1 and 3 increased in
the intima, as both intimal thickness and age increased. Elastic fibers
in the intima increased predominantly in the apex as age increased.
There was no apparent tendency of the volume of elastic fibers in
the outer wall related to age. Deposit of ß-lipoproteins in the
outer wall intima increased as age increased, but not in the apical
intima.

EM findings: Late in the first decade, the endothelial cells

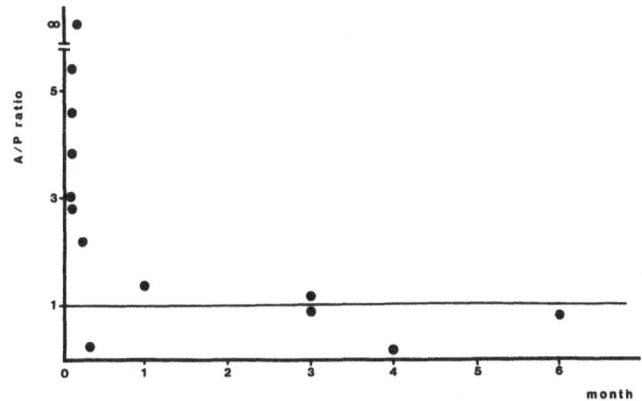

FIG. 1 Ratio of intimal thickness in apical to proximal outer wall
(A/P) at IMA in cases of younger than 6 months of age.

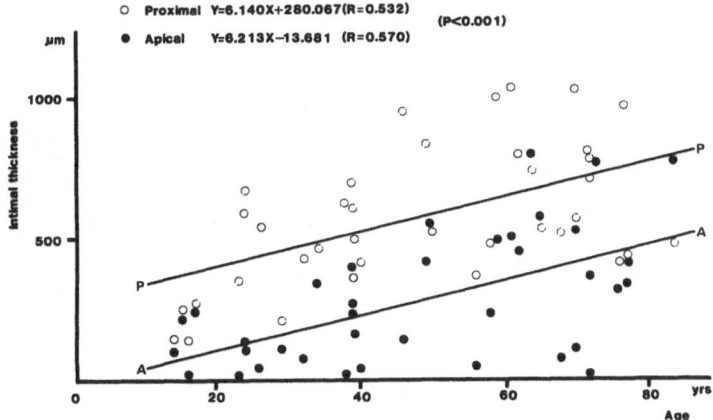

FIG. 2 Intimal thickness of apical and proximal outer walls at
branchings of IMA (n=37).

on the apex showed apparent bundles of stress fibers in cytoplasms with well developed subendothelial basement membranes (BM). There were no marked differences in the figure of the intimal SMC nor in the amounts of extracellular matrices between the apical and outer wall intimas. In the second decade, predominant findings in the apical intima were the occurrence of synthetic SMC accompanied with a bunch of collagen and elastic fibers and increase of BM and BM-like substances beneath the endothelium. In the third decade, apical intima covered with flat endothelial cells had a remarkable increase of collagen fibers, giving a dense appearance. Intimal SMC embedded among collagen fibers were elongated and showed contractile phenotype, being rich in cytoplasmic filaments (Fig. 3). Contrary to the apical intimas, the outer wall intimas had a loose appearance due to the accumulation of a matrix abundant in GAGs, and sparse in collagen and elastic fibers. Intimal SMC were thick due to being equipped with rich rough surfaced endoplasmic reticuli (RER), so they were regarded as synthetic phenotype (Fig. 4). Endothelial cells covering mucinous intima of outer walls appeared to bind uncertainly to the underlying tissues, as if floating on the mucinous intimas without the existence of anchoring structures. After the fourth decade, the outer wall intima exhibited frequent denudation of endothelial cells, leading to enhancement of insudation and the accumulation of blood constituents in the increased matrices of the inner layer of the intima. There was infiltration of lymphocytes and macrophages, as well as deposition of fibrin threads. Subsequently, cellular and fibrous components in the inner layer of the intima looked to have been dispersed by the accumulation of edema fluid. Lipid droplets appeared in synthetic SMC in the intima, to form foam cells. In the depth of intimas collagen

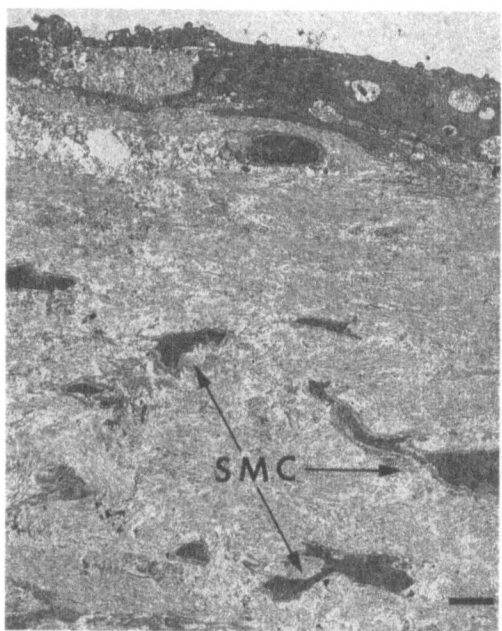
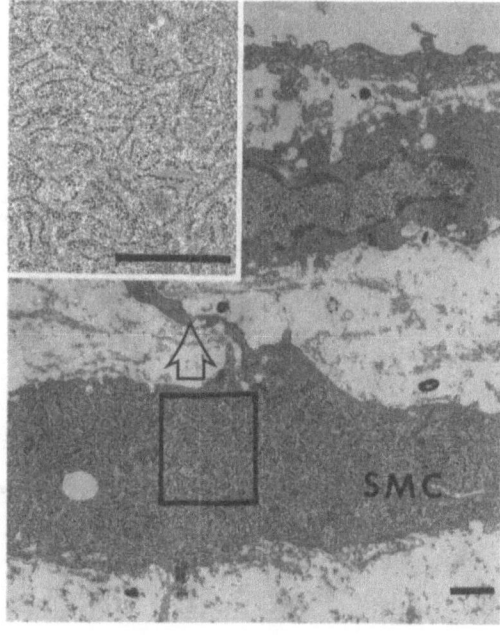

FIG. 3 IMA apex shows densely collagenous intima with contractile SMC. 25 year old female.   Bar: 1μ

FIG. 4 IMA outer wall mucinous intima still has synthetic SMC. The same case to FIG. 3.

fibers increased and SMC showed contractile phenotype.

Observation of subendothelial BM, comparing between the apical and outer walls, under a scanning electron microscope revealed that thick fibrils consisting of BM were both parallel and in the direction of blood stream in both the apex and outer wall in the first decade. In cases past the third decade, fibrils of BM in the outer wall became thin and disarrayed, resulting in loose, spongy BM, while the fibrils in the apex structures similar to those in the first decade.

2. Effects of collagen gel on cell growth and phenotype of SMC

The number of the SMC plated on the gel reached a plateau at a lower density than did the cells plated directly on plastic dishes. The amount of cAMP was increased and DNA synthesis (1443 ± 57 in experimental group, 2419 ± 241 DPM/10^4 cells in control group on 5th day) was suppressed in the cells cultivated on collagen gel (Tab. 1). Electron microscopy disclosed that cellular areas covered with thin filaments increased by the 10th days after seeding on the gel (Tab. 2).

TABLE 1 Effects of type 1 collagen gel on cell growth and cAMP production in atherosclerotic intimal SMC

Day	Number of cell (10^4/dish)		cAMP (pmol/cell $\times 10^4$)	
	Cultures on gel	Cultures on dishes	Cultures on gel	Cultures on dishes
1	10.3±1.2	8.9±0.9	3.23±0.31	3.15±0.23
3	20.9±1.1	27.2±1.2	6.35±0.34	3.35±0.60
5	25.5±1.6	43.3±1.9	10.50±1.26	5.38±0.22
7	27.4±1.4	45.8±2.8	11.60±0.33	8.38±1.16

TABLE 2 Areas rich in thin filaments in atherosclerotic intimal SMC cultured on type 1 collagen gel for 10 days

collagen concentration	n	%area
2.0 mg/ml	57	16.5±1.2
1.0	24	14.3±2.3
0	18	8.0±1.0

3. Pattern of lipid deposition on the arterial wall of cholesterol fed rabbits

Early lipid deposition, caused by dietary induced hypercholesterolemia, in arterial walls of rabbits has been observed in so-called high shear stress regions, such as the apex of bifurcations, contrary to human arteries. Distribution of lipid depositions on histological serial sections from branchings from aortic arches of rabbits which had received with the atherogenic diet for two weeks, were copied on dental paraffin plates, in order to learn the 3-dimensional pattern of lipid deposition on paraffin models of flow dividers. Careful observation of lipid depositions in the flow dividers on reconstructed models disclosed that the oval shaped linear deposit developed symmetrically, running from approximately 0.3 mm to 1.4 mm from the ridge on either side. From the center, the 2 linear deposits close in, fusing at both ends to form an oval fashion on the whole (Fig. 5).

Apical portions of flow dividers spared of lipid deposition showed flat endothelial cells with well developed subendothelial BM, BM-like substances, and collagen fibers in intact rabbits not on cholesterol diets (Fig. 6). Special areas where lipid deposition is expected in

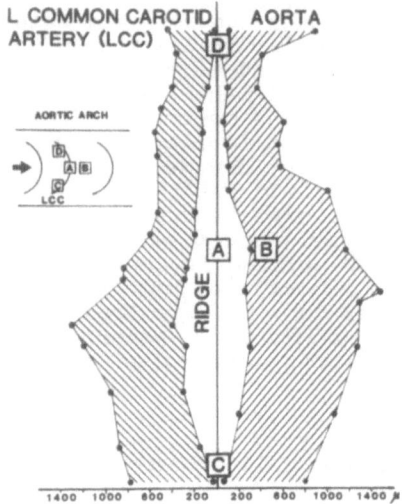

L COMMON CAROTID ARTERY (LCC)   AORTA

AORTIC ARCH

RIDGE

FIG. 5 Lipoprotein deposition ///// on a flow divider of a rabbit fed chol. for 2 weeks.

early atherosclerotic rabbits showed swollen endothelial cells with large vacuoles and the development of poor BM and BM-like substances beneath the endothelium even in intact rabbits (Fig. 7). During the experimental period with feeding of the cholesterol diet, no remarkable chagnes were found in the apical endothelial cells and subendothelial spaces. The areas apart from the apex where lipid deposition was apt to occur were covered by endothelial cells with opened intercellular junctions and lipid inclusions had increased subendothelial spaces due to an increase in the number of intimal SMC and extracellular matrices.

DISCUSSION

Long standing mechanical stimuli produced by blood flow on the arterial wall could develop microarchitecture which may be favorable or resistant to atherosclerosis.

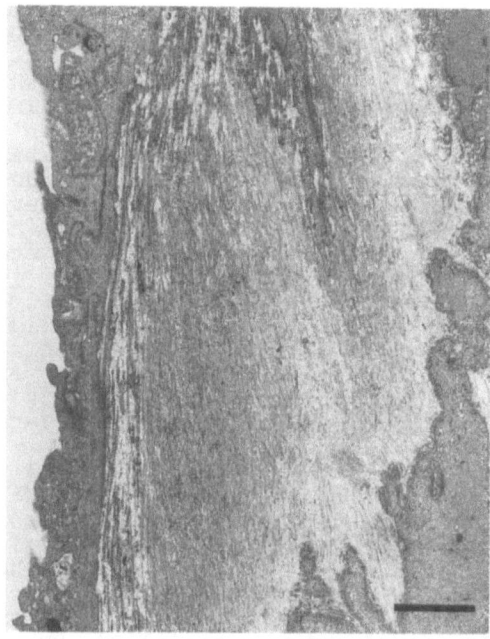

FIG. 6 Apex of a flow divider at LCC branching of an intact rabbit shows fibrous intima.

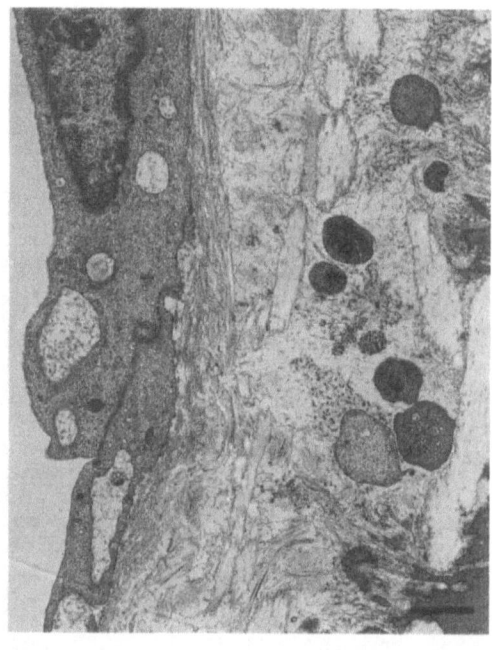

FIG. 7 Area 300μ apart from the apex of the same divider in FIG. 6 has vacuolated endothelial cells.

High shear stress affecting on flow dividers could induce not only stress fibers in endothelial cells, but well developed subendothelial basement membranes and dense intimal collagen fibers including types 1 and 3. Although the effects of stress fibers in endothelial cells on permeability of lipoproteins through endothelial cells still remain obscure, collagen fibers may change phenotype of intimal smooth muscle cells from synthetic to contractile, which have been confirmed as lesser responders to growth factors in vitro [4], resulting in low proliferative activity of SMC in the arterial wall. Cyclic AMP has been well known to be a substance regulating cell proliferation and production of cytoskeleton[5]. Type 1 collagen increased the amount of cAMP in SMC in vitro.

Contrary to those in high shear stress regions, SMC in low shear stress regions remained thier synthetic type even in cases beyond the third decade. A large accumulation of glycosaminoglycans in the outer wall intima might be induced by synthetic SMC, although mechanisms of GAGs production by SMC in low shear stress regions have not been clarified. Endothelial cells covering mucinous intima appeared to have a loose and fragile attachment to the subendothelial layer, that leading to easy denudation of endothelial cells. Blood constituents permeated and accumulated in the intimal matrices rich in GAGs. Not only do GAGs act as a molecular sieve, but they form both soluble and insoluble complexes with lipoproteins to precipitate in the intima[6]. GAGs make the LDL particles large electronegative aggregations which are taken up by macrophages, devoid of feedback control[7]. Particularly intimal synthetic SMC have shown high ability to ingest lipoproteins to form foam cells. These results may explain different vulnerability of arterial wall to atherosclerosis between high and low shear stress regions.

Dietary induced hyperlipidemic rabbits showed special narrow areas of lipid deposition. Apical portion spared of lipid deposition, and shoulders of flow dividers, preferential for lipid deposition, showed apparent morphological differences from each other, even in intact, healthy rabbits. These morphological differences could give the idea that endothelial cells located in specific narrowed areas might be particularly vulnerable due to a certain range of shear stress, for additional toxic substances such as hyperlipidemic LDL and peroxide lipids.

CONCLUSION

Long standing mechanical stimuli produced by high shear stress of blood flow may develop the microarchitecture in the arterial wall which may be strongly resistant to atherogenic stimuli. Shear stress within a certain range of strength may cause atherosclerosis. Persistence of synthetic smooth muscle cells in low shear regions may bring about microarchitecture which is favorable to atherosclerosis, such as loose endothelial attachment to subendothelial tissue, accumulation of GAGs in the intima and frequent occurrence of foam cells.

Acknowledgment: This work was supported by Research Grant for Cardiovascular Diseases (60C-2) from the Ministry of the Health and Welfare.

REFERENCES

[1]Fukushima T, Azuma T (1982) Biorheology 19:143-154
[2]Ku DN, Giddens DP, Zarins CK, Glagov S (1985) Arteriosclerosis 5: 293-302
[3]Caro CG, Fitz-Gerald JM, Schroter RC (1969) Nature 223:1159-1161
[4]Chamley-Campbell J, Campbell GR, Ross R (1979) Physiol. Rev. 59:1-61
[5]Dedman JR, Brinkley BR, Means AR (1979) Regulation of microfilaments and microtubules by calcium and cyclic AMP. In: Greengard P and Robinson GA(eds) Advances in Cyclic Nucleotide Research vol. 11. Raven Press, New York, pp 131-174
[6]Srinivasan SR, Dolan P, Radhakrishnamurthy B, Berenson GS (1975) Biochim. Biophy. Acta 388:58-70
[7]Berenson GS, Radhakrishnamurthy B, Srinivasan SR, Vijayagopal P, Dalferes ER (1985) Proteoglycans and potential mechanisms related to atherosclerosis. In: Lee KT(ed), Atherosclerosis. New York Acad Sci., pp 69-78

The Relationship Between Intimal Thickening and the Hemodynamic Environment of the Arterial Wall

M.H. FRIEDMAN

Applied Physics Laboratory, The Johns Hopkins University, Laurel, MD 20707, USA

ABSTRACT

The time-varying shear rates at the walls of human arteries are estimated from laser Doppler anemometer measurements in flow-through casts of human aortic and coronary bifurcations, through which physiologically realistic, fluid dynamically scaled, pulsatile flows are passed. These shear rates are then correlated against morphological measurements at corresponding sites in the vessels from which the casts had been made. These correlations suggest that the dependence of intimal thickening rate on mural shear is complex and changes over time; in particular, the intimal thickness at sites exposed to high or more unidirectional shear stresses increases quickly to a modest value, growing slowly thereafter, while the thickness at sites exposed to low or more oscillatory shears rises more slowly but, after time, reaches higher values. This behavior can be the result of competing shear-dependent processes. This explanation of the experimental results is supported by a mathematical model of intimal thickening that incorporates a selection of the biological processes that take place in the arterial wall as it responds to its hemodynamic environment. A best parsimonious fit to the data is obtained when, at sites exposed to relatively high shear, smooth muscle cells accumulate more rapidly in the intima but express extracellular matrix at a slower rate.

INTRODUCTION

For some years, we have been studying the interaction between hemodynamics and the arterial wall, and the mediation of this interaction by arterial geometry. There is a considerable body of indirect evidence that hemodynamic factors are involved in the initial formation and localization of atherosclerotic lesions. It is therefore important to elucidate the response of the vascular wall to its hemodynamic environment.

METHODS

To advance knowledge in this area, realistic hemodynamic data are obtained by laser Doppler anemometry at multiple sites in transparent flow-through casts of minimally involved human aortic [1] and coronary artery [2] bifurcations. The vessels are obtained at autopsy, fixed under physiological pressure, and infused with silicone rubber to form a luminal mold around which the cast is formed. Minimally involved vessels are selected so that the lumen and the flow field have not yet been altered by the presence of raised lesions.

The pulsatile flow waves used in these investigations are physiologically realistic, and the flow magnitude and pulse frequency are fluid dynamically scaled to reproduce the in vivo state. Both rigid and compliant casts have been prepared for these investigations. For either kind of cast, a working fluid is selected whose refractive index matches that of the cast; this makes it possible to form a well-defined scattering volume in the flow in spite of the irregularity of the vessel wall.

Mural shear rates estimated from time-varying velocities measured at multiple sites close to the walls of the casts are correlated against the morphology of corresponding sites in the original vessels. Wall shear rates are estimated from the velocity data by dividing the measured velocities by the perpendicular distance from the velocity measurement site to the wall. In the aortic bifurcation casts, this distance ranged between 0.5 and 0.9 mm. An advantage of this approach is that the hemodynamic environment and morphologic response of individual sites are obtained. The sites selected are primarily along the lateral walls of the parent and daughter vessels and along the flow divider, in the approximate plane of the bifurcation, where the circumferential component of the fluid velocity is small. The measurements on the tissue include intimal, medial and adventitial thickness; the sites are also scored for sudanophilia.

RESULTS AND INTERPRETATION

In analyzing the data, shear rate has been selected as the primary hemodynamic variable, at least in part because turbulence and extensive separation were not seen in any of the casts. The vascular response that was examined in greatest detail is the thickening of the arterial intima, since it is believed that local thickening of this layer can be a precursor to focal atherosclerosis. Altogether, shear rate and morphology data were obtained at over 160 sites in ten aortic bifurcations and their casts, and at fourteen sites in a left main coronary artery bifurcation and its cast.

For each of the aortic bifurcations, linear regressions were computed between intimal thickness and seven measures of wall shear rate [3]. These included:

1. the time-average (mean) shear rate;
2. the time-average of the logarithm of the absolute shear rate;
3. the maximum instantaneous shear rate;
4. the pulse shear rate [4], which is the difference between the maximum and minimum shear rates and measures the flow acceleration in systole;
5. max $\{I_+, I_-\}/(I_+ + I_-)$, where $I_+(I_-)$ is the magnitude of the impulse acting on a unit area of the wall during antegrade (retrograde) flow. This quantity measures the unidirectionality of the flow at the wall.

These measures are highly correlated with one another; that is, a site exposed to a relatively low maximum shear is also exposed to a relatively low mean shear, less flow acceleration, and a less unidirectional impulse. In the discussion to follow, the terms "high shear" and "low shear" should be understood to have the broader meanings suggested by these correlations.

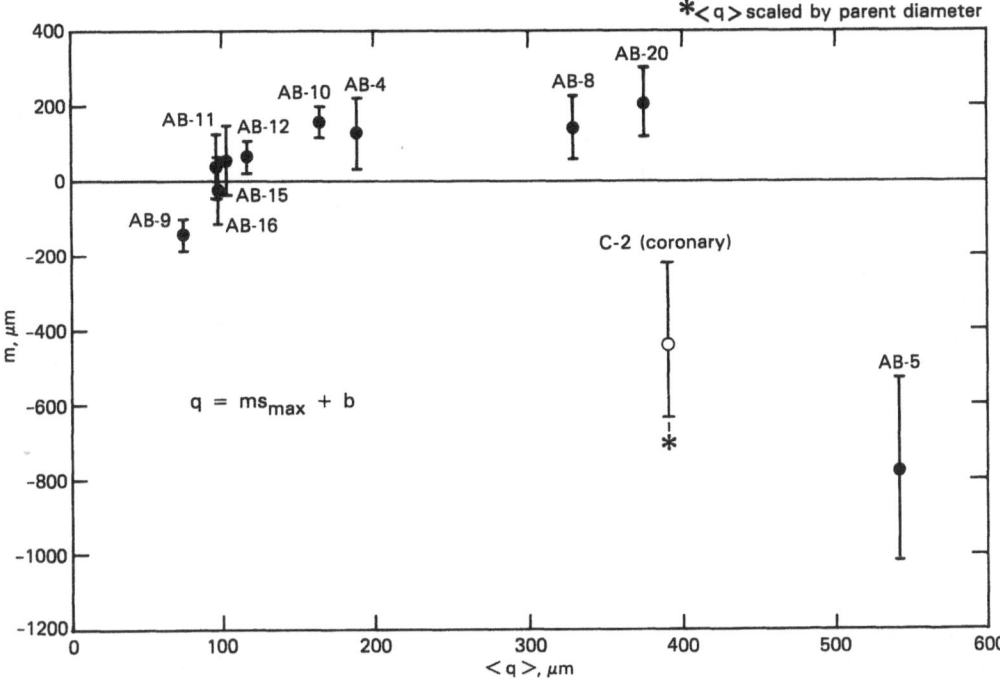

FIG. 1. Variation with mean intimal thickness of the slopes of linear correlations between thickness and shear rate, for ten aortic bifurcations and a left main coronary artery bifurcation. The coronary artery datum was made consistent with the aortic bifurcation data by assuming that intimal thickness can be scaled according to the diameter of the parent vessel at the branch.

The slopes of the regression lines were related to the mean intimal thickness in the branch [5]. Figure 1 shows the results of these regressions when the shear rate measure used was maximum instantaneous shear rate. To lessen the effect of differences among the experimental flow rates in the several casts, and the differences between the experimental flow in a given cast and the in vivo flow in the vessel from which it had been made, the maximum shear rates were normalized by dividing each one by the average of the maximum shear rates obtained in that cast. Because of the high correlation among the shear rate measures, the results summarized in Fig. 1 were not qualitatively different when other measures were used.

Referring to Fig. 1, when the intima is thin, the slopes of the thickness-shear rate correlations are naturally near zero. When the intima is moderately thick, the slopes of the correlations are positive; that is, the sites at which the intima is thickest are those exposed to relatively high shears. For the aortic bifurcation having the largest mean intimal thickness, and for the coronary artery bifurcation, the slope was decidedly negative.

Each of the correlations in Fig. 1 describes the relation between shear rate and intimal thickness in a different individual, a snapshot taken when the subject died. What we would like to do is to combine these snapshots to make a movie that will give us a sense of how the thickening process proceeds over time. To do this, we regard

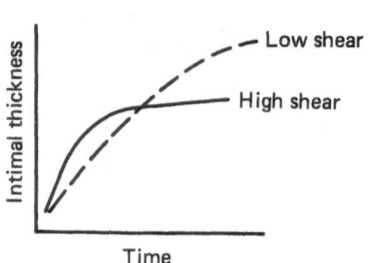

FIG. 2. Sketch of the variation of intimal thickness with time, for two different shear rates, as inferred from the correlations between intimal thickness and wall shear rate in ten human aortic bifurcations.

mean intimal thickness as a measure of "biological age". Then, the behavior illustrated in Fig. 1 can be thought of as representing the chronology of the thickening process in a single vessel. The data in Fig. 1 then imply that the slope of the thickness-shear rate relation changes over time, first assuming positive values, and then becoming increasingly negative.

This implies that curves of thickness versus time at different shear rates cross, as shown schematically in Fig. 2. Specifically, the intimal thickness at sites exposed to high or more unidirectional shear stresses initially increases relatively quickly to a modest value, growing more slowly thereafter; in contrast, the intimal thickness at sites experiencing lower or more oscillatory shears rises more slowly at first, but ultimately becomes larger. Thus the dependence of intimal thickness and thickening rate on mural shear changes over time.

A MODEL OF INTIMAL THICKENING UNDER SHEAR

The behavior shown in Fig. 2 can be the result of competing shear-dependent processes at and in the vessel wall. The plausibility of this explanation is supported by a biologically simple mathematical model of early intimal thickening that we have developed to explore this possibility more fully. The model conforms with what is known about the biological processes that take place in the arterial wall and the response of arterial wall cells to hemodynamics. Most of this knowledge has been gained from experiments using cells in culture. The results of fitting the model to our experimental data support the notion that multiple shear-dependent processes can account for the behavior shown in Fig. 2.

A cartoon of the version of the model that gave the best parsimonious fit to our experimental data is shown in Fig. 3. The salient features of this version are:

1. the rate of smooth muscle cell accumulation in the intima (J_s in Fig. 3) is more rapid at sites exposed to relatively high shear;
2. the rate constant for extracellular matrix production by smooth muscle cells (k_e in Fig. 3) is lower at the high-shear sites;
3. the latter shear dependence is stronger than the former;
4. monocyte-derived macrophages can leave the intima until the matrix level reaches a critical value, after which the macrophages remain in the intima as foam cells.

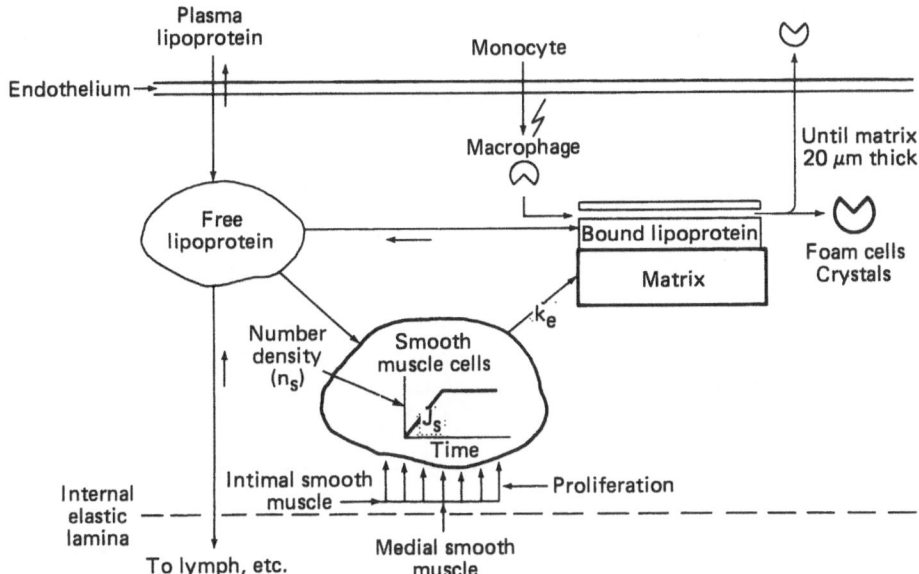

FIG. 3. Best parsimonious model of shear-dependent intimal thickening. The parameters on stippled backgrounds vary with wall shear. The heavily outlined compartments contribute to intimal thickness.

Other processes that were considered for inclusion in the model, but whose retention could not be justified statistically, were the chemotaxis of monocytes by smooth muscle cells and the lysis of matrix by macrophages. The addition of a shear dependence to the inhibition of smooth muscle cell proliferation could not be justified on statistical grounds, nor could a shear-dependent monocyte entry rate.

This version of the model predicts that the early stages of thickening are dominated by smooth muscle accumulation. Since this proceeds more rapidly where the shear is high, young intimas are thicker at high-shear sites. As time proceeds, increasing amounts of matrix are produced, particularly where the shear is low. The threshold for foam cell formation is reached first at these sites, and the combination of foam cells and increased matrix leads eventually to more intimal thickening where the shear is low.

The model assigns a nondimensional biological age, T, to each vessel, based on the intimal thickness measurements and the values of the parameters of the model. In Fig. 4, the values of T for each specimen are correlated against the ages of the subjects at death. The biological ages of the females are almost all less than those predicted from their chronological ages, and the opposite is true for the males; womens arteries age more slowly than those of men. This is consistent with sex differences in the incidence of the usual endpoints of vascular disease.

Models like the one presented here do not prove mechanism, but they do allow us to interpet the outcome of the natural in vivo experiment, carried out over a period of decades in a living artery, in terms of knowledge gained from laboratory experiments in cell biology. They serve as a valuable synthesizing tool, and in conjunction with fluid mechanical investigations and measurements of

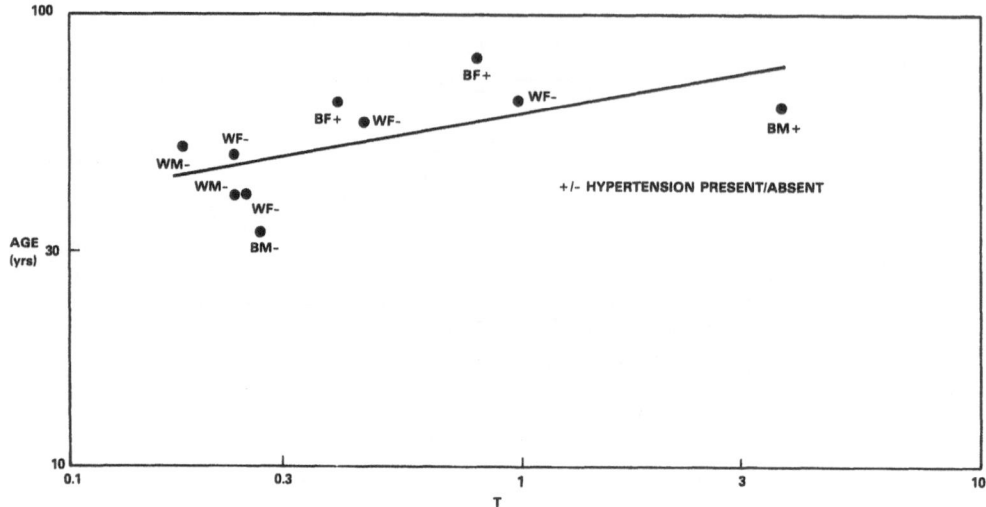

FIG. 4. Age of each vessel when acquired vs. nondimensional biological age of the vessel obtained from the model in Fig. 3. Indicated on the figure are sex, race and hypertensive status (+/-) of each subject.

human pathology, can further our understanding of the role of hemodynamics in atherogenesis.

Acknowledgments: My colleagues in the experimental program are C. B. Bargeron, O. J. Deters, G. M. Hutchins and F. F. Mark. I would also like to acknowledge P. F. Davies advice during the development of the intimal thickening model. The fitting of the model to the experimental data was carried out by S. Favin. This research is supported by Grant HL-34626, National Institutes of Health.

REFERENCES

[1]Friedman MH, Hutchins GM, Bargeron CB, Deters OJ, Mark FF (1981) Atherosclerosis 39:425-436
[2]Friedman MH, Bargeron CB, Deters OJ, Hutchins GM, Mark FF (1987) Atherosclerosis, in press
[3]Friedman MH, Deters OJ (1987) J. Biomechanical Engineering 109:25-26
[4]Friedman MH, Hutchins GM, Bargeron CB, Deters OJ, Mark FF (1981) J. Biomechanical Engineering 103:204-207
[5]Friedman MH, Deters OJ, Bargeron CB, Hutchins GM, Mark FF (1986) Atherosclerosis 60:161-171

The Role of Haemodynamics in the Proliferative Lesions of Atherosclerosis

W.E. STEHBENS

Department of Pathology, Wellington School of Medicine and the Malaghan Institute of Medical Research, Wellington 2, New Zealand

ABSTRACT

Atherosclerosis, a degenerative disease of blood vessels, is universal in man and is not species-specific. Popular theories of its aetiology are only concerned with some aspects of the disease and do not explain the pathogenesis and the complications. Present evidence substantiates the view that the topography of the disease can be explained by local haemodynamic factors and indicates also that haemodynamically-induced vibrational stress is capable of producing the disease and its complications even in the absence of elevated serum lipids. This fatigue hypothesis is the most plausible explanation of the disease and its complications.

INTRODUCTION

Atherosclerosis is a chronic degenerative disease universal in man with the only variable being the severity of individual involvement. It occurs in varying severity in many lower animals and therefore not being species-specific it follows that the cause must also pertain to these other species. Currently four hypotheses of the aetiology of the disease warrant consideration.

THROMBOGENIC THEORY

The thrombogenic hypothesis postulates that thrombi forming within the vessels are incorporated within the intima and become atheromata. This is untenable because (1) all available experimental evidence indicates that thrombosis is secondary to intimal discontinuity which then becomes the primary lesion and the thrombosis is a secondary phenomenon, (2) the distribution of thrombi differs from that of atherosclerosis and (3) the concept does not explain the pathogenesis of the disease and all its complications. Nevertheless, the incorporation of thrombi into the vessel wall in advanced disease can contribute to mural thickening and further encroachment on the lumen.

INTIMAL INJURY THEORY

The intimal injury theory[1] postulates that mitogenic factors from platelets adherent at the site of a hypothetical endothelial defect stimulate the proliferation of intimal smooth muscle cells to produce the intimal thickening that precedes lipid deposition. This is an hypothesis pertinent to only one step in the pathogenesis. It does not explain the complete pathogenesis of the disease and its complications. The endothelial defect is the primary lesion, the hypothetical injury is the cause and the mitogenic factor is but one of the possible mediators of cellular proliferation. Moreover endothelial injury must be more prevalent in superficial subcutaneous veins and yet no progressive lesion develops as a consequence irrespective of blood lipids. Evidence from in vivo studies in experimental animals indicates that platelets do not adhere to intact endothelium even in stagnant vessels despite the enhancement of platelet stickiness[2], so it is most improbable that platelets adhere at forks of large arteries in the absence of severe endothelial injury. No evidence of platelet sticking or thrombosis has been observed at the cerebral arterial forks of foetuses and neonates when the initial intimal proliferation develops. Endothelium is highly sensitive to injury but the concept of consistent injury at very specific anatomical sites in arteries is difficult to sustain. Furthermore since microthromboembolism occurs after trivial endothelial injuries, and if such microthrombi progress to intimal proliferation and then to atherosclerosis rather than resolving, survival of mammalian life would be doubtful.

An important feature of this theory is the implicit recognition that fibro-musculo-elastic proliferation of the intima is an integral part of atherosclerosis and that it precedes the accumulation of lipid.

LIPID HYPOTHESIS

The lipid hypothesis merely theorizes simplistically about the reason for and means of lipid accumulation in the vessel wall. The pathology of the cholesterol-fed animal and that of familial hypercholesterolaemia have been misrepresented for these diseases are lipid storage disorders with irreconcilable differences from spontaneous athero-sclerosis[3-5]. Epidemiological evidence never proves a cause and effect relationship and only provides correlations that require verification by other means or substantiation by experimental evidence or pathological confirmation in man. As the national mortality rates have been shown to be fallacious due to substantial but unquantifiable diagnostic error[6] and the pathological evidence required for plausibility of the epidemiological evidence has been misrepresented, the lipid hypothesis is lacking in scientific basis. The results of large-scale intervention trials undertaken for the prevention of coronary heart disease have not only been disappointing but have failed to take into account the large diagnostic error associated with such studies. The majority of investigators in the field of atherogenesis are poorly acquainted with the pathology and its natural history and as a consequence the validity of the lipid hypothesis has been accepted on reaffirmation.

After it was demonstrated that the chronic administration of egg yolk or cholesterol induced lipid-containing lesions in rabbit arteries and veins, the lipid hypothesis emerged. Subsequently the assumption has been promulgated that atherosclerosis is a disease primarily concerned with lipid metabolism and typified by an inability of the vessel wall to either dispose of or metabolize lipid accumulation in the intima due to an excessive influx of cholesterol or more recently of low density lipoproteins. The lipid hypothesis has dominated thinking and research in atherosclerosis and haemodynamics was relegated to a lesser role as merely a localizing factor. Other factors such as age, sex, smoking, hypertension etc., have all been assigned causal roles though obviously this is not possible because the cause (or causes) must be present in every human and every lower animal with atherosclerosis. Though cause has been misused by epidemiologists and extrapolation from coronary heart disease to atherosclerosis is invalid, the more simplistic elements of the lipid hypothesis have been disseminated by vested interests with inconsistencies and fallacious data conveniently ignored.

FATIGUE HYPOTHESIS

The fourth hypothesis is the fatigue or haemodynamic theory. Early this century atherosclerosis was considered to be a degenerative disease essentially due to "wear and tear" because it occurred with increasing severity with age and the topography of lesions was in large part determined by non-specific haemodynamic factors. For example the severity of the disease is greater in the systemic circulation than in the pulmonary circulation and is least severe in the venous circulation which correlates with the respective blood pressure in these circulations. An increase in blood pressure is associated with an increase in the severity of the disease in each of these circulations and hypotension is usually associated with longevity. Atherosclerosis is more severe in the abdominal aorta and iliac arteries than in the proximal aorta because of the augmented systolic and pulse pressures distally and varies in severity from vascular bed to vascular bed. In each circulatory tree it is most severe in the large vessels. Atherosclerosis is particularly prone to occur about sites of branching, unions and curvatures and in the carotid siphon and is localized in intimal cushions beyond the lesser curvatures[2]. It is said to be augmented by increased functional demand and affects the vessel wall from within out, each layer being affected and not merely the intima. Consequently haemodynamics was believed to be important in the localization of the disease.
Macroscopic lipid staining is of dubious value in localizing atherosclerotic lesions due to limited penetrability of lipid stains and the lipid that stains macroscopically in advanced lesions does not necessarily reflect the initial site of early lesions. Moreover it is now widely accepted that there is a pre-lipid phase of atherosclerosis and clues to aetiology are best sought in the earliest demonstrable microscopic lesions. For these reasons detailed histological study of serial sections of a large number of arterial forks from humans and other animals revealed that the intimal thickening at arterial forks occurred initially in the foetus as small intimal proliferations at specific anatomical sites that suggested haemodynamic localization. These localized zones of intimal proliferation (pads or cushions) occur in the entrance to the daughter branches immediately beyond the lateral angles and also over the crescentic flow divider where the blood impinges and divides into the two streams that enter the daughter branches. In flow studies of experimental glass models of forks, periodic vortex shedding has been generated at the bifurcation and this is believed to be akin to a jet edge effect and responsible for the intimal thickening over the flow divider. The lateral pads have been attributed to the vibrational effects in the boundary layer separation[2].
These and other observations led to the concept that atherosclerosis was due to haemodynamically-induced engineering fatigue of the vessel wall. The complications of the disease can also

be explained on the basis of loss of tensile strength and histologically and ultrastructurally all degenerative changes in the vessel wall could be manifestations of loss of cohesion of the vascular tissue.

EXPERIMENTAL MODELS

Since the complications of atherosclerosis usually take at least 50 years to become manifest, it followed that to test the fatigue hypothesis it was necessary to accelerate the disease by using models known to be associated with severe vibrational stress (viz. arteriovenous fistulae and aneurysms). The third model selected was the U-shaped bend in which the acute bend at the base of the U is often noticeably pulsatile. In glass models of U-bends vortex shedding occurs at low Reynolds numbers.

In the first model, the arteriovenous fistula, the anastomosed vein is subjected to intense vibrational stress and the wall develops intimal proliferation and the full gamut of changes of atherosclerosis including aneurysmal dilatation, tortuosity, intimal tears, dissection, mural thrombosis, calcification and lipid accumulation despite the absence of dietary manipulation[8]. The progression of the lesions is similar morphologically to the human disease and it has its human counterpart in the arteriovenous shunt used for haemodialysis.

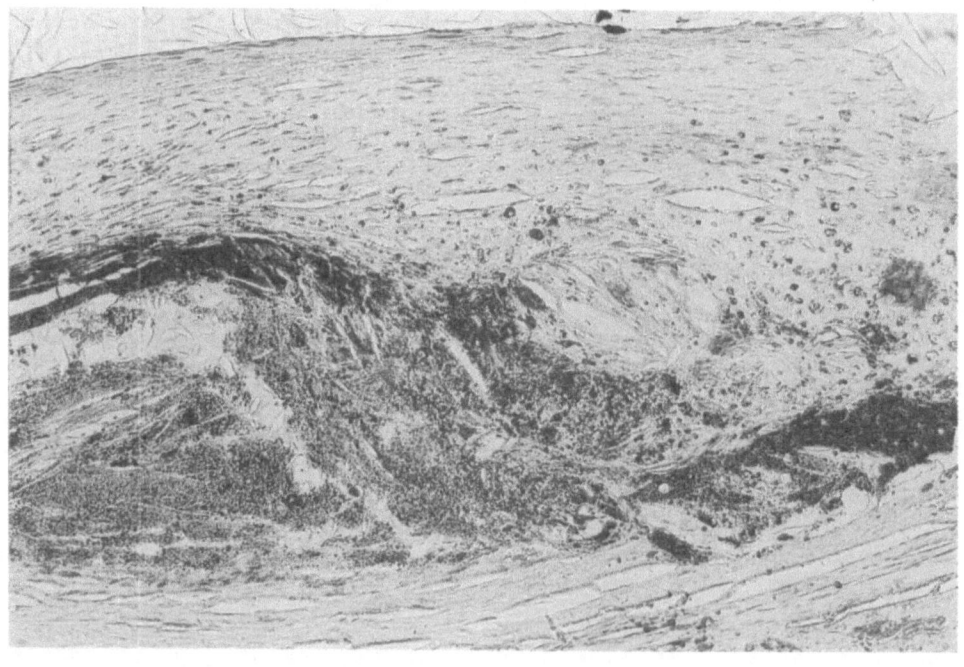

Figure 1. Frozen gelatin-embedded section of portion of the wall of an experimental fusiform aneurysm from a rabbit on a stock diet. Note the advanced atherosclerosis and the abundant lipid accumulaltion. Fett rot 3B and Haematoxylin. (X 42)

Since it is known that berry aneurysms appear to develop atherosclerosis at an accelerated rate, three types of aneurysm were produced by microvascular surgery in rabbits on a stock diet. Again atherosclerosis developed in the aneurysms from the early intimal proliferation progressing to advanced atherosclerotic disease with dilatation, thrombosis, calcification and lipid accumulation. Morphologically the lesions were identical to the human disease (Figure 1).

The third model was the lesion developing on the distal aspect of the lesser curvature of bends such as in the carotid siphon of man. Consequently U-shaped loops were produced in the common carotid arteries of rabbits and sheep and intimal proliferation similar to that of atherosclerosis developed in an identical site on the lesser curvatures of the bends[9]. In sheep, lipid deposits occurred despite the herbivorous diet but as yet sufficient time has not elapsed for the advanced lesions of atherosclerosis to be developed in this model. There is a need for longer term experiments on more animals.

GENERAL DISCUSSION

It is apparent therefore that haemodynamics can induce vascular changes identical to those of atherosclerosis in the absence of elevated serum lipids. Feeding a cholesterol rich diet to rabbits with experimental arteriovenous fistulae or saccular aneurysms combines the haemodynamic stress and the hypercholesterolaemia, so much emphasized by the current dogma, but the lesions produced still exhibit the characteristic features of the storage disease superimposed on haemodynamically induced changes. It is therefore apparent that haemodynamics must be more than merely a localizing factor. The evidence suggests that it can accelerate atherogenesis and to postulate involvement of some other hypothetical factor in the absence of firm evidence is unscientific.

Lipid is only one prominent feature of atherosclerosis in its advanced stages and the many other features have been virtually ignored by protagonists of the lipid hypothesis viz. ectasia, tortuosity, calcification, bizarre-shaped smooth muscle cells, abnormal basement membranes of both endothelium and smooth muscle with patchy separation from the plasma membranes[10], abundant matrix vesicles derived primarily from viable or degenerative muscle cells (Figure 2), abnormal collagen fibres at times resembling those in hereditary connective tissue disorders associated with fragility, loss and destruction of elastica, medial thinning and the complications. These changes can all be produced experimentally. It would appear that the abundant matrix vesicles (cell debris) have an affinity for lipid and calcium salts no doubt due to altered permeability characteristics of the limiting membranes. The breakdown of tissues to form pools of acellular fat-rich debris could be due to the further effect of vibrational stress on the accumulations of lipid containing vesicles and foam cells in the atherosclerotic intima. Selecting one facet of this complex disease (viz. lipids) and concentrating most effort and finance on it, though invaluable to the progress of knowledge of lipid metabolism, has long hindered the ultimate elucidation of the aetiology and pathogenesis of atherosclerosis.
Exception may be taken to this mechanical concept of atherogenesis, but the facts are that (1) the circulatory system is not immune to the fundamental laws of hydrodynamics (2) vibrational stress and fatigue failure with compensatory repair provides a logical explanation for the complications (3) the disease can be produced by altering blood flow in experimental animals on a stock diet and (4) that surgeons are regularly though not intentionally producing the disease in venous

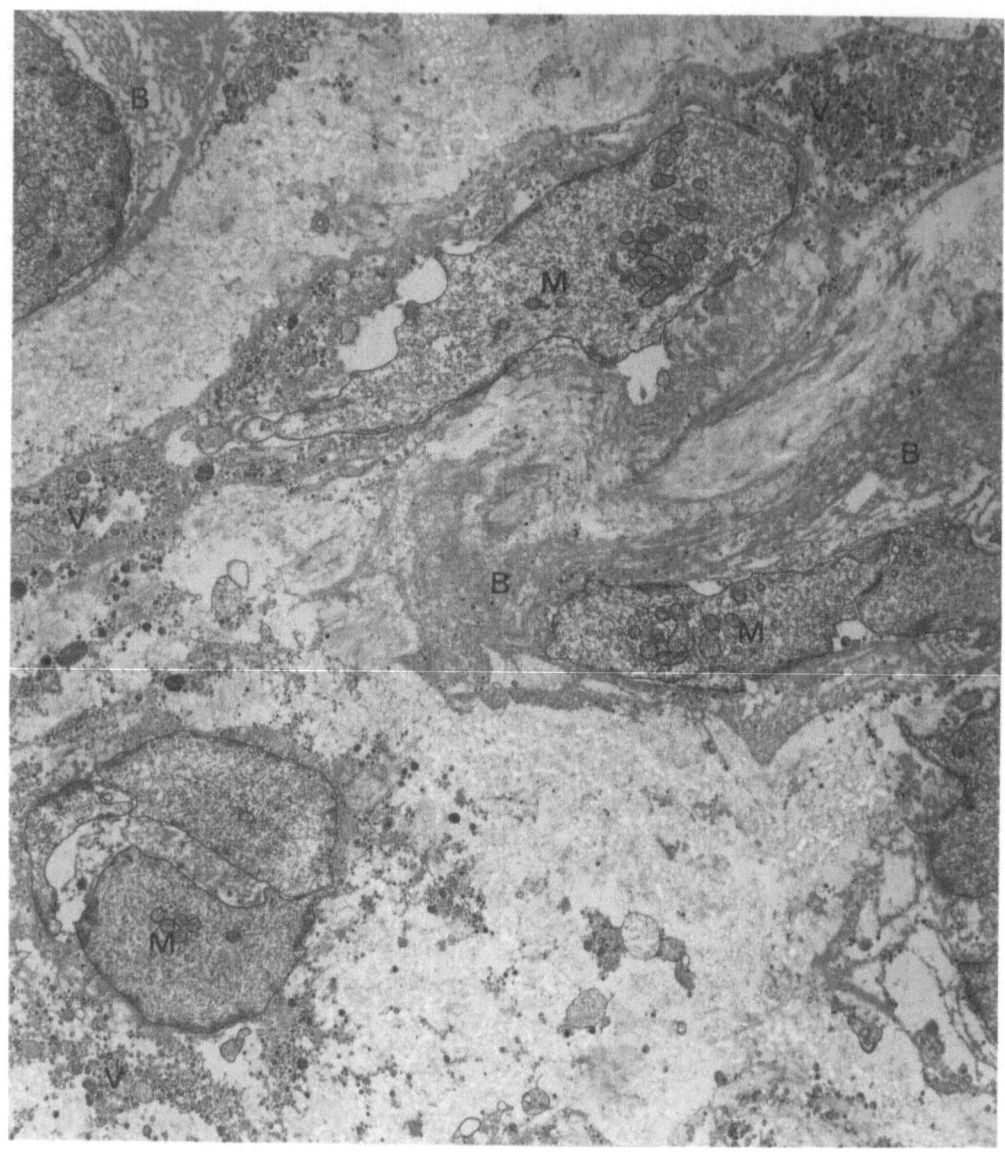

Figure 2. Electron micrograph of the wall of an experimental fusiform aneurysm showing well separated smooth muscle cells (M) with abundant dystrophic basement membrane material (B) and patchy separation from the smooth muscle cells. Note the abundant matrix vesicles (V). (X 11,250).

by-pass grafts and the veins of therapeutic arteriovenous shunts in humans whereas the veins so affected, would have demonstrated only mild sclerotic changes during the remainder of the subjects' lives if the veins had not been subjected to the severe haemodynamic stress consequent upon the surgical procedures.

It must be concluded that atherosclerosis can be produced by haemodynamic means in the absence of elevated serum lipids and that these experimental models discussed can provide invaluable tissue for experimental studies of the underlying mechanisms.

Acknowledgements: This work has been supported by the Medical Research Council and the National Heart Foundation and the Wellington Medical Research Foundation.

REFERENCES

[1]Ross R, Glomset J (1976) N Engl J Med 295:369-377, 420-425
[2]Stehbens WE (1979) Hemodynamics and the Blood Vessel Wall. C.C. Thomas, Springfield
[3]Stehbens WE (1986) Progr Cardiovasc Dis 29:107-128
[4]Stehbens WE (1986) Progr Cardiovasc Dis 29:221-237
[5]Stehbens WE, Wierzbicki E (1987) Progr Cardiovas Dis accepted for publication
[6]Stehbens WE (1987) Lancet i:606-611
[7]Stehbens WE (1958) Intracranial Aneurysms and Atherosclerosis, Thesis, University of Sydney
[8]Stehbens WE (1974) Proc Roy Soc Lond B 185:357-373
[9]Stehbens WE (1986) Exp Mol Path 44:177-189
[10]Stehbens WE (1975) Arch Path 99:582-591

Secondary Flow and Atherogenesis

N. Ohyama, A. Nishiyama, and T. Okamura

The Fourth Department of Internal Medicine, The Jikei University School of Medicine, Tokyo, 105 Japan

ABSTRACT

   Hemodynamic factors appear to affect atherosclerosis. Secondary flow in the aorta was studied by subjecting rabbits to constant pressure perfusion fixation and observing endothelial arrangement by scanning electron microscopy.
   Endothelial orientation is oblique in a lateral—medial direction on the dcrsal and ventral sides in the ascending, arch and descending segments. The direction of blood flow in these regions is oblique. This oblique flow is thought to be the result of longitudinal flow and secondary flow. The oblique orientation of the endothelial cells suggests the existence of secondary flow.

INTRODUCTION

   Atherosclerosis is caused by multiple factors. The role of lipidmetabolism has been emphasized. However, the incidence of atherosclerotic lesion is high in branching and curving regions of arteries and hemodynamic factors seem to affect atherosclerosis. Secondary flow is thought to occur where the blood flow changes direction. Blood changes direction as it proceeds from the ascending aorta through the arch to the descending aorta, so that secondary flow is thought to occur in these portions. In this study, we observed the arrangement of endothelial cells in the ascending, arch, descending and thoracic aorta using scanning electron microscopy, in relation with the direction of blood flow in these portions.

EXPERIMENT METHOD

   Female Japanese white rabbits, weighing 2.5—3.0 kg, were used. Prior to sacrifice, they were anesthetized with 30 mg/kg of pentobarbital sodium. A vasodilator, 6 mg/kg of isosorbide dinitrate, was injected intravenously according to the method of Moro in order to prevent retraction of the aorta after sacrifice(1). After a median incision the chest opened by manual fracure of the ribs. The heart was then exposed and the left ventricle punctured by an 18 gauge scalp vein infusion set. The heart was perfused and rinsed for 6 minutes with an 8% sucrose solution buffered with 0.1 M phosphoric acid, containing 500 units/kg of heparin. Almost simultaneously with procedure, the cervical arteries, pulmonary arteries and veins and abdominal aorta were ligated to poduce pressure and volume loading of the aorta.

Constant pressure perfusion fixation using a 2% gultaraldehide solution
buffered with 0.1 M phosphoric acid was then carried out for 1 hour.
The perfusion solution had a ph of 7.4, an osmotic pressure of 450 mosm
and administered at a perfusion pressure of 132 mm Hg and a temperature
39 c. In addition, the fixative was injected into the thoracic and
abdominal cavities to achieve fixation from the adventitial side of the
aorta. After perfusion fixation the aorta was removed and immersed in
the fixative for 24 hours for further fixation.

Specimens 7 mm in length were excised from the following four parts
of the aorta: the ascending segment just central to the branching of
the brachiocephalic trunk; the arch segment halfway between the
brachiocephalic trunk and the branching portion of the left subclavian
artery; the descending segment just distal to the branching part of the
left subclavian artery; the thoracic segment at the middle 1/3 of the
thoracic aorta. After dehydration the specimens were dried at the
critical point. Each specimen was split into four parts of equal width
parallel to the longitudinal axis. In this way, the aortic endothelial
arrangement on the inner coat of the segment could be observed for the
entire circumference. After vacuum sputtering with carbon and gold,
each specimen was termed 1.dorsal 2.medial 3.ventral and 4.lateral side
(Fig.1), and the arrangement and morphology of the endothelial cells
were observed and photographed by scanning electron microscopy.

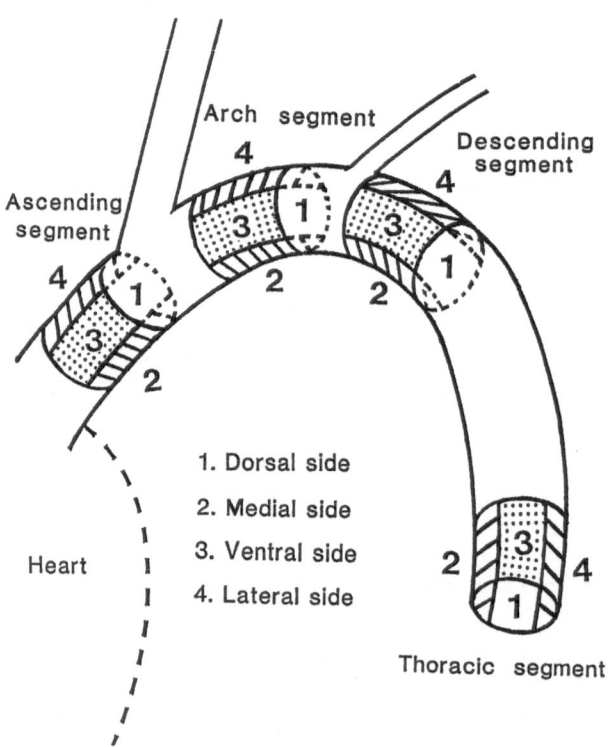

Figure 1 Sampled areas and segments of the aorta

RESULT (Fig.2)

Orientation of endothelial cells in each segment of the aorta was as follow:
1)Dorsal side of the aorta
The orientation of the endothelial cells in the ascending, arch and descending segment were orientated obliquely to the longitudinal axis, from lateral to medial sides, while the orientation of the endothelial arrangement of the thoracic segment was almost parallel to the longitudinal axis.
2)Medial side of the aorta
The orientation of the endothelial cells was almost parallel to the longitudinal axis in the arch and thoracic segments, while the orientation was slightly oblique in a ventral—dorsal direction in the ascending and descending segments.
3)Ventral side of the aorta
The endothelial cells in the ascending, arch and descending were orientated obliquely to the longitudinal axis from the lateral to medial sides, while the orientation of cells in the thoracic segment was parallel to the longitudinal axis.
4)Lateral side of the aorta
The orientation of the endothelial cells was almost parallel to the longitudinal axis in the arch and thoracic segments, while the orientation was slightly oblique to the logitudinal axis in a dorsal—ventral orientation.

DISCUSSION

Secondary flow occurs when flow changes direction. The dynamics of this flow was demonstrated theoretically by Dean in 1921. Since then secondary flow under different flow conditions (laminar flow, pulstile flow, etc.) has been studied theoretically and experimentally(2).
We believe that when fluid flows through a curved tube, the centrifugal force moves the central flow of fluid from the axial region to the lateral region along the aorta. The fluid then flows centrifugally from the medial side to the lateral side. Simultaneously, the fluid returns centripetally from the lateral side to the medial side along the wall of the tube. This is the secondary flow.
The aorta changes its direction by almost 180 degrees as the blood proceeds from the ascending aorta through the arch and the descending aorta to the thoracic aorta. The aorta is thus a curved tube, so the secondary flow is thought to occur in this portion.
Endothelial cells observations are shown in Fig.2. The endothelial arrangement is oblique to the longitudinal axis in a lateral—medial orientation on the dorsal side and ventral side in the ascending, arch and descending segment. The orientation of the endothelial cells in the descendimg aorta is shown in Fig.3, the left side is ventral, the right side is dorsal, the upside is lateral and the downside is medial. On the dorsal side the endothelial arrangement is oblique to the longitudinal axis in a lateral—medial orientation and on the ventral side the endothelial arrangement is oblique to the longitudinal axis in a lateral—medial orientation. The endothelial cells are thought to be arranged to the direction of blood flow(3,4), so the direction of blood flow is not parallel to the longitudinal axis of the aorta, but is oblique to the longitudinal axis in the lateral—medial direction on the dorsal and ventral side in the descending segment. This oblique flow is thought to be generated by the longitudinal flow and the secondary flow. Secondary flow is thought to occur in this segment. The oblique orientation of the endothelial cells suggests the existence

| | Ascending segment | Arch segment | Descending segment | Thoracic segment |

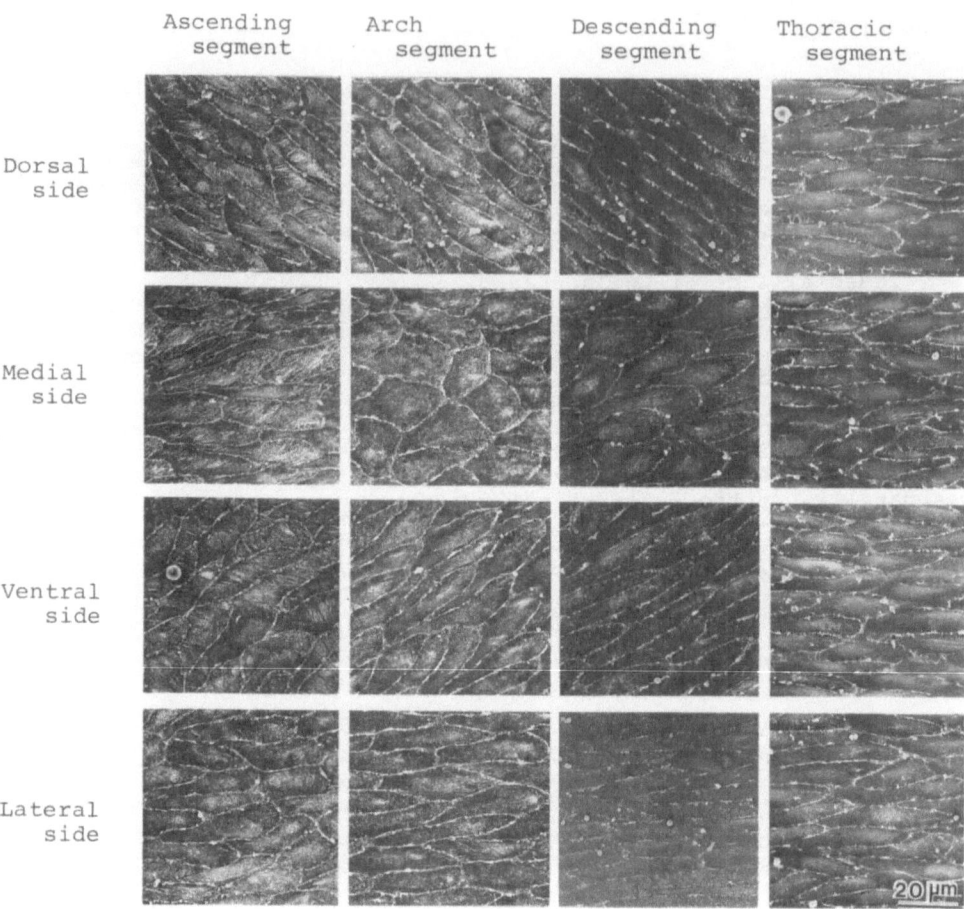

Figure 2 Arrangement of endothelial cells

of the secondary flow. The oblique orientation of the endothelial arrangement in the ascending and arch segment also suggests the existence of the secondary flow.

In the thoracic segment, endothelial arrangement is almost parallel to the longitudinal axis on the dorsal, medial, ventral and lateral side, suggesting that the direction of blood flow in this segment is almost parallel with the longitudinal axis. Secondary flow is thought to disappear in this segment.

As stated above, the secondary flow is thought to occur between the ascending and descending segment in the aorta. Atheroma present between the ascending and descending segment in the aorta in the rabbit might be affected with secondary flow in this region.

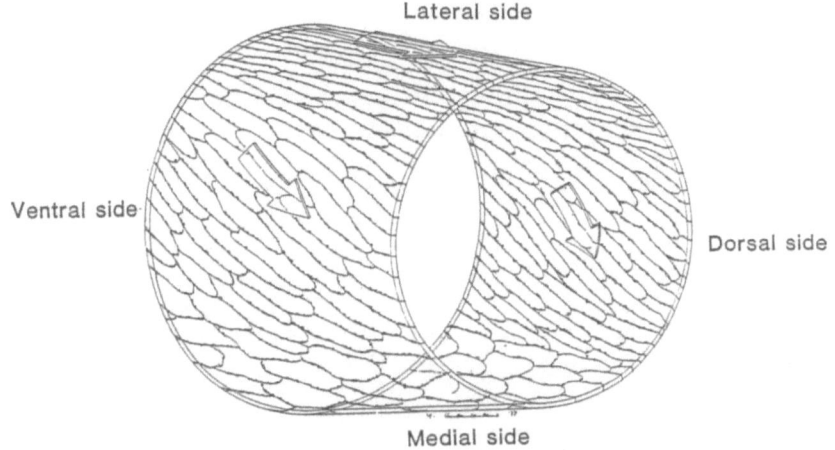

Figure 3 Three dimentional presentation
of the endothelial arrangement

CONCLUSION

　1.Secondary flow was suggested from the endothelial
arrangement in the aortic arch
　2.Secondary flow in the aortic arch might turn the occurrence
of atherosclerosis in this region

REFERENCE

　(1) Moro A., Studies of relationship between endothelial
arrangement of rabbit aorta and aortic blood flow. Tokyo Jikei
Medical Journal. 100 895—906.1985. (2) Dean W.R., Note on the motion
of a fluid in a curved pipe. Phil. Mag.7, 208—223 1927. (3) Flaherty
J.T.,et.al Endothelial nuclear patterns in the canine arterial tree
with particular reference to hemodynamic events. Circ.Res.30 23—33,
1972. (4) Dewey C.F.Jr. Effects of fluid flow on living vascular cells.
J.Bioch.Engng. 106 31—35,1984.

Chapter 2
Fluid Mechanics of Blood Flow in Atherogenesis

The Utility of Correlations Between Model Flow Studies and Vessel Pathology in Describing Atherogenesis

D.P. Giddens[1], C.K. Zarins[2], D.N. Ku[1], and S. Glagov[3]

[1]George W. Woodruff School of Mechanical Engineering, Georgia Institute of Technology, Atlanta, GA 30332-0405, USA
[2]Department of Surgery, University of Chicago, Chicago, IL 60637, USA
[3]Department of Pathology, University of Chicago, Chicago, IL 60637, USA

The list of hemodynamic factors which have been speculated to be associated with atherogenesis is long indeed. Among them are high wall shear stress, low wall shear rate, high pressure, locally low pressure, turbulence and oscillating wall shear. While studies of effects of each of these flow related phenomena upon the arterial wall undoubtedly contribute to general biological knowledge, such investigations may be but remotely related to the question of atherogenesis. Surprisingly, it has only been recently that the distribution of lesions in given anatomical regions of human subjects has been correlated with quantitative fluid dynamic measurements, thus allowing a sharper focus upon the potentially relevant hemodynamic atherogenic factors.

Because atherosclerosis initially is highly focal and since in susceptible bifurcations several candidate atherogenic flow phenomena may be found in close proximity, correlative studies using flow models and human pathology are essential to identifi cation of the role of hemodynamics in atherogenesis. The detailed flow measurements required, particularly with regard to the undoubtedly critical near-wall region, are such that hemodynamic investigations in the living system only are inadequate, so that researchers must turn to model studies as a complement to in vivo measurements. Life size models may in some circumstances be too small to allow necessary spatial resolution of the velocity field, and hence optimum studies may require models which are scaled upward in size.

Variability among individuals, in terms of vascular geometry, flow conditions and lesion distribution, is a major confounding problem in the attempt to correlate fluid dynamic factors with localization of disease. We must keep in mind the dangers inherent in averaging a nonlinear process. The fluid dynamic equations of motion are well known to be nonlinear, so that flow behavior determined in two bifurcations of different branch angles will not be the average of the flow behavior in a bifurcation whose angle is the average of the two branch angles. Perhaps not so obvious, however, is the likelihood that the process of plaque development is also nonlinear (although we have no known set of differential equations to describe the process), and it might well be that the average dis tribution of atherosclerotic lesions in the two hypothetical bifurcations is not the same as the lesion distribution in the single average bifurcation. These possibilities speak strongly for an experimental approach in which thorough and detailed studies performed in average models to elucidate strong correla tions from large numbers of specimens are complemented by perhaps more limited measurements in models of individual vessels.

Flow visualization is an extremely useful, perhaps necessary, adjunct to measurements of the velocity field. However, flow visualization alone is not sufficient in studying fluid dynamics, and investigations which do not progress beyond the qualitative description provided by flow visualization are incom plete. Despite the importance of obtaining quantitative data for velocity, wall shear and other flow field variables, care must be taken to avoid an obsession with numerical values. For example, while it may be very significant whether a wall shear stress value is 5 dynes/cm^2 or 25 dynes/cm^2, it may not matter to the artery wall whether the value is 25 or 30 dynes/cm^2.

The past decade has seen significant advances in the ability to model blood flow in arteries. Study of steady flow in rigid tubes of idealized geometry provided great insight into hemodynamics, and the advent of laser Doppler anemometry allowed detailed noninvasive measurements of the velocity field to be performed in laboratory models. However, investigators quickly realized the importance of modeling the relevant geometry of vessels, particularly in view of the fact that atherosclerosis often prefers to develop in branches and bifurcations; and experimen talists began to model specific atherosclerosis-prone bifurcations such as the carotid and coronary arteries. Although not trivial, it is now well within the state of the art in experimental hemodynamics to model either life-like arteries of specific individuals or to construct scaled up models for improved spatial resolution and to map the velocity field using LDA instrumentation.

While steady flow studies were vital to the progression of knowledge, arterial flows are inherently pulsatile. Although many features of steady flow are to be found in pulsatile situations, it is now clear that important differences can also arise. Regions of flow stasis and virtually permanent flow separation found in steady flow may become strongly dynamic when physiological pulsatile conditions are imposed. Changes in wall shear magnitude and direction are common at walls which in steady flow have virtually zero wall shear values, and particle residence times in the neighborhood of these surfaces may be altered as well. The importance of pulsatility depends, of course, upon the frequency parameter; but for the arteries involved in atherosclerosis, these values are generally sufficiently large to invalidate an assumption of quasi-steady flow. Thus, a guiding philosophy has evolved such that steady flow experiments are employed as a preliminary step to pulsatile investigations using physiologically relevant flow waveforms. A concommitant problem, how ever, has developed: how can the massive amounts of data which can be gathered in pulsatile experiments be analyzed and consolidated to allow meaningful interpretation? It is, after all, the task of the experimentalist not to just collect data of good quality but to analyze and interpret it as well. Thus, although presently it is possible to perform elaborate and accurate experiments in pulsatile flows, there remain many unanswered questions regarding basic understanding of pulsatility.

Experimental techniques have advanced to the point where problems which have previously been considered to be secondary can now be addressed. Of particular interest are the questions of wall motion and the non Newtonian behavior of blood. These points may be especially relevant to atherogenesis since it is the interaction of blood with the vessel wall which is crucial to uncovering basic atherogenic mechanisms. Investigators are just beginning to make inroads into modeling wall motion and blood rheology, and much is yet to be learned. It is useful to take extreme cases in initial studies so that upper boundaries can be set upon effects which might occur under real physiologic conditions. We must, however, be cautious in our interpretation of these experiments since our knowledge of actual wall properties and motion and of blood rheology in vivo is at best limited, making it difficult to devise experiments which can elucidate subtle effects. Nonetheless, tackling these problems is now very much appropriate, and their relevance to atherogenesis must be examined carefully.

While the control and resolution afforded by model studies are essential to hemodynamic research, the study of animal models and, indeed, of human subjects is likewise vital. Not only do parameters necessary to design laboratory model studies derive from in vivo investigations, but results from the fluid dynamics laboratory must be validated under biological conditions. The interaction of the real living system with the imposed experimental conditions can have profound effects.

From a practical viewpoint, experimentalists are limited to performing a relatively small number of investigations with models. Unless the experimental results and interpretations are underpinned by a theoretical framework, the research is not only incomplete - it is of limited value. The comparison of theory and experiment allows confidence in both sets of results; but more importantly, it allows extrapolation of the experimental findings to situations not examined in the laboratory, thus providing insight into more general understanding. Theoreticians can now compute pulsatile two-dimensional flow fields and steady three-dimensional flows for many (but not all) geometries and conditions which are physiologically interesting. As computational methods and computer speed and power improve, the calculation of pulsatile flow in branching vessels using the full equations of motion will be possible and practical.

The papers contained in this session reflect advances made in the ability to address more and more difficult, and relevant, problems in arterial fluid mechanics. Certain relationships between flow behavior and localization of atherosclerosis in humans are now well established, although not all questions have been answered by any means. Experimentalists are now tackling the subtitles of vessel wall motion and blood rheology and their effects upon the near wall fluid behavior. Attention is being focused upon the flow field as an environment which has a direct effect upon the living artery.

Finally, any relationship of fluid dynamics to atherogenesis can be discovered only through study of the human lesion. Cell cultures and animal models can contribute vital knowledge, but it is human disease that is the central issue. The significance of hemodynamics in atherogenesis will ultimately relate to the fluid-wall interaction in the human artery, whether this be by a transport process, a direct or indirect biochemical interaction, or through a direct mechanical effect such as alteration of endothelial function or smooth muscle cell proliferation by mechanical stimulation. Thus, studies of the flow field and cor relations with disease localization must be viewed as a means to narrow the list of candidate hemodynamic atherogenic mechanisms, rather than as an end to prove specific mechanisms.

Flow Patterns and Preferred Sites of Atherosclerosis in Human Coronary and Cerebral Arteries

T. Karino, T. Asakura, and S. Mabuchi

McGill University Medical Clinic, Montreal General Hospital, Montreal, Quebec H3G 1A4, Canada

ABSTRACT

Using transparent segments of arteries prepared from humans postmortem, flow patterns and the exact anatomical locations of atherosclerosis in major arteries of the human coronary and intracranial cerebral circulations were studied in detail by means of flow visualization and cinemicrographic techniques. It was found that in both coronary and cerebral arteries, atherosclerotic plaques and wall thickenings were localized exclusively on the outer wall (hip) of one or both daughter vessels at major bifurcations and T-junctions, and at the inner wall of curved segments where flow was either slow or disturbed and formation of secondary and recirculation flows were dominant.

INTRODUCTION

Atherosclerosis is a degenerative disease which affects relatively large arteries by the progressive thickening and eventual hardening of the vessel wall through the formation of atheromatous plaques rich in cholesterol. The disease has been found to develop not randomly and not everywhere in the circulation, but is localized in particular areas in the arterial tree such as bifurcations, T-junctions, and curved segments of arteries, strongly suggesting the involvement of hemodynamic factors in the pathogenesis and further progression of atherosclerosis. Hence, to elucidate the possible correlation between blood flow and the localization of the sites of atherosclerosis, we have been carrying out a series of fluid mechanical investigations using various models of branching vessels and isolated transparent natural blood vessels. In this paper, we summarize our latest findings on the detailed flow patterns and the exact sites of atherosclerosis observed in major arteries of the human coronary and intracranial cerebral circulations.

METHODS

Preparation of Transparent Arterial Segments

Isolated transparent segments of human coronary arterial trees and cerebral arterial networks containing the whole or parts of the circle of Willis were prepared as follows by a modification of the method described by Karino and Motomiya [1].

Coronary arterial trees. The human hearts were obtained at autopsy from subjects in whom the major cause of death was not coronary artery disease. The aorta was cut at about 5-7 cm downstream of the aortic valve and cannulated with a 10 cm long plastic cylinder having a diameter approximately the same as the inner diameter of the aorta to provide an inlet to the coronary arteries. The aortic valve was sealed by inserting a tightly fitting plastic disk into the aorta proximal and adjacent to the valve cusps and tying the surrounding aortic tissues over it. The end of the plastic cylinder was connected to a head tank via flexible plastic tubing. The aorta and the coronary arteries were perfused with isotonic saline to wash out the blood. The left and right coronary arteries and their major branches having diameters greater than 1.5 mm were exposed and separated from the heart to the point of cannulation by dissecting the heart muscles and removing the surrounding tissues. After cannulating all the major branches with blunt syringe needles, and ligating or coagulating all the microvessels, the aorta and the coronary arteries were firmly fixed onto a 3-dimensional stainless steel frame to maintain the original geometrical configuration of the heart and the arteries. The arterial tree, still attached to the heart, was then fixed by perfusing it with a mixture of 2% glutaraldehyde and 4% formaldehyde in isotonic saline at the physiological mean perfusion pressure of ~ 100 mm Hg, and at the same time, immersing it in the same fixing solution. The arterial tree, together with the aorta, was then isolated from the heart, dehydrated with ethanol and suspended in oil of wintergreen containing 5% ethanol to render the vessel transparent. Special care was taken to maintain the geometrical configurations (shape orientations, curvatures, lengths and diameters) as closely as possible to the in vivo diastolic conditions by filling the left ventricle with pieces of cotton gauze, perfusing the arteries at the physiological transmural pressure and supporting the arterial tree in a 3-dimensional frame throughout the entire process of preparation. Finally, the whole arterial tree, mounted on a supporting frame, was installed in a transparent glass chamber filled with oil of wintergreen.

Circle of Willis. The human brain was obtained at autopsy from subjects in whom the major cause of death was not a cerebrovascular episode. After cannulating the branches of the arterial network of the circle of Willis, the whole network was firmly fixed onto a 3-dimensional supporting frame, perfused with isotonic saline to wash out the blood cells and fixed under the mean physiological pressure. The whole network was then isolated from the brain, dehydrated and rendered transparent. Finally, it was installed in a transparent glass chamber filled with oil of wintergreen containing 5% ethanol.

Experimental Procedure and Analysis

The transparent blood vessel, mounted on a supporting frame and suspended in oil of wintergreen (containing 5% ethanol) in a transparent glass chamber, was firmly installed on the vertically mounted stage of a microscope and was illuminated with either low intensity light from a tungsten filament lamp, or high intensity light from a 200 W d.c. mercury arc lamp. Steady and pulsatile flow was obtained using a head tank system in combination with an oscillatory flow pump. Suspensions of 15 to 150 μm diameter polystyrene microspheres (density: 1.06 g/cm^3, the size depending on the vessel diameter) in oil of wintergreen containing 5% ethanol (density: 1.16 g/cm^3, viscosity: 0.026 g/cm sec) were subjected to steady or pulsatile flow through the vessel. The behavior of individual suspended tracer microspheres flowing in a steady or pulsatile fashion through various regions of the transparent artery was observed through a zoom lens (1× to 5×) attached to a cine camera, and photographed on 16 mm cine films using a Hycam 16 mm camera at speeds from 500 to 3000 frames/sec. The developed films were subsequently projected onto a drafting table and the movements of individual tracer particles were analyzed frame by frame with the aid of a stop-motion 16 mm movie projector to obtain the detailed flow patterns and distributions of fluid velocity and shear rate (or shear stress).

RESULTS

In each of five human coronary arterial trees and more than twenty arterial networks of the human circle of Willis prepared and studied, atherosclerotic plaques and wall thickenings were found to be localized almost exclusively on the outer wall (hip) of one or both daughter vessels at major bifurcations and T-junctions, and along the inner wall of curved segments where wall shear stresses are expected to be low. Figures 1 and 2 illustrate some examples of such cases observed in the human coronary arteries and intracranial cerebral arteries, respectively. Furthermore, when flow patterns were studied in detail in such vessels, it was discovered that both in steady and pulsatile flow, these sites were the very places where flow was either slow (low shear region) or disturbed and formation of secondary and recirculation flows were dominant. In no instance were atherosclerotic plaques and wall thickenings found in high shear regions such as downstream of flow dividers (inner walls) of bifurcations and T-junctions where the formation of initial atherosclerotic lesions has been reported in experimental animals fed high cholesterol diets [2-4].

In the left main coronary artery (LMC), formation of a recirculation zone was observed in three vessels right at the entrance of the artery. In all three cases, eddies were formed along the lower wall due to a sudden change in flow direction at the sharp-angled lower leading edge of the main coronary artery which stemmed off the aortic sinus. Also as illustrated in Figure 3, in three cases the strong deflection of the main flow from the LMC at the flow divider of the left anterior descending branch (LAD) and the left circumflex branch (LCx) resulted in the formation of recirculation zones in one or both daughter vessels around the outer wall (hip) of the bifurcation at the very sites where atherosclerotic plaques and wall thickenings were localized. In the LAD, atherosclerotic lesions were found along the inner (lower) wall of the gently curved segment of the proximal portion of the LAD which overlay the myocardium where the fluid velocity and wall shear stress were relatively low compared to that at the outer wall. In the right coronary artery, as shown in Figure 4, most of the atherosclerotic lesions were confined to the curved segments along the inner wall where flow was either disturbed with formation of a recirculation zone or very slow. It was also noted that in both left and right coronary arteries, the frequency and degree of severity of atherosclerotic lesions tended to decrease with increasing distance from the origin of each artery from the aortic sinus.

In intracranial cerebral arteries, the results revealed several important facts which suggested the direct involvement of local flow patterns in the localization of atherosclerosis.

It was found that in each of the five middle cerebral artery bifurcations studied, atherosclerotic thickening of the vessel wall was localized around the hips of the bifurcation. When the flow patterns were studied in detail in these vessels, it was discovered that a standing recirculation zone was formed along the outer wall of one or both daughter vessels (depending on the Reynolds number in the parent vessel and the flow ratios in the two daughter vessels) at the exact locations where the

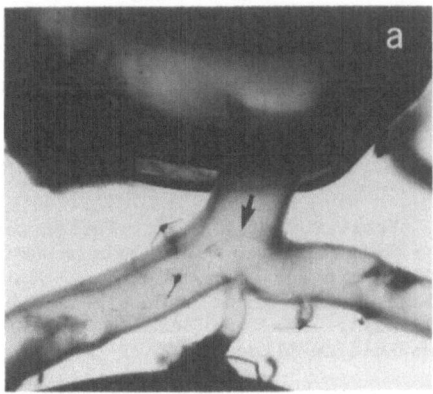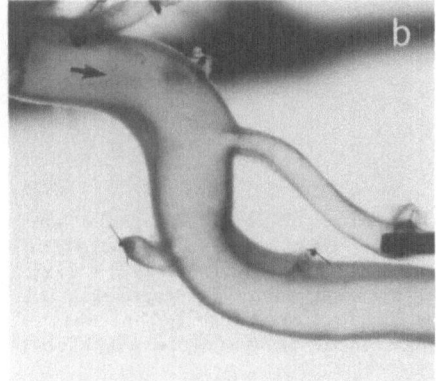

FIG.1 Photographs of isolated transparent human coronary arteries taken from a 61 year old man, showing the exact location of atherosclerotic wall thickenings at (a) the branching site of the left main coronary artery, and (b) a curved segment in the right coronary artery.

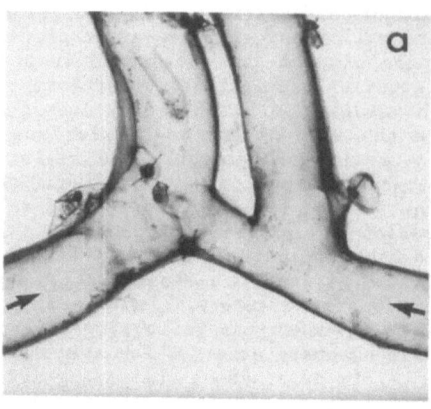 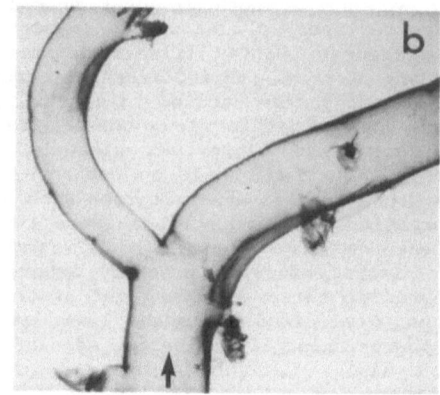

FIG.2 Photographs of isolated transparent human cerebral arteries taken from an 83 year old man, showing the exact location of atherosclerotic wall thickenings at (a) the junction of the anterior communicating artery and left and right anterior cerebral arteries, and (b) the first bifurcation of the middle cerebral artery.

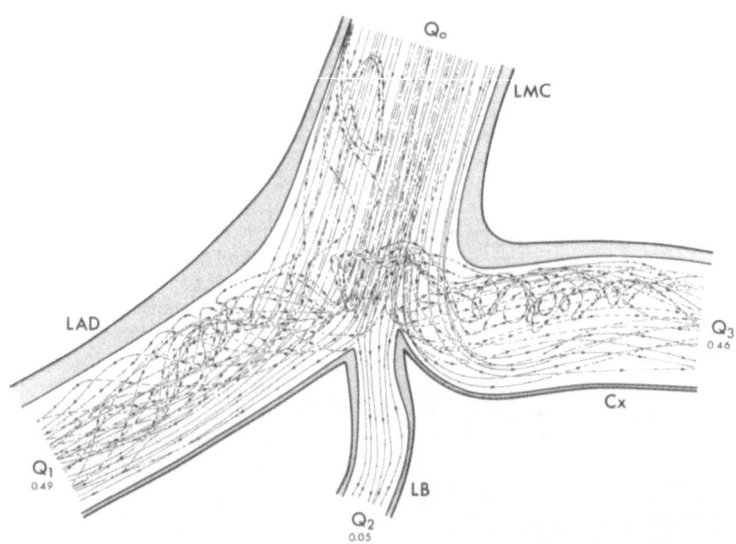

FIG.3 Tracings of particle paths showing the formation of a recirculation zone and secondary flows at the trifurcation of the left main coronary artery (shown in FIG. 1) in steady flow at Re_o = 772, Q_o = 334 ml/min and $\bar{U}_o$ = 416 mm/sec. The solid lines are the paths of particles in or close to the common median plane, and the dashed lines are the paths which are far away from the common median plane (projection of the particle paths on the common median plane).

atherosclerotic thickening of the vessel wall occurred. Furthermore, under the normal physiological range of flow rates and flow ratios tested, there was an apparent positive correlation between the longitudinal length of the regions of disturbed flow and that of the atherosclerotic wall thickening. Figure 5 shows the detailed flow

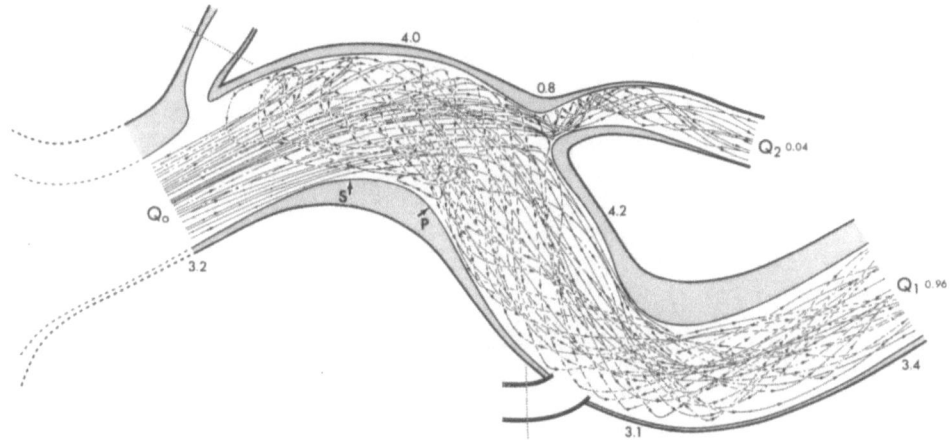

FIG.4 Tracings of particle paths as in FIG.3 showing the formation of recirculation zones and secondary flows at a curved segment of the human right coronary artery (shown in FIG. 1) in steady flow at $Re_o = 994$, $Q_o = 335$ ml/min and $\bar{U}_o = 686$ mm/sec.

patterns observed in steady flow in one of the bifurcations having an almost perfectly symmetric structure and spatial arrangement of the daughter vessels. As evident from Figure 5, even when the flow in the parent vessel was distributed equally to the two daughter vessels, the region of disturbed flow (formed along the outer walls of the bifurcation) was much longer in the right side branch where the region of atherosclerotic wall thickening was also longer than that in the left side branch where the wall thickening was confined to only a very narrow area. Furthermore, the size of the backflow region remained almost unchanged even when the flow rate in the left daughter vessel was reduced to 21% of the inflow rate in order to facilitate the formation of a large recirculation zone in that branch. The region of disturbed flow was still confined to a narrow area adjacent to the site of wall thickening, suggesting a strong correlation between the size of the regions of disturbed flow and that of the atherosclerotic lesions found at such sites. In pulsatile flow, the complex spiral secondary flows and the recirculation zones oscillated periodically and the locations of the stagnation and separation points situated on the outer walls of the bifurcation moved back and forth along the vessel wall. However, the general flow patterns remained the same as those observed in steady flow. This was true for all five vessels studied. A similar observation was made at an arterial bend located further downstream from the middle cerebral artery bifurcation shown in Figure 2b. Here, a recirculation zone was formed along the inner wall of the bend slightly downstream from the apex at the very site of the atherosclerotic wall thickening.

CONCLUSION

We have described our latest findings on the exact sites of atherosclerosis and detailed flow patterns existing in such regions in human coronary and intracranial cerebral arteries in relation to the localization of atherosclerosis in the human circulation. The results demonstrated convincingly that the flow separation and formation of secondary flows and standing recirculation zones, previously observed in various models of branching vessels [5,6], do occur also in natural blood vessels in both steady and pulsatile flow. Furthermore, it was confirmed repeatedly that preferred sites for the formation of atherosclerotic plaques and wall thickenings were

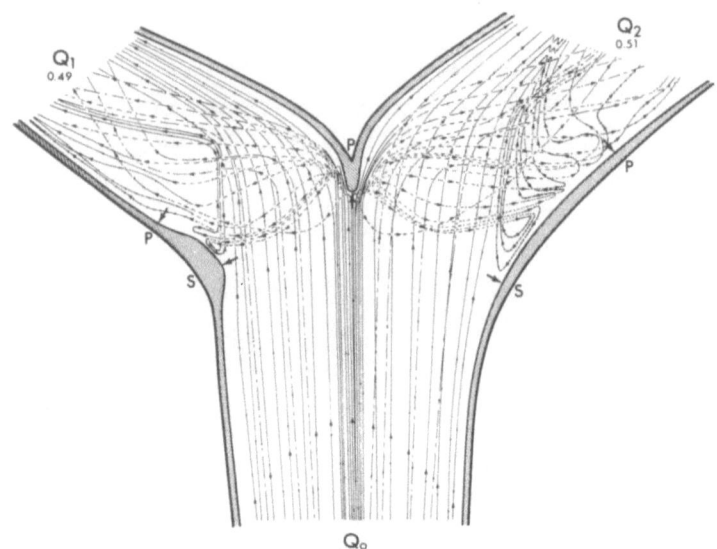

FIG.5 Detailed flow patterns at the middle cerebral artery bifurcations taken from a 73 year old woman, showing the formation of secondary flows and recirculation zones along the outer walls of the bifurcation in steady flow at Re_o= 452, Q_o= 147 ml/min and $\bar{U}_o$= 325 mm/sec. The arrows at S and P denote the respective locations of the separation and stagnation points.

localized not at flow dividers (high shear region) as observed previously by several investigators in experimental animals by feeding them diets containing high levels of cholesterol [2-4], but almost exclusively on the outer wall (hip) of one or both daughter vessels at major bifurcations and T-junctions and along the inner wall of curved segments where flow was either slow (low shear region) or disturbed with formation of secondary and recirculation flows. These results indicate that there is a strong correlation between the sites of flow disturbance and the preferred sites for the genesis and development of atherosclerosis in man.

Acknowledgment: This work was supported by Grant HL-29502 from the National Heart, Lung and Blood Institute, N.I.H., U.S.A., Grant MT-7084 from the Medical Research Council of Canada, and the Quebec Heart Foundation.

REFERENCES

[1]Karino T, Motomiya M (1983) Biorheology 20:119-127
[2]Roach MR (1977) The effects of bifurcations and stenoses on arterial disease. In: Hwang NHC, Norman NA (eds) Cardiovascular Flow Dynamics and Measurements. University Park Press, Baltimore, pp 489-539
[3]Roach MR, Cornhill JF, Fletcher J (1978) Atherosclerosis 29:259-264
[4]Roach MR, Fletcher J (1979) Atherosclerosis 32:1-10
[5]Karino T, Kwong HHM, Goldsmith HL (1979) Biorheology 16:231-248
[6]Karino T, Goldsmith HL (1985) Biorheology 22:87-104

Early Atherosclerosis and Pulsatile Flow in the Human Carotid Bifurcation

D.N. Ku[1], C.K. Zarins[2], D.P. Giddens[1], and S. Glagov[3]

[1]George W. Woodruff School of Mechanical Engineering, Georgia Institute of Technology, Atlanta, GA 30332-0405, USA
[2]Department of Surgery, University of Chicago, Chicago, IL 60637, USA
[3]Department of Pathology, University of Chicago, Chicago, IL 60637, USA

Three regions in the human arterial system are predisposed to the development of intimal thickening, including the formation of atherosclerotic plaques, which may lead to reductions in blood flow, causing clinical symptoms. These three regions include the coronary arteries, the infrarenal abdominal aorta and arteries to the lower limbs, and the carotid bifurcation. Together these three sites cause most of the clinical problems associated with atherosclerosis. Because these lesions localize in such a predictable manner and are usually well-defined in their axial extent, hemodynamic factors may play an important role in the preferential localization of atherosclerosis.

The human carotid bifurcation is particularly well-suited for identifying which of several possible hemodynamics variables are most consistently associated with the presence or absence of intimal disease. The approach of our group is to utilize specimens which are controlled pressure-fixed to obtain data on the axial and circumferential distribution of early, asymptomatic, non-stenosing, intimal lesions. This data is then related to flow patterns, flow velocities profiles, and shear stresses obtained from in vitro model bifurcations subjected to pulsatile flow.

Methods

The carotid bifurcation specimens were obtained at autopsy from patients age 27 to 73 years with no history of symptomatic cerebral vascular disease. Each transected vessel was canulated and distended with warm, buffered Formalin (3.8%) at an interluminal pressure of 100 mm Hg. Tissue samples were obtained at standard levels and processed through parafin, sectioned at 5 micrometers, and stained with H&E, or with the Weigert van Gieson procedure for differential staining of connective tissue fiber and cells. Each section was projected onto a digitizing tablet and the contours of the lumen, the internal elastic lamina, and the outer limit of the media were traced with a microcomputer. This analysis allowed us to obtain the intimal area at that cross-section.

A plexiglas bifurcation model was used for the fluid dynamic studies and were constructed from biplanar angiograms. The working fluid was a mixture of water and glycerine which was pumped from an upstream tank through an electronically controlled shaker valve. The pulsatile waveform used for the present study was a replica of a carotid flow pattern obtained by noninvasive ultrasound Doppler velocimetry in a 22 year old man with no evidence of arterial stenosis.

The time varying flow divisions between the internal and external carotid artery was modeled to provide 45% of the flow through the external carotid during peak systole and only 30% flow through the external over the entire pulsatile cycle. The time varying resistance to the external carotid was achieved through the use of a Starling resistor which mimics the physiologic situation very closely.

Velocity measurements were obtained with a DISA laser Doppler anemometer (LDA). The sample volume formed by the intersection of the helium-neon laser beams is approximately 1.08 x 0.12 mm in the water-glycerine mixture. Wall shear stress was calculated from the velocities measured near the model walls using the relation $\tau=\mu(du/dy)$. The velocity gradient at the wall was estimated by computing the slope of a linear regression curve that employed three values of velocity obtained close to the wall.

Results

While shear stress in the proximal common carotid artery follows the upstream flow waveform and exhibits no peculiar tendencies the wall shear stress ranges from 3 to 29 dynes/cm^2 in this region. The inner wall near the flow divider experiences shear stresses which are unidirectionally positive throughout the cardiac cycle. The wall shear stresses in this region range from 17 to 50 dynes/cm^2.

Along the common-internal artery outer wall, the wall shear stress oscillates between positive and negative values during systole. This oscillation occurs in a well-defined area at the outer wall of the carotid sinus. The wall shear stress begins to shift in the negative direction as the point of arterial bifurcation is approached. At X_c = -0.25D, the wall shear stress becomes negative in late systole at a phase of 60°. Shear stress versus time at this axial position is shown in Figure 1.

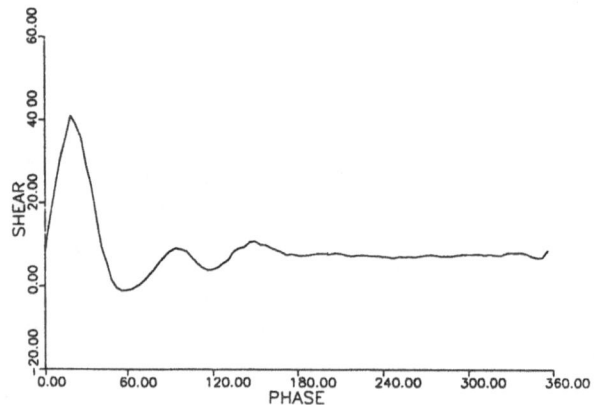

Figure 1

Negative wall shear stress becomes larger up to X_1 = .22D and reaches a maximum value of 11 dynes per square cm at ϕ = 11°, then falls to a minimum value of -6 dynes/cm^2 at ϕ = 45°.

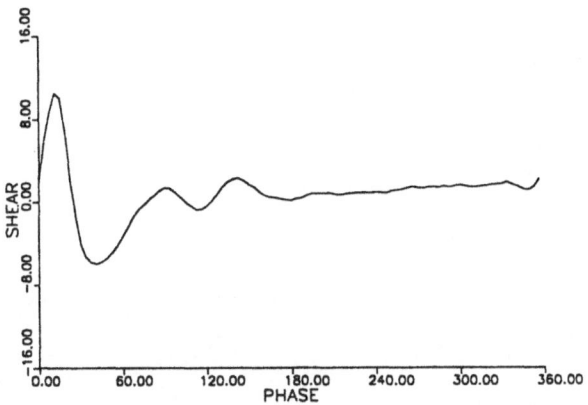

Figure 2

The time-averaged mean value over the entire cycle at this point is 0.8 dynes/cm^2.

Between stations $X_1 = 0.9D$ through $X_1 = 1.57D$, a second relative minimum can be seen to develop. This is shown in Figure 3 which illustrates shear stress versus time at station $X_1 = 1.12D$.

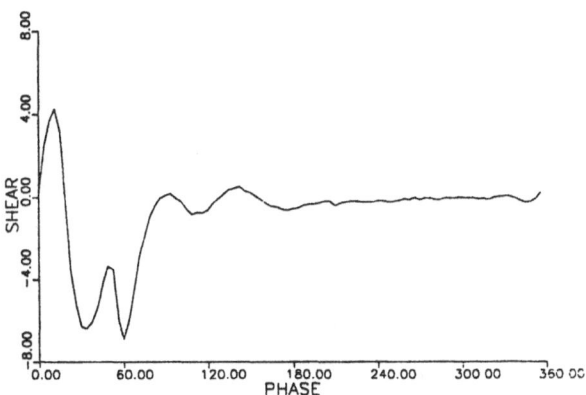

Figure 3

This second local minimum dominates in this region and arises from a slowly moving vortex which is actually moving upstream in the retrograde direction. The upstream movement of the vortex is due to its presence in the separation zone which has a convective velocity in the negative, retrograde direction.

Thus, the first relative minimum occurs from the development of a separation region causing the initial negative shear stresses. The second minimum occurs from the augmentation of this reverse flow with the convection of a secondary vortex.

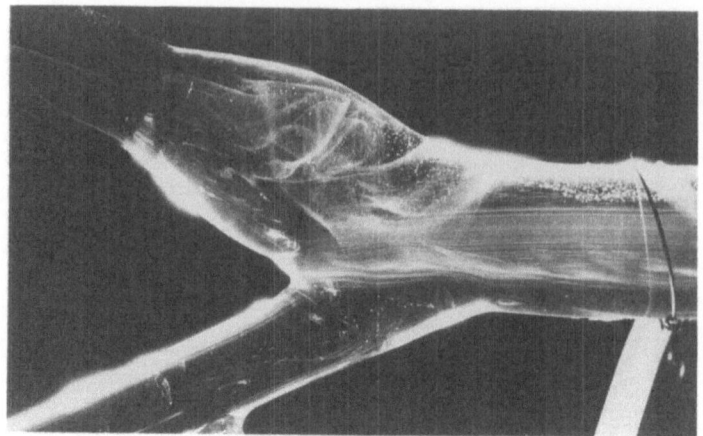

Figure 4

This vortex is eventually convected into the distal internal carotid artery. Because of the narrowing in cross-sectional area from the carotid sinus into the distal internal carotid, all of the velocities are increased. This acceleration of flow into the internal carotid compresses the vortex and causes it to rotate with a greater angular speed. These vortices are seen as high frequency spikes between ϕ = 56 and 90° in Figure 5.

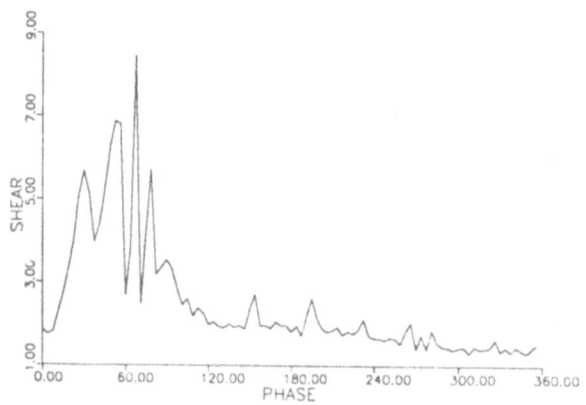

Figure 5

This figure illustrates the circumferential wall stresses versus time at station X_i = 3.2D along the side walls in the distal internal carotid. The spikes are indicative of the breakup of circumferential vortices into coherent structures at the end of systole.

Lesion localization and specimens. Each of the specimens examined histologically showed intimal thickening or plaque formation. Luminal surfaces on intimal thickenings including atherosclerotic plaques, were concave on transverse cross section. None of the lesions were ulcerated or surmounted by thrombi. Quantitative determinations of intimal thickness at the outer wall where plaques were most prominent are listed in Table I. Additionally, the intimal area at each level is shown in this table.

Table I

	Outer Wall Intimal Thickness (mm)	Intimal Area (mm^2)
Common Carotid	0.12 ± 0.03	2.2 ± 0.3
Proximal Internal Carotid	0.63 ± 0.17	7.1 ± 1.5
Midpoint Carotid Sinus	0.49 ± 0.10	4.9 ± 0.8
Distal Internal Carotid	0.08 ± 0.04	0.9 ± 0.4

In the common carotid and distal internal carotid the wall intimal thickening was minimal at approximately 0.1 mm. This minimal thickening was circumferential and showed no predominance at either the inner wall or outer wall. Intimal thickness was significantly greater in the proximal internal carotid and the midpoint of the carotid sinus at the outer wall. This significance was determined using student's t-test with a p-value of <0.05 at the midponit of the carotid sinus and a p-value of <0.01 at the proximal internal carotid. Intimal area was also more prominent in the proximal internal carotid and midpoint of the carotid sinus. In the bulb region, intimal area ranged from 4.9 mm^2 - 7.1 mm^2. This compares with a common carotid and distal internal carotid area of 0.9-2.2 mm^2. The intimal thickness at the flow divider in a wall was small and ranged from .14 - .19 mm comparable to the common carotid and distal internal carotid arteries.

Correlation of shear stress with intimal thickness. Twenty measurement locations were considered for intimal thickness and compared with both maximal shear stress and minimal shear stress. Linear correlations were performed which revealed an inverse relationship with r values between 0.63 to -0.69. Upon plotting the data of shear stress versus intimal thickening, we observed a strong inverse relationship which could best be represented by the reciprocal of maximum and mean shear stresses. The correlation between intimal thickening and the reciprocal of maximum shear stress obtained during the cycle resulted in an r-value of 0.90, p < 0.0005 and the correlation using the reciprocal of the mean shear stress gave an r-value of 0.82, p < 0.001. This would indicate that intimal thickening correlates strongly with low levels of mean shear stress. Observation of the flow patterns in the region of maximum intimal thickening reveal that plaque tended to occur in those areas where there were oscillatory shear stresses in which the shear stress oscillated between positive and negative directions. An oscillatory shear index was developed to quantify the degree of oscillations at a point from the shear stress time curve and this oscillatory shear index (OSI) yielded a significant correlation with intimal thickening with an r-value of 0.82, p < 0.001. Representative values for the mean shear stress and oscillatory shear index are given in Table II. Figure 6 illustrates mean shear stress versus intimal thickening at the various sites.

Table II

	Outer Wall Mean Shear Stress (Dynes/cm^2)	Oscillatory Shear Index
Common Carotid	7	0
Proximal Internal Carotid	-0.5	0.32
Midpoint Carotid Sinus	-0.7	0.35
Distal Internal Carotid	20	0.

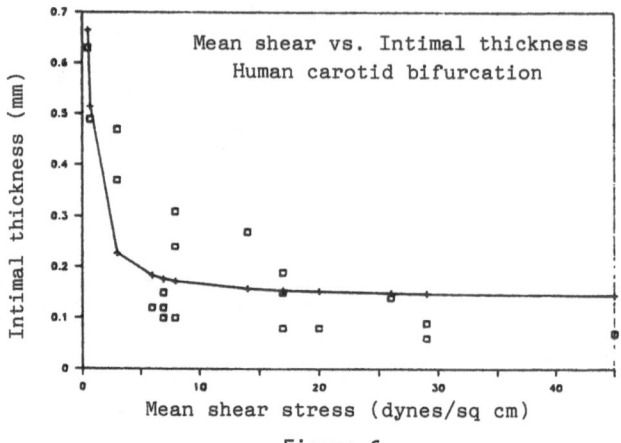

Figure 6

The solid line indicates the best fit relationship between the
reciprocal of mean shear stress and intimal thickening.

Discussion

Under conditions of pulsatile flow, the inner wall of the carotid
bifurcation and the distal internal carotid artery are subjected to
relatively high shear stresses. The outer wall of the carotid sinus,
however, is a region of relatively low shear stress. Pulsatility
generates a changing region of flow reversal and separation that
disappears during early systole but redevelops during late systole
into a separation region larger than predicted by steady flow
modeling. Pulsatile flow conditionally causes significant fluctuations in the magnitude of all shear stress which were not predicted
during steady flow. For example, maximum shear stress in the common
carotid during the peak of systole was approximately twice as large as
that measured during steady flow with a Reynolds number comparable to
that seen at peak systole. Thus, representation of hemodynamics with
in vitro models demands that pulsatile flow be used in order to obtain
accurate and realistic measurements of shear stress and shear stress
versus time.

Our finding that intimal thickness bears an inverse relationship
to the magnitude of shear stress is consistent with our previous
studies in the carotid bifurcation. The outer wall, where atherosclerosis is most prominent initially is a site of low, time-average mean
shear stress and oscillatory shear stress. Both low mean shear stress
and oscillatory shear stress contribute to an increased fluid residence time in the carotid sinus. The increased fluid residence time
may result in modification of the mass transport of atherogenic substances between lumen and wall or in interference with endothelial
metabolism. Blood-borne cellular elements such as platelets and
macrophages, said to play a role in atherogenesis, would be expected
to have an increased probability of deposition or adhesion in regions
of increased residence time.

The development of oscillating shear stress patterns which are
complex and include convected vortices may in itself cause an

increased ingress of plasma constituents through the endothelial monolayer by effects on the stability of intercellular junctions.
Changing shear stress patterns may cause a disorientation of intercellular overlapping borders and allow for a localized increase in
permeability.

Several factors influence internal velocity profiles and may cause
marked individual variations in the shear stress patterns in a given
individual carotid bifurcation. Two elements show great anatomic and
physiologic variation. One variation is the branch angle which has a
large standard deviation around the mean. Extrapolating from model
studies of others, carotid bifurcations with relatively large branch
angles may have a larger outer wall area subjected to oscillating
shear stress patterns, and possibly more extensive intimal plaque
formation.

The carotid pulse waveform could also be significant a contributing factor. Different pulse shapes would affect the formation and
size of the separation region, the extent of flow reversal, and the
size and position of the zone of increased residence time. The relationship of pulse waveform and heart rate to the development of atherosclerosis is presently under investigation.

The observation that low mean shear stresses and oscillatory shear
stress directions with an increased local residence time of fluid elements to the localization of carotid atherosclerosis may be extended
to the abdominal aorta and the coronary arteries, two sites of important clinical disease. In the abdominal aorta, the relatively
straight segment is subjected to oscillations in shear stress at the
wall which are presently being quantified. Similarly, the coronary
arteries are theoretically subjected to oscillatory shear stress
patterns which may localize depending on an individual's anatomy. The
degree of importance of the various hemodynamic factors on atherogenesis at these other areas of important clinical disease remains to be
explored.

In conclusion, comparison of detailed, pulsatile hemodynamic measurements with quantitative morphologic studies of the distribution of
atherosclerosis in the human carotid bifurcation revealed that low
mean shear stress and marked oscillations in the direction of wall
shear stress may be critical factors in the development and localization of atherosclerotic plaques. Furthermore, the results imply that
high unidirectional shear stress may exert a protective effect against
the induction of lesions. We are presently studying these relationship in other accurate models of vessel geometry and corresponding
pressure-fixed specimens.

Flow Separation and Horseshoe Vortex in a Tube with Side Branches During Pulsatile Flow

An *in vitro* Visualization Experiment Using a Dog Abdominal Aorta

T. FUKUSHIMA, T. HOMMA, and K. HARAKAWA

Institute of Cardiovascular Diseases, Shinshu University School of Medicine, Matsumoto, 390 Japan

ABSTRACT

Steady and pulsatile flow experiments were performed using a dog abdominal aorta that was made transparent and its glass model. Visualized flow patterns in both models were qualitatively similar. In front of the apex of each flow divider at branching sites, there appeared a bound vortex, the so-called horseshoe vortex. When the rate of flow to a branch decreased, separation of the flow occurred at the proximal outer wall of the branch artery. The region around the separation point experiences rather low wall shear stress while the horseshoe vortex will produce a high wall shear stress around the apex. An increase of the flow rate to the branch causes the flow to separate from the opposite wall of the branch orifice in the main trunk.

INTRODUCTION

Atherosclerotic plaques tend to develop in certain regions in the arterial tree, such as the neighbourhood of branch orifices and the inside wall of bends. The abdominal aorta with its major branches, the coronary arteries, and the cerebral arteries are well-known predilection sites for atherosclerosis. Several hemodynamic theories of atherogenesis have been proposed in association with the focal nature of atheromatous lesions, since disturbances of blood flow are known to take place in these regions[1,2]. Factors such as high or low wall shear stress, boundary layer separation, and turbulence have been implicated as initiating factors. To isolate the hemodynamic factors associated with disease processes, a considerable amount of work has been done on the character of flow in large arteries using blood vessel models. However, it is still not possible to pick out the dominant hydrodynamic factor associated with atherogenesis[2].

The various types of arterial junction may be grouped into threee main types[3]. One of these may be called the Y-junction and the most characteristic example is the bifurcation of the abdominal aorta into the two illiac vessels. The reverse condition of the Y-junction, where two or more branches join to form a single trunk, for instance the fusion of the two vertebral arteries to form the basilar artery on the medulla, is the second type. The third is the side-branch, where a single branch, usually of much smaller dimensions, leaves the parent trunk at an angle which depends on the anatomical position. In the large vessels, this is the most common type and contains a great many variations.

In this study we investigated disturbances of flow in the abdominal aorta at side-brances, and the present study is thus concerned with the third type.

MATERIALS AND METHOD

The abdominal aorta with its major branches, such as the celiac, superior mesenteric and right and left renal arteries, was obtained from healthy mongrel dogs.   After removing the surrounding tissue and ligating small branches and connecting pipes to the proximal and distal aorta and the major branches, the aorta was supported in a frame.   The vessel was then made transparent by fixing, dehydrating, and treating with methyl salicilate under a transmural pressure of 100 mmHg to ensure its in vivo configuration, a procedure developed by Karino and Motomiya [4]. Thus obtained, the transparent aorta was mounted firmly in a glass chamber filled with methyl salicilate, the kinematic viscosity of which was 2.6 cSt at 20°C.   The same liquid was used to perfuse the aorta as a substitute for blood, and a suspension of graphite powder with specific gravity of 2.3 was used to trace the flow by injecting the suspension through a fine needle. We may call this suspension a dye solution in what follows because the suspension appears as such. The inlet portion of the abdominal aorta was connected to a reversed Y-shaped connector and the dye solution was injected by the needle inserted in one of the two branches of the connector.   The other branch was used to supply the test fluid.

As shown in Fig.1, the glass model of the abdominal aorta consisted of five pipes: a main trunk of 26mm in internal diameter representing the aorta, two pipes of 10mm in internal diameter representing the celiac and superior mesenteric arteries, and two pipes of 8mm in internal diameter corresponding to the left and right renal arteries.   Not only the diameter ratios of the daughter vessels to the main trunk but the spatial arrangement of these vessels was made similar to those in the living body.   The flow system and visualization technique have been reported in previous papers [5,6].

RESULTS

Flow Patterns in Glass Model T-junctions

Figure 1 shows typical flow patterns produced in the glass model at a Reynolds number of 1600 calculated at the entrance of the aorta. Four branch arteries received the same flow division, a sixth of the total flow rate.   Each daughter vessel received part of the main flow passing through a certain limited area in a cross-section of the main trunk proximal to the branching site of the celiac artery.   The cross-section was divided into six areas as shown schematically in the top left of FIG.1.   All the liquid particles passing through area A, called the wall layer, and those through area B flowed into the celiac artery. The superior mesenteric artery was supplied with part of the main flow passing through area C.   Similarly, the renal arteries were fed with the streams through areas D and E.   The dorsally deflected central flow passing through F was received by the distal abdominal aorta beyond the branching site of the renal arteries.

As shown in the photographs of FIG.1, the dye solutions injected at points a, b, c, d, and e, whose locations over the cross-section are indicated in the top left figure, demonstrated patterns of complicated spiral flow in the model of the abdominal aorta.   The celiac artery received streams flowing in the wall layer. Therefore, a dye stream along the dorsal wall stagnated at the point S opposite the celiac orifice, and then divided into two streams, each continuing circumferentially to the upstream point (or corner) of the celiac orifice.   This circumferential tracing of the dye streaks was the line of flow separa-

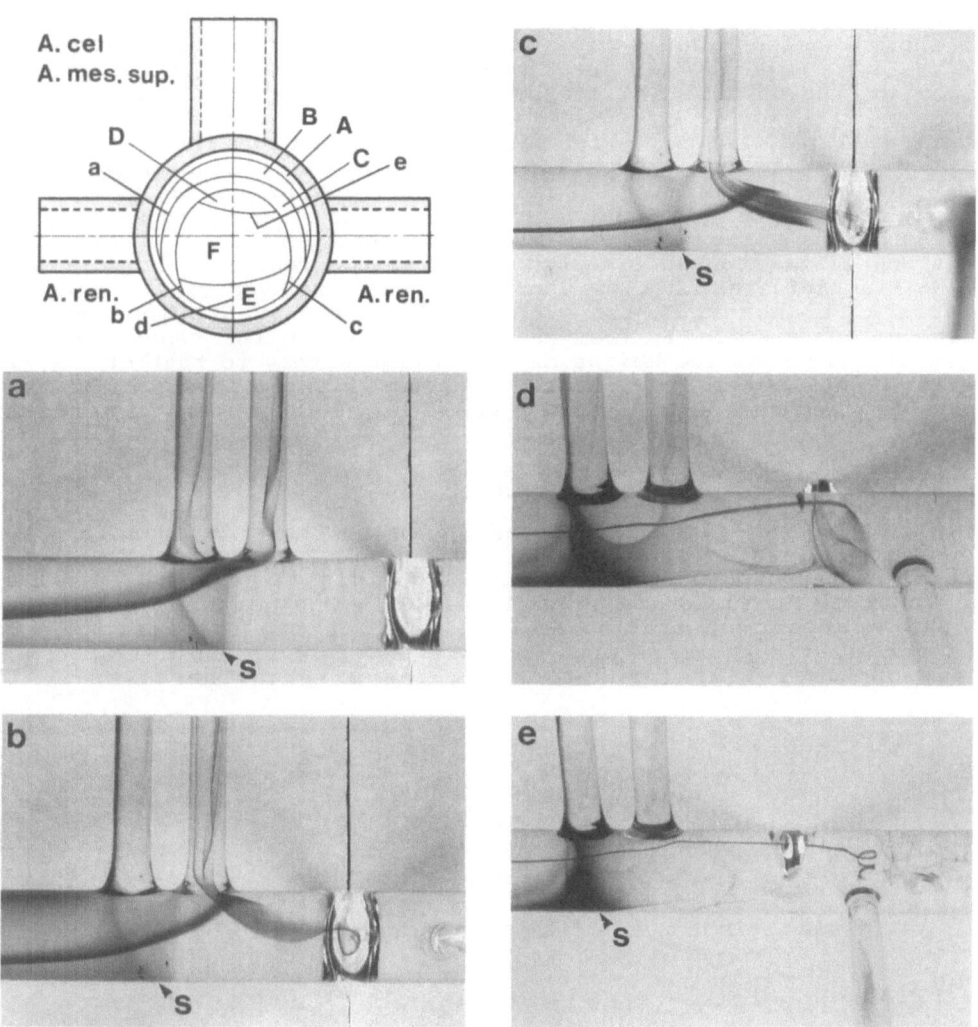

FIG.1   Patterns of steady flow in a glass model of the abdominal aorta.

tion, which occurred due to the flow to the celiac and superior mesenteric artery.
     The dye streak starting at point a displayed complicated pattern,
with the spiral flow entering the celiac and superior mesenteric arteries (FIG.1-a).   Injection of the dye solution at points b and c
clearly demonstrated generation of a bound vortex at the branching site
of the superior mesenteric artery (FIG.1-b, c).   The vortexes visualized
by the two dye streaks from points b and c formed a pair.   The vortex
trailed into the distal aorta and the mesenteric artery.   When a
streak of dye started, for instance, from point c, it began to diverge
as the orifice of the mesenteric artery was approached.   The dye was
taken into the vortex core formed near the downstream edge of the mesenteric orifice and moved in a helical fashion both upstream and downstream.

The streak of dye solution injected at point d near the dorsal
wall showed a slight deflection while it passed by the separation region
over the dorsal wall. The streak then rolled up into a vortex which was
produced on the dorsal wall of the abdominal aorta (FIG.1-d).   Similarly the dye solution injected at point e showed a vortex formation on the
ventral wall (FIG.1-e).   Fluid particles captured by these ventral and
dorsal vortexes moved in a helical fashion to the orificies of the left
and right renal arteries.   However, the ventral vortex was shed repeatedly downstream while the dorsal vortex was relatively stable.   The
shedding of the vortex produced flow disturbance like turbulence in the
main trunk distal to the branching site of the renal arteries (FIG.1-e).

No stagnant area of flow separation was observed at the corners of
the arerial branches. On the other hand, in the separation region ex-
tending circumferentially from the dorsal wall to the ventral wall and
longitudinally from the height of the celiac artery to that of the renal
arteries, there was a slow stream which had a direction opposite to the
main flow and fed finally into the celiac and superior mesenteric
arteries.

<u>Flow</u> <u>Patterns</u> <u>in</u> <u>Dog</u> <u>Abdominal</u> <u>Aorta</u>

Flow patterns qualitatively simlilar to those in the glass model
were observed in the dog abdominal aorta during steady flow at an inlet
Reynolds number of 640 with the same flow division.   Some of the corresponding flow features are shown in FIG.2.   The pattern of dye streak
in FIG.2-a resembled that in FIG.1-a, indicating the formation of a
bound vortex at the distal site (or flow divider) of the celiac orifice.
At the proximal site (or corner) of the orifice there was no flow

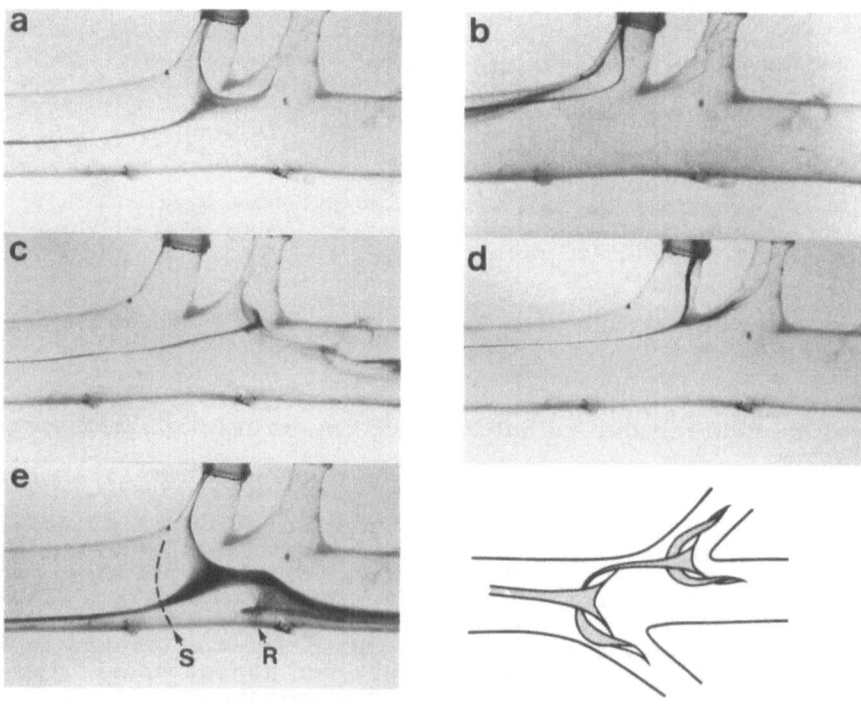

FIG.2 Patterns of steady flow in a dog abdominal aorta.

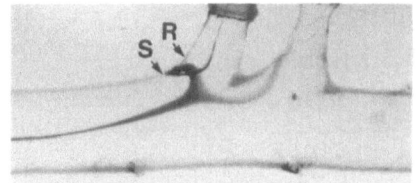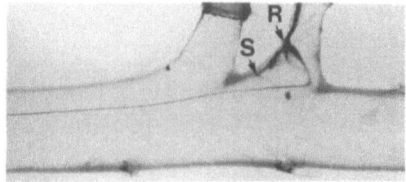

FIG.3 Flow separation, produced by decreasing flow rate to a branch,
       at the corners of the branch arteries during steady flow.

separation. The dye streak along the aortic wall upstream of the celiac
bifurcation smoothly turned the corner of the orifice with no sign of
the separation bubble there(FIG.2-b).
     A similar vortex formation was also visualized at the flow divider
of the aorta-superior mesenteric artery bifurcation as shown in FIG.2-c.
We can see a similar pattern of dye streaks in the glass model in FIG.1-
b and c.   In FIG.2-d, the dye streak was divided into two when it
reached at the flow divider, and these ran parallel to the walls of
branch arteries.   Thus no separation bubble was observed at the corner
of the superior mesenteric artery bifurcation.
     Although flow separation did not occur at the corners of the celiac
and superior mesenteric arteries, it occured at the dorsal surface as
shown in FIG.2-e.   The separation point is indicated by the letter S
and the rear end of the separation region by the letter R.   The dashed
line drawn on the photograph shows the separation line, along which
movement of fluid particles occurred to the celiac corner.   After the
dye streak was spread and divided into two near the celiac flow divider,
the dye stream directed downstream turned round and moved circumferentially toward point R on the dorsal surface.
     Thus the qualitative nature of flow in the abdominal aorta was
similar to that obtained in the glass model, although the Reynolds
number in the glass model was approximately twice that in the aorta.
     Figure 3 shows the flow separation that occurred at the branching
corners of the celiac and superior mesenteric arteries when the flow
rates to the branches were reduced.   The branch-trunk flow division
ratios were 0.074 and 0.062 at the aorta-celiac and -superior mesenteric junctions, respectively.   The division ratio at which initial
flow separation took place was 0.15 in both the celiac and superior
mesenteric branches at a Reynolds number of 610.   The values decreased
to 0.12 when the Reynolds number was 470.

     Pulsatile flow experiments showed results qualitatively similar
to those obtained during steady flow as in FIGs 2 and 3.   The pulsatile
flow wave adopted in the study is shown in FIG.4.   The velocity profiles, which are also shown in FIG.4, were calculated on the assumption
of fully developed flow in a uniform cylindrical tube [3].   The related pulsatile flow parameters were as follows: the Reynolds number of
the mean flow was 360, the Womersley number was 6.0, and the velocity
ratio of the peak U_p to the mean U_m, was 1.8.   When the flow division
ratios of the celiac and superior mesenteric arteries were a sixth of
the total flow, a bound vortex was produced at each divider of the two
arteries during the phase of 110 to 250 degrees. Flow separation did
not occur on the dorsal wall during the pulse cycle with these flow
division ratios, but it did occur during steady flow as shown in FIG.2.
This result suggests that the effect of an arterial branch was restricted to a narrow region around the branch orifice during pulsatile
flow.

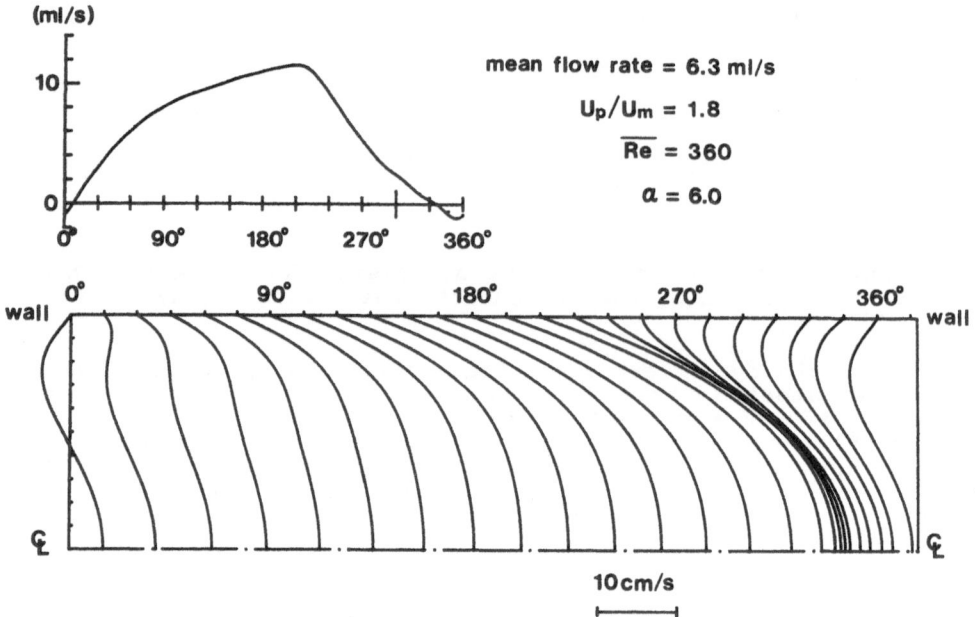

FIG.4   Pulsatile flow wave and velocity profiles.

        Figure 5 shows the patterns of dye streaks obtained during pulsa-
tile flow with a flow division ratio of 0.07 at the celiac juntion,
keeping other parameters unchanged.   The photographs on the left taken,
at the phase of 125 to 149 degrees, show the development of vortex
formation at the flow divider of the superior mesenteric artery.   The
flow pattern observed in the bottom photograph persisted until the 210-
degree phase.   The flow did not separate from the wall at the corner of
this artery. As expected from the results of steady flow experiments,
the reduction of flow rate to the celiac branch produced separation of
flow at the outer wall of the celiac artery as shown in the right of
FIG.5.   The tracer particles of the dye solution moving along the
ventral wall in a plane containing the axes of the aorta and the two
branches separated from the wall, indicated by the letter S in the
bottom photograph.   From the top to the bottom, the photographs show
the movement of tracer particles close to the aortic ventral wall.
The mass of particles indicated by the letter P moved downstream and
separated from the wall at point S, leaving a streak-line entering the
celiac artery.
        Figure 6 shows the effect of flow reduction, a division ratio of
0.07, to the superior mesenteric artery.   The photographs on the left
demonstrate the successive changes of the dye streak, showing the vortex
formation at the branching site of the celiac artery.   The photographs
on the right represent the development of the dye streak, part of which
entered the separation region at the corner while the remainder flowed
into the superior mesenteric artery along the outer wall.   A fraction
of the dye solution, as indicated by an arrow-head, deflected at the
flow divider, moved on the wall surface against the outer wall, and
then reversed toward the separation point S.   The point indicated by
the letter R represents the rear of the separation region maximally
extended during the pulsatile flow.

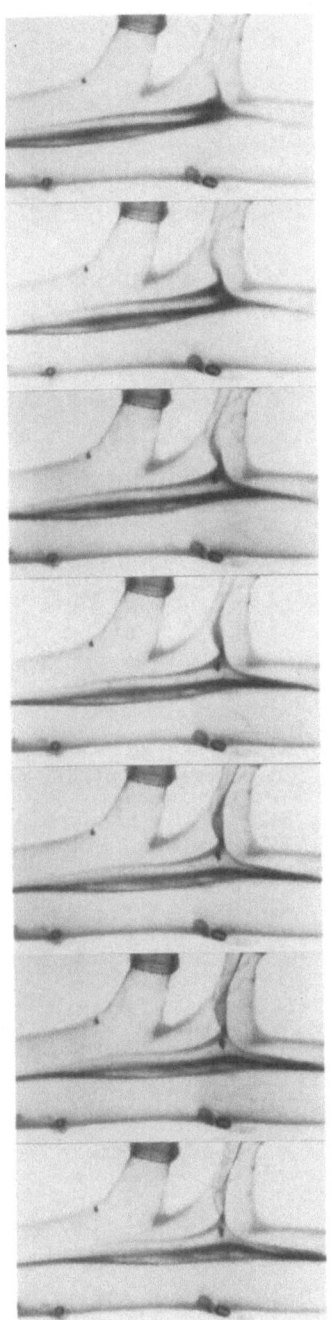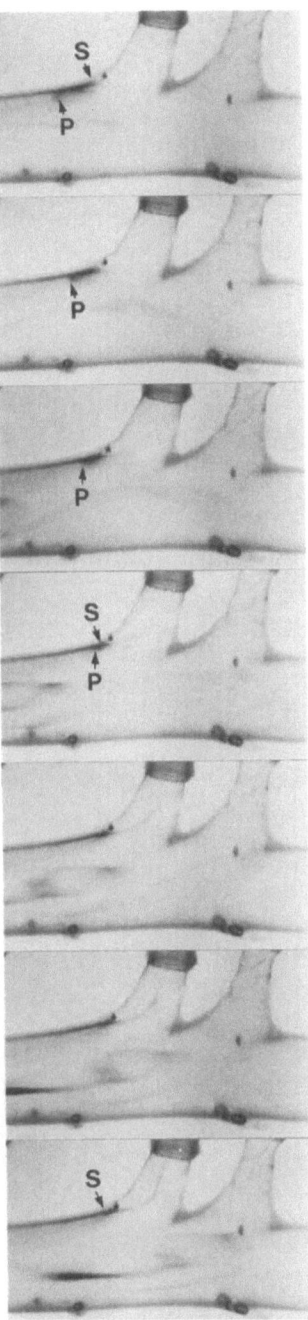

FIG.5 Horseshoe vortex at the flow divider of the superior mesentric artery(photographs on the left) and flow separation at the corner of the celiac artery(photographs on the right). Branch-trunk(inlet) flow rate ratios are 0.07 at the aorta-celiac junction and 0.17 at the aorta-superior mesentric junction.

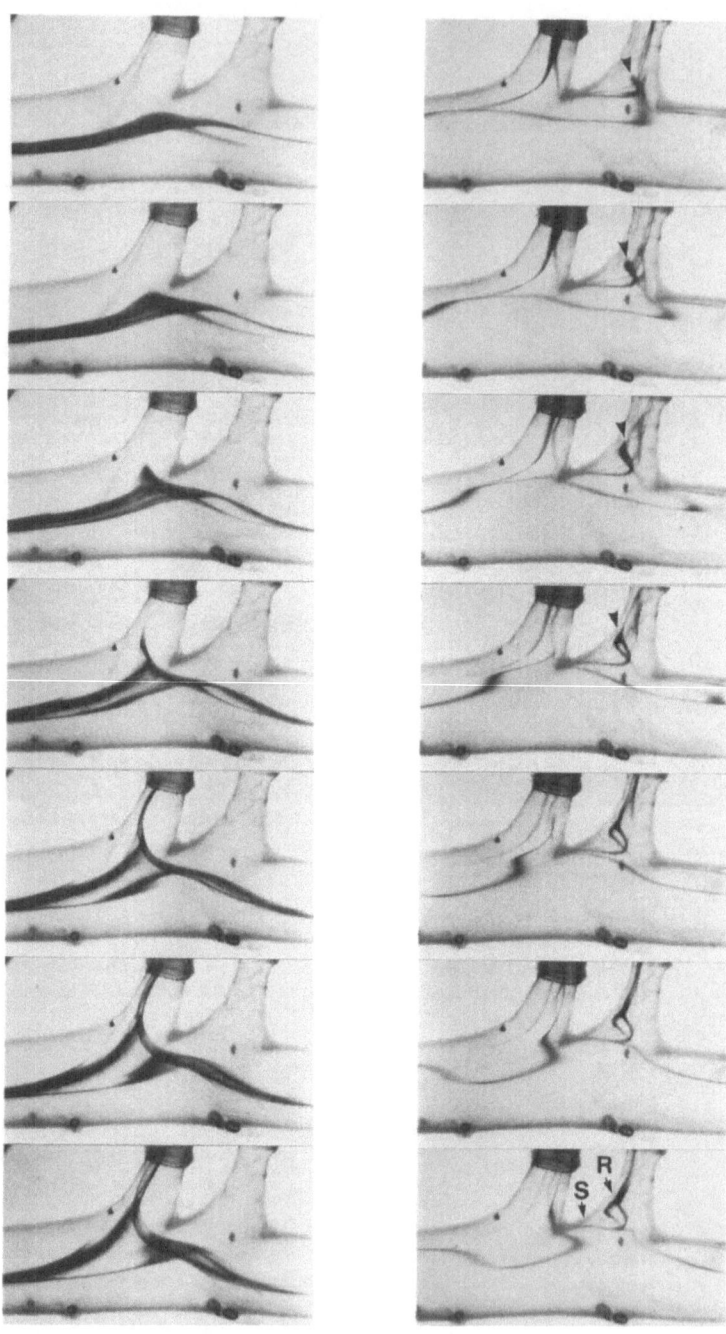

FIG.6 Horseshoe vortex at the flow divider of the celiac artery (photographs on the left) and flow separation at the corner of the superior mesentric artery(photographs on the right). Branch-trunk(inlet) flow rate ratios are 0.17 at the aorta-celiac junction and 0.07 at the aorta-superior mesentric junction.

DISCUSSION

The present visualization study revealed that the complicated pattern of flow produced in a tube with side branches has a character similar to that around wall-based obstacles[5,6,7]. The vortex formation in a tube with a small side branch has been reported by Pinchak and Ostrach[8] during steady flow. The branch-trunk diameter ratios were from 1/16 to 3/16 and the Reynolds number ranged 100 to 1000. They gave the details of the dye streak trapped by the vortex, and described the helical flow obtained in the main trunk just downstream of the branch orifice by postulating a vortex-sink flow of inviscid fluid at the branch orifice. The same flow pattern has also been obtained in our previous study using the same glass model as in the present study [5]. The branch-trunk diameter ratios were 4/13 and 5/13. The previous study also visualized the vortex formation in a tube with a Y-shaped bifurcation or a obstacle protruding inside from the wall. These results as well as those of the present study prove that the vortexes observed in the arterial models were similar in nature to the so-called laminar horseshoe vortex[5,6,7].

We visualized the flow patterns in the dog abdominal aorta made transparent by the method of Karino and Motomiya[4]. At the sites of the arterial branches, the generation of the horseshoe vortex was demonstrated during both steady and pulatile flows. Karino and Motomiya[4] showed a γ-shaped path-line of tracer particles at the aorta-celiac junction during steady flow, which may be produced by the particles beeing trapped by the horseshoe vortex. The horseshoe vortex was produced in the pulsatile flow during the time interval when the net flow was relatively large. However, the reversal flow which occurred near the wall during deceleration, as shown in FIG.3, transiently destroyed the flow pattern. It is known that a horseshoe vortex system produces high wall shear stress[7]. This fact may account for the poor incidence of atherosclerosis around the apex of the flow divider.

A reduction of flow rate to a branch artery induced the flow to separate from the wall at the corner during steady and pulsatile flows. The same phenomena of flow separation have been also reported by Lutz et al.[9] in a glass model. The separation region at the outer wall of the celiac artery was more stagnant than that of the superior mesenteric artery, as seen especially during steady flow in FIG.2. This might be related to the difference between the velocity profiles of flows moving toward the flow dividers[9]. The measurements showed that the velocity profile toward the divider of the superior mesenteric artery is skewed and high velocities occur near the ventral wall. As demonstrated on the right of FIG.5, the time required for clearance of tracer particles near the separation point of the celiac artery was considerably greater than elsewhere in the aorta. This observation means that the areas around the separation point experience rather low wall shear stresses. Moreover, the direction of the stress may not be unidirectional. These hemodynamic features may be related to the preference of this site for atherosclerosis, although the mechanism is not clear.

Acknowledgment: This work was supported by a Research Grant for Cardiovascular Diseases(60C-2) from the Ministry of the Health and Welfare and Japan Heart Foundation Research Grant for 1985.

REFERENCES

[1]Caro CG, Pedley TJ, Schroter RC, Seed WA (1978) The Mechanics of the Circulation. Oxford University Press, Oxford, pp 86-105

[2]Nerem RM (1981) Arterial fluid dynamics and interaction with the vessel walls. In: Schwartz CJ, Werthessen NT, Wolf S(eds) Structure and Function of the Circulation, Vol.2, Plenum Press, New York, pp 719-835

[3]McDonald DA (1974) Blood Flow in Arteries. Edward Arnold (Publishers) Ltd., Oxford, pp 92-95

[4]Karino T, Motomiya M (1983) Biorheology 20: 119-127

[5]Azuma T, Fukushima T (1976) Biorheology 13: 337-355

[6]Fukushima T, Azuma T (1982) Biorheology 19: 143-154

[7]Baker CJ (1979) J Fluid Mech 95(2): 347-367

[8]Pinchak AC, Ostrach S (1976) J Appl Physiol 41: 646-958

[9]Lutz RJ, Hsu L, Menawat A, Zrubeck J, Edwards K (1983) J Biomechanics 16: 753-766

Flow Studies in True-to-Scale Models of Human Renal Arteries

D. LIEPSCH[1], A. POLL[1], and S. MORAVEC[2]

[1] Hal B. Wallis Research Facility of the Eisenhower Medical Center, Rancho Mirage, CA 92270, USA
[2] Institut für Biotechnik u. Fachhochschule München, D-8000 München, Federal Republic of Germany

ABSTRACT

The flow behavior in rigid and elastic models of human renal arteries have been studied using glycerol-water and a blood-like viscoelastic fluid. The studies were done at steady and pulsatile flow. The differences between Newtonian and non-Newtonian blood-like fluids were especially visible at unsteady flow in the flow separation zones. Here the flow consists of high local convective parts. The studies were limited to the abdominal aorta downstream of the renal arteries where most sclerotic plaques are formed. The flow was visualized by using dyes and a birefringent solution. The disturbed flow can easily be localized with these methods. The velocity profiles were measured with a laser-Doppler-anemometer. The velocity gradients increased in the pulsatile flow between the main forward and reverse flow. These lead to higher shear stresses which can activate blood platelets and change the surface of the membrane of red cells. We found about a 15% flow increase during pulsatile flow with a representative Reynolds number of 250 for the polyacrylamide mixture compared to glycerol-water.

INTRODUCTION

Atheromatosis and thrombosis predominantly occur in the femoral, popliteal and renal arteries. At bends and bifurcations of human arteries, deposits and blockages are often found as well as eddies and secondary flows. The flow is disturbed. A higher pressure drop occurs. The flow separation distal to bifurcations is strongly dependent on the geometry, branch-to-trunk flow rate ratio, pulsatility, and also elasticity of the vessel wall and the non-Newtonian flow behavior of blood in such low shear regions. These flow parameters are studied separately in a rigid and elastic human model of the abdominal aorta with two renal arteries. Several flow visualization studies and velocity measurements which can not be all mentioned here have been carried out using models with enlarged diameters or anatomically accurate molds of arteries [1,2,7,8,9,10]. None of these studies however were carried out using non-Newtonian fluids similar to human blood over a wide shear rate range. Earlier studies in a 90°-T-junction with such fluids showed a quite different flow behavior especially of the secondary flow [4,5]. The influence of the elastic wall and the pulsatility on the flow separation zones were also studied in these models.

Models and Methods

Two rigid polyester resin models and an elastic 1:1 true-to-scale silicone rubber model were used for the flow visualization studies and for the laser-Doppler-anemometer measurements. The preparation technique has been described several times [3,5]. The silicone rubber model has an equal wall thickness of

1 mm. The flow was visualized with dyes and also using a birefringent solution. This method has the advantage of allowing a picture of the whole flow field to be taken. The length of the disturbed flow, beginning of disturbances, flow separation and reattachment points can be localized. This method is described in detail by Liepsch [4]. Having localized the disturbed areas, the velocity distribution is measured with a laser-Doppler-anemometer. The velocity measurements were done with a one and two-component laser-Doppler-anemometer for steady and pulsatile flow. A detailed description of the system and the experimental set-up is given in Liepsch [4] and Moravec [6].

RESULTS

Studies were done with a glycerol-water solution (η = 5.2 mPas, ρ = 1126 kg/m^3 at 21°C) and a polyacrylamide mixture (0.05 weight % aqueous AP30 and 0.04 weight % AP45 mixed in a rate 3:1, to this mixture is added 0.01% Mg Cl$_2$ and to all of them 4% isopropanol) which consists of long chain molecules with a similar flow behavior like blood in a shear rate range from 0.3 to 400 inverse seconds. Only the elastic component is higher compared to human blood. The measurements were done with a Couette viscosimeter. The fluid shows a viscoelastic and thixotropic flow behavior. The representative viscosity of such a fluid is η_r = 4.5 mPas for an entrance Reynolds of Re = 250, and a density ρ = 990 kg/m^3.

Figure 1 shows the Newtonian flow behavior using a birefringent solution (diluted Vanadiumpentoxide) in a rigid model prepared by Sabbah et al. [9] at an entrance Reynolds number Re = 1365 at steady flow. 17.5% of the flow goes in

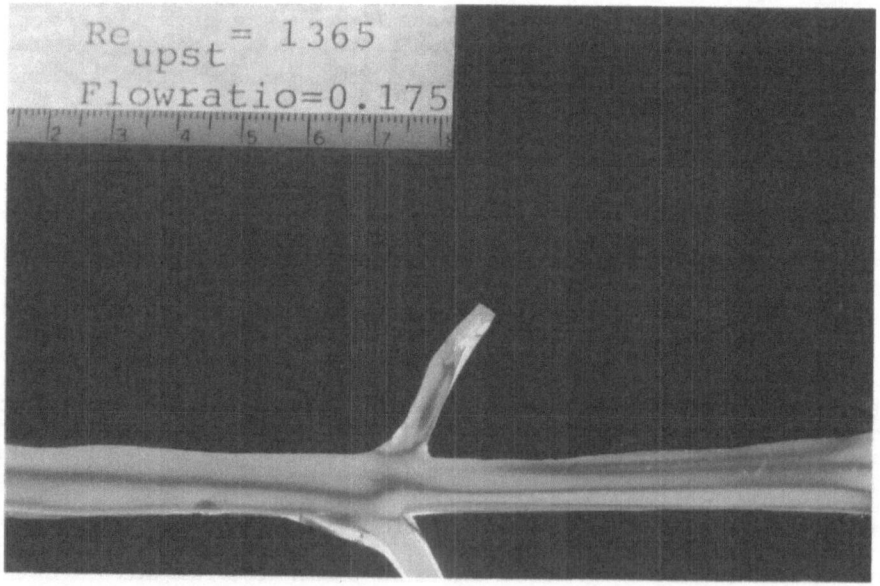

FIG. 1 Abdominal aorta and renal arteries of a acrylic glass model. The right renal branch of the artery is shown at the bottom of the figure. The proximal Reynolds number in the aorta is Re = 1365, the flow in the renal arteries is 17.5% each. The used birefringent solution is a diluted Vanadiumpentoxide solution with a viscosity of ν = 1.3 x 10^{-6} m^2/s.

Velocity distribution U(r) and velocity
fluctuations Ũ'(r) at steady flow: Re = 495
Separan solution; V̇1;V̇3;V̇4 = 1;0.25;0.25

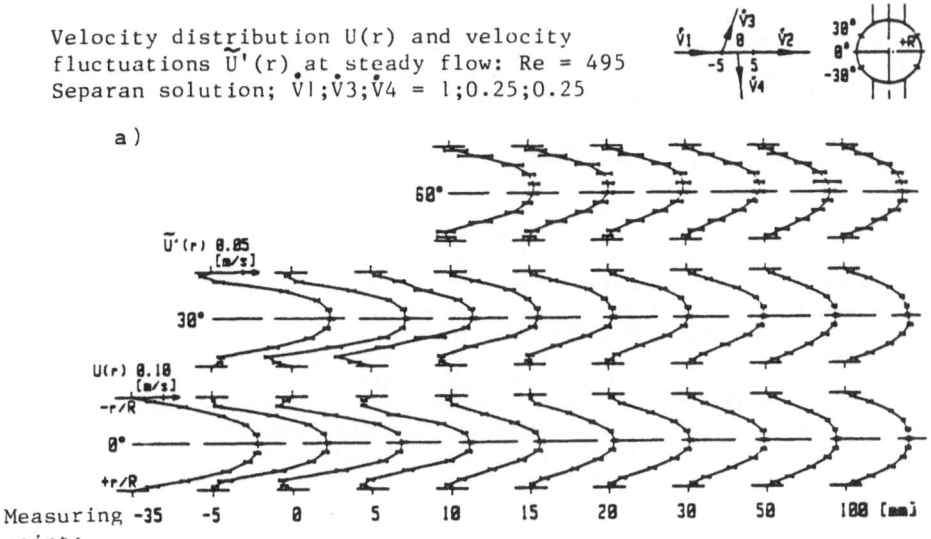

FIG. 2a Velocity distribution U (r) and velocity fluctuations Ũ' (r) at steady
flow: Re = 495 Separan solution; V1, V3, V4 = 1;0.25;0.25. Viscosity η = 4.5
mPas.

Velocity distribution U(r) and velocity
fluctuations Ũ'(r) at steady flow: Re = 495
Glycerol-water; V̇1;V̇3;V̇4 = 1;0.25;0.25

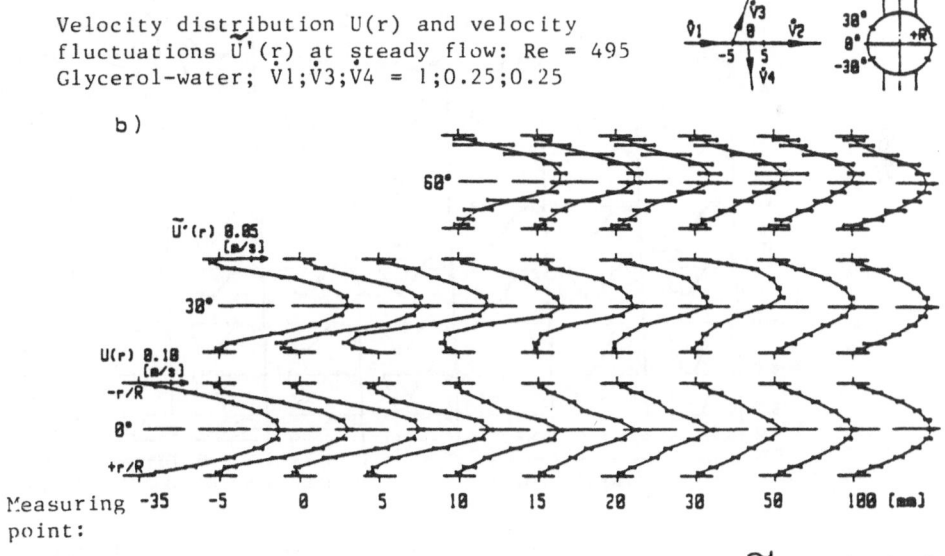

FIG. 2b Velocity distribution U (r) and velocity fluctuations Ũ' (r) at steady
flow: Re = 495 Glycerol-water; V1;V3;V4 = 1;0.25;0.25. Viscosity η = 5.2 mPas.

each of both renal arteries. Only small separation zones downstream in the abdominal aorta can be seen marked by the black line close to the wall. Also small velocity fluctuations are indicated by another black line which is divided in two lines. Detailed studies with different flow ratios and entrance Reynolds numbers are recorded on a video-tape. To get detailed information of the velocity distribution, laser-Doppler-anemometer measurements were carried out. Figures 2a and 2b show the velocity measurements in a simplified rigid model of the abdominal aorta and the renal arteries. The entrance flow has a Reynolds number 495; 25% of the whole flow is directed in each renal artery. Velocity fluctuations can be seen already in the abdominal aorta at steady flow downstream of the branches. Besides the velocity also the velocity fluctuations are recorded in the measured plains 0°, 30° and 60°. The measured points are indicated at the abscissa from -35 to 100 mm. Differences in the 60° plain between the glycerol water solution (Figure 2b) and the non-Newtonian Separan solution (Figure 2a) are observed. The differences between both fluids are much higher with increasing entrance Reynolds numbers.

Small velocity fluctuations were observed at nearly every measuring point with the Separan solution, whereas with the glycerol water solution the velocity fluctuations are relatively high. Velocity fluctuations distal to the branches were especially evident for pulsatile flow. Figure 3 shows the velocity distribution for pulsatile flow with the same Reynolds number and the same two solutions.

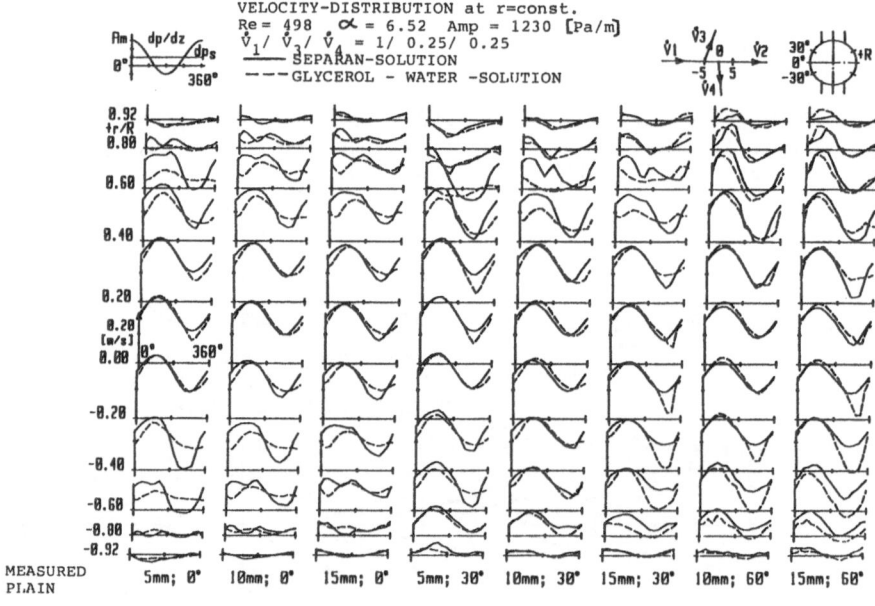

FIG. 3 Velocity distribution for pulsatile flow at r = const with an aqueous Separan mixture and an aqueous glycerol solution.

The local velocity profiles were recorded over 14 cycles. The average velocity
was always plotted. The flow around the tube axis shows very small disturbances
close to the branches at all measured points over the whole pulse cycle with the
polyacrylamide solution. With the glycerol-water solution, higher disturbances
along the tube axis can be observed. Both fluids show negative velocities or
small oscillations around zero close to the wall at the measured point 5 mm
downstream of the branches over the whole pulse cycle. Dead water regions can
be created at these points. The disturbed flow regions with the Newtonian fluid
extend from the wall to the tube axis whereas with the non-Newtonian fluid
reverse flow only can be observed close to the wall. The flow disturbances are
much larger with the Newtonian fluid compared to the non-Newtonian fluid.
Therefore flow studies with non-Newtonian blood-like fluids cannot be neglected.

   For the pulsatile flow, beside the Reynolds number and the Womersley
parameter, the amplitude of the pressure drop (Pa/m) is important. Figure 4
demonstrates (in a straight rigid tube) theoretical velocity distributions over
a whole pulse cycle at phases ω t 0°, 40°, 80°, 120°, 160°, 200°, 240°, and 280°
for a sinusoidal wave form. The Reynolds number is 500 and the Womersely
parameter is 6.5.

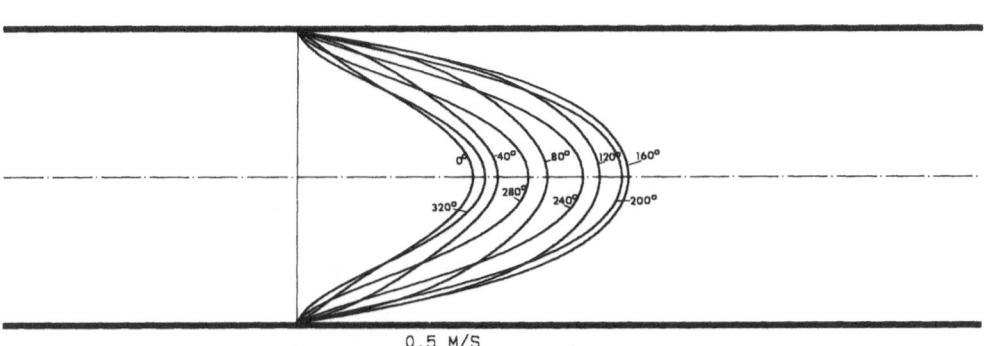

```
                    0.5 M/S
     TUBE DIAMETER        : 10 MM
     AVERAGE REYNOLDS No: 500
     WOMERSLEY PARAMETER: 6.52
     KINEMATIC VISCOSITY: 4.61 *10^-6 M^2/S
     OSCILLATING dp/dx   : 1230 Pa/M
```

FIG. 4 Numerical calculation of the pulsatile flow in a straight rigid tube for
an average Reynolds number over a whole cycle Re = 500 and with a Womersley
parameter α = 6.5. The pressure difference of the pulse was $\pm$ 20 mm mercury.

ACKNOWLEDGMENT: We would like to thank Deborah Sloss for preparation of the manuscript and the Deutsche Forschungsgemeinschaft for support under contract L:256-13/15.

REFERENCES

[1]Karino T, Kwong HB, Goldsmith HL (1979) Biorheology 16: 231-248.
[2]Ku DN, Giddens DP (1983) Atherosclerosis 3: 31-39.
[3]Liepsch D, Zimmer R (1978) Biomed Tech 23: 227-230.
[4]Liepsch D (1986) Stroemungsuntersuchungen an Modellen menschlicher Blutgefaess Systeme. Fortschrittberichte VDI, Reihe 7: Stroemungstechnik Nr. 113, VDI-Verlag
[5]Liepsch D (1984) Biorheology 23: 395-433.
[6]Moravec ST (1986)Stroemungsuntersuchungen mit newtonschen und viskoelastischen Fluessigkeiten in Modellen menschlicher Nierenarterien unter Verwendung eines Laser-Doppler-Anemometers. Ph.D. Thesis TU Muenchen
[7]Niimi H (1983) Clin Hemorheol 3: 223.
[8]Rodkiewicz CM (1981) CISM Courses and Lectures, No. 270, Wien: Springer.
[9]Sabbah HN, Hawkins ET, Stein PD (1984) Atherosclerosis 4: 28-33.
[10]Stehbens WE (1975) Q J Exp Physiol 60: 181-192.

Unsteady, Separated Laminar Flow in Non-Uniform Vessels

T.J. Pedley[1], M.E. Ralph[1], and O.R. Tutty[2]

[1]Department of Applied Mathematics and Theoretical Physics, University of Cambridge, Cambridge, England
[2]Department of Aeronautics and Astronautics, University of Southampton, Southampton, England

ABSTRACT

Regions of flow separation appear to be important sites for athero-genesis. Here we show that flow unsteadiness, even at low frequencies, has a significant effect on the location of and wall shear stress in separated eddies. Experimental and computational results are presented for (i) flow past a time-dependent, asymmetric indentation in a two-dimensional channel, and (ii) oscillatory flow through a fixed expansion Trains of vorticity waves are observed downstream of the indentation or expansion, each wave associated with a separated eddy which somtimes itself divides into two. The wall shear stress in the eddies is <u>much larger</u> than in steady or parallel flow. Also, in each case the flow eventually becomes three-dimensional.

Certain sites in the arterial system are particularly prone to atherogenesis; examples include the inner bend of the aortic arch, the carotid sinus, the curved coronary arteries, bifurcations (both natural and the junctions with coronary by-pass grafts) and stenoses. Many of these sites occur where there is rapid expansion of vessel cross-sectional area or sharp streamwise curvature of the wall, with the consequence that <u>steady</u> flow through the system would be associated with a sharp adverse pressure gradient at the wall and hence with flow separation. Moreover, when the motion is steady, regions of separated flow are invariably associated with low fluid velocities, in nearly stagnant eddies and hence with <u>small</u> values of wall shear stress.

However, blood flow in arteries is pulsatile, with the consequence that both the pressure gradients and the wall positions vary with time. Even in parallel-sided vessels the ratio of the amplitude of the wall shear oscillation to the mean is much greater than the same ratio for volume flow rate [1]. In non-parallel vessels flow separation still occurs wherever there is rapid expansion or curvature, but the unsteadiness means that the motion in the eddies can be dramatically altered. Recent work by Ku, Giddens et al. [2,3] on the carotid bifurcation has demonstrated how the wall shear changes sign over a considerable area, well-correlated with zones of atheromatous plaque formation. These auth ors have explained one reason for the relatively high level of reversed wall shear in a time-dependent eddy, based on the backwards acceleration of already sluggish flow near the wall when the pressure gradient reverses direction [4]. Sobey [5] had earlier given a more detailed explanation of this effect as it occurs in wavy-walled tubes.

In this paper we present experimental and computational results on variety of relatively low-frequency flows in two-dimensional non-uniform channels which reveal (a) that new separated eddies may appear at locations where they are absent in steady flow, and (b) that the peak magnitude of the reversed wall shear in these eddies is <u>several times larger</u> than any value occurring for steady flow or for unsteady flow in a

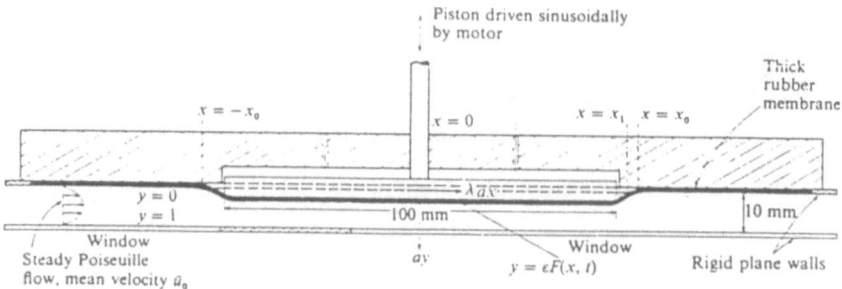

<u>Fig.1</u>. Sketch of the experimental channel mid-plane, with dimension-
less variables marked. From [7].

corresponding parallel-sided channel. This counter-intuitive result may
have profound implications for atherogenesis.

We consider first flow in a channel, width a , of which part of one
wall moves in and out sinusoidally with period T from the flush to an
indented position, the upstream flow being steady Poiseuille flow with
average velocity $\bar{u}_0$ (fig.1). Governing parameters are Reynolds number
Re = a $\bar{u}_0$/ν (where ν is the fluid kinematic viscosity, Strouhal number
St = a/$\bar{u}_0$T and the maximum ratio ε of indentation height to a . Numerica
computations of the flow have been made [6], and computed streamline
patterns for various times during one oscillation period are shown in
fig.2, for the case Re = 507, St = 0.037, ε = 0.38. This is one of the
cases studied experimentally [7], and agreement is qualitatively excellent and quantitatively good. During each cycle, "vorticity waves" are
generated downstream of the indentation and propagate downstream, the
wave-front propagating more rapidly than the wave crests/troughs; these
facts are well-explained by a small-amplitude inviscid theory [7].
From the present point of view, the interesting observations are the occurrence of separated-flow eddies beneath the crests/above the troughs.
The region of most rapid circulatory motion within an eddy moves to
the downstream end of the eddy, and a second co-rotating eddy often
develops upstream with a counter-rotating region at the wall ("eddy-
doubling"). The dimensionless wall shear on the plane wall of the
channel is plotted as a function of position, for various times, in fig.
We note that, while the wall-shear in Poiseuille flow is 6 on this scaling, and the maximum wall shear in two-dimensional Womersley flow at
α = 10.9 (α^2 = 2πReSt), and with amplitude determined from the piston
motion by conservation of mass is 12, the maximum shear under wave B
(see fig.2) is negative (corresponding to the reversed flow under the
fast vortex) and has value 36.

The second flow to be considered is oscillatory <u>flow</u> past a <u>fixed</u>
(and still asymmetric) indentation, with a geometry similar to that of
fig.1. The experiments were done by Sobey [8], and the corresponding
computations have only recently been performed [9]. Once more waves are
generated downstream of the indentation during each cycle, but in this
case the crests propagate only a little way downstream before moving upstream again, although the wave front still moves rapidly downstream.
Again, however, eddies are formed under the wave-crests, and they have a
similar structure to those in the previous case. The computed streamlines and wall vorticity are shown in figs.4,5 for the case in which the
edge of the indentation has sharp, right-angled corners, and Re = 500,
St = 0.024, ε = 0.5. The maximum wall-shear magnitude is comparable
with that shown in fig.3.

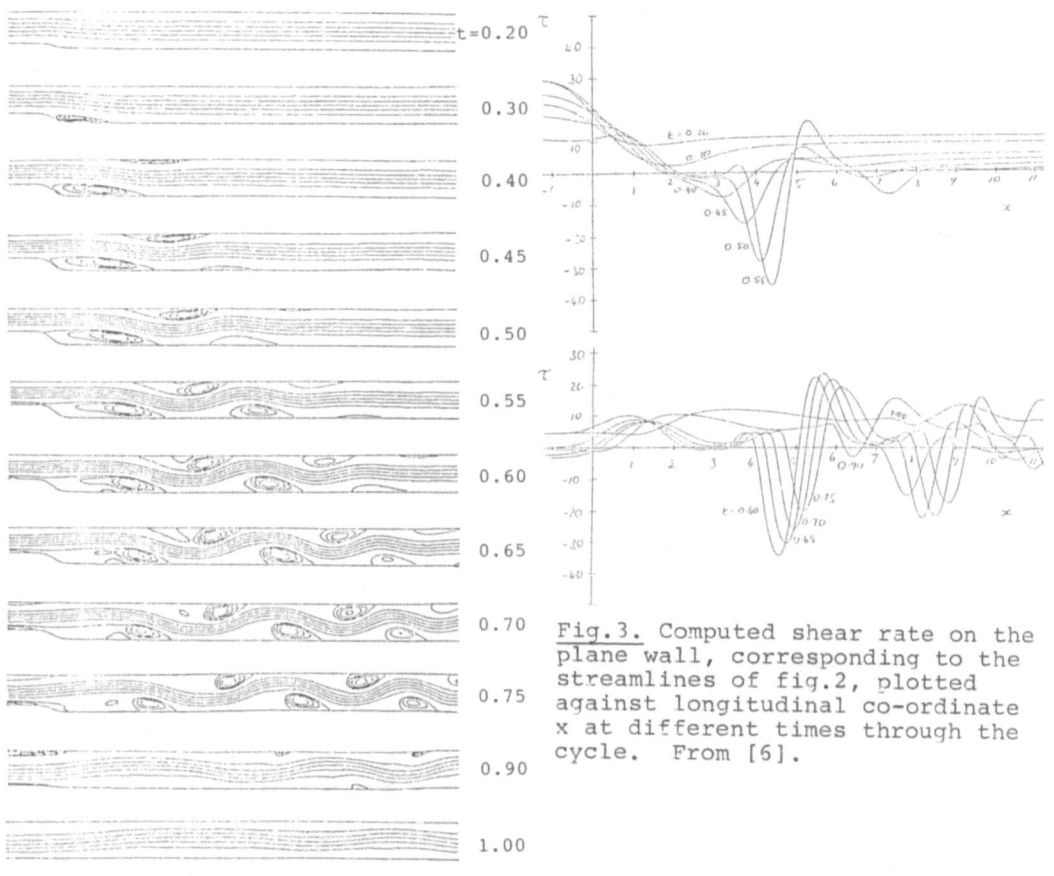

Fig.3. Computed shear rate on the plane wall, corresponding to the streamlines of fig.2, plotted against longitudinal co-ordinate x at different times through the cycle. From [6].

Fig.2. Computed instantaneous streamline plots corresponding to the experiments in [7]: Re = 507, St = 0.037, ε = 0.38. Times are given in fractions of a cycle period. From [6].

Other flows that have been considered are oscillatory flows in symmetric or asymmetric wavy-walled tubes and channels [e.g.5,10]. Since the walls are already wavy we do not see the same development of vorticity waves, but non-quasi-steady flow patterns and enhanced wall shear stress are observed.

Finally, it should be borne in mind that the computations reported above are for two-dimensional flows (or axisymmetric: see [10]); the experimental flows are nominally two-dimensional too. Many other studies are also concerned with either two-dimensional or axisymmetric pipe flows. However, most sites of interest in the arterial system are in fully three-dimensional geometries, such as curved tubes and bifurcations, with relatively strong cross-stream velocities. In such circumstances fluid flows into and out of separated flow zones,which cannot be regarded as closed, stagnant eddies, even when the flow is steady. Also, even in nominall-two-dimensional flows, strong cross-stream velocities may be observed in the separated eddies when they are stable and laminar [8,11], and the eventual breakdown into turbulence of some of the flows examined above

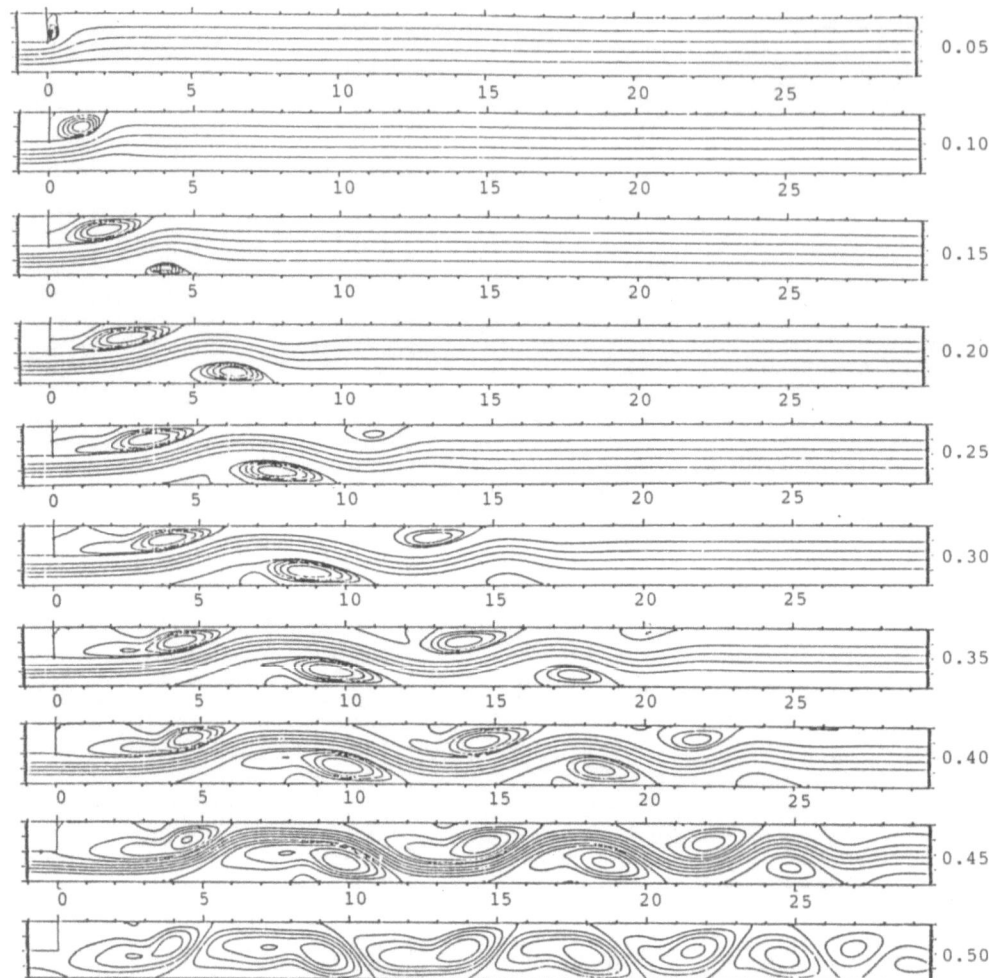

Fig.4. Computed instantaneous
streamline plots corresponding
to the experiments in [8]:
Re = 500, St = 0.024, ε = 0.5.
Times are given in fractions of
a cycle period. From [9].

takes place via a three-dimensional instability [7,8]. The interaction
between three-dimensionality and time-dependence in determining the wal
shear in separated eddies has not yet been examined in fluid-mechanical
detail, and is an important task for the future.

The numerical and experimental work described here was supported
by the Science and Engineering Research Council of the U.K.

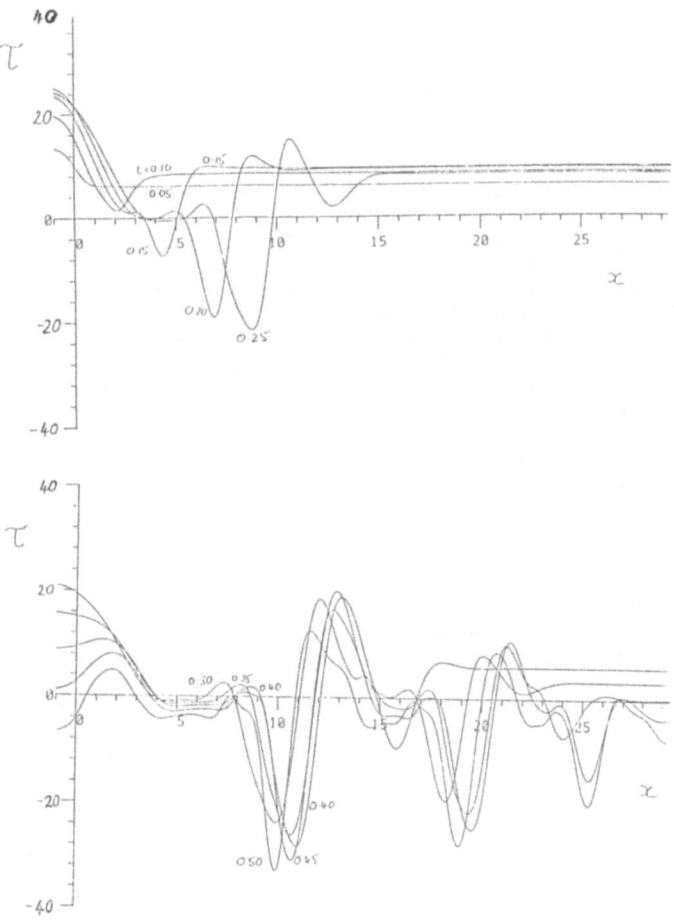

Fig.5. Computed shear rate on the plane wall, corresponding to the streamlines of fig.4, plotted against longitudinal co-ordinate x at different times through the cycle. From [9].

REFERENCES

[1] Pedley, T.J. (1976) Viscous boundary layers in reversing flow. J. Fluid Mech. 74: 59-79.
[2] Ku. D.N., Giddens, D.P., Zarins, C.K., Glagov, S. (1985) Pulsatile flow and atherosclerosis in the human carotid bifurcation: positive correlation between plaque location and low and oscillating shear stress. Arteriosclerosis 5: 293-302.
[3] Ku, D.N., Phillips, D.J., Giddens, D.P. & Strandness, D.E. (1985), Hemodynamics of the normal human carotid bifurcation: in vitro and in vivo studies. Ultrasound in Med. and Biol. 11: 13-26.
[4] Giddens, D.P., Ku, D.N. (1987) A note on the relationship between input flow wave form and wall shear rate in pulsatile, separating flows. J. Biomech. Engg. 109: 175-176.
[5] Sobey, I.J. (1983) The occurrence of separation in oscillatory flow. J. Fluid Mech. 134: 247-257.
[6] Ralph, M.E. & Pedley, T.J. (1987) Flow in a channel with a moving indentation. J. Fluid Mech, accepted.
[7] Pedley, T.J. & Stephanoff, K.D. (1985) Flow along a channel with a time-dependent indentation in one wall: the generation of vorticity waves. J. Fluid Mech. 160: 337-367.
[8] Sobey, I.J. (1985) Observations of waves during oscillatory channel flow. J. Fluid Mech. 151: 395-426.
[9] Tutty, O.R. & Pedley, T.J. (1987) Computations of oscillatory flow in a non-uniform channel. In preparation.
[10] Ralph, M.E. (1986) Oscillatory flows in wavy-walled tubes. J. Fluid Mech. 168: 515-540.
[11] Bertram, C.D. & Pedley, T.J. (1983) Steady and unsteady separation in an approximately two-dimensional indented channel. J. Fluid Mech. 130 315-345.

Effects of Phase Relationships on Wall Shear Stress in Curved and Straight Elastic Artery Models

J.M. Tarbell, M. Klanchar, and A. Dutta

Department of Chemical Engineering, The Pennsylvania State University, University Park, PA 16802, USA

ABSTRACT

Wall shear stress, diameter and flow waveforms were measured in elastic curved and straight tube physical models under sinusoidal flow conditions with up to 11% diameter variation. The straight tube experiments were simulated with a theoretical model. Both the experiments and the theoretical model predict extreme sensitivity of wall shear stress to the phase angle between wall shear stress and diameter. Under fixed flow waveform conditions, the experiments showed as much as a five-fold increase in wall shear stress over a 20-40 deg change in phase angle. The onset of strong wall shear stress reversal was also observed in this sensitive phase angle range. Even greater effects were predicted by the theoretical model which covered a broader range of phase angle variations. These results suggest that wall elasticity may play an important role in determining wall shear stress distributions in large arteries.

INTRODUCTION

Wall shear stress (WSS) is believed by many to play a role in atherogenesis. Since artery walls are elastic, and 10% variations in artery radius have typically been observed in vivo [1,2], it would seem important to consider the influence of radial wall motion on WSS. Chang and Tarbell [3] simulated elastic curved tube flows numerically and found relatively minor effects of wall motion on WSS distribution for 10% diameter variations when flow and diameter oscillations were in phase. Chang [4] measured flow rate and pressure drop in elastic curved and straight tube models under aortic flow conditions and found the impedance modulus to follow rigid straight tube theory fairly well when flow and diameter variation were in phase. However, when the diameter waveform lagged the flow waveform significantly (up to 60 deg) there was a marked increase in the modulus of impedance. Liepsch et al. [5] measured axial velocity profiles by LDA in pulsating flow through rigid and elastic models of a 35 deg bifurcation and observed significant differences in velocity profiles during flow deceleration. They did not report phase relationships. Mark et al. [6] estimated WSS in a compliant cast of the aortic bifurcation and found significant elevation of peak WSS in the compliant cast relative to a rigid cast. They did not discuss phase relationships.

The basic hypothesis of the present work is that wall motion may affect WSS magnitude and distribution significantly and the phase relationships among flow, diameter, and WSS may be influential.

EXPERIMENTAL METHODS

Curved and straight tube physical models were constructed from a 300 cm length of constant diameter latex rubber tubing (inside diameter 1.6 cm, thickness/diameter = .03, wave speed about 500 cm/sec) and positioned in a flow loop with a long straight flow development section upstream of the measurement site. A sinusoidal flow with a mean Reynolds number (Re) of 1400, peak Re of 2380 and unsteadiness parameter of 12.5 was maintained in all experiments. The magnitude of the diameter variation and the phase angle between flow and diameter variation were altered through a distal flow resistor. Diameter variations up to 11% of mean diameter were obtained in some experiments. WSS was measured with a flush-mounted hot-film anemometer probe (TSI, Model 1268W) glued to the latex tube wall and free to move with the wall. Diameter variation was measured with a linear variable displacement transducer and flow with two electromagnetic flowmeters mounted on rigid tubing at the proximal and distal ends of the elastic tubing. The hot film probe and the displacement transducer were placed within a few cm of each other at a distance of 270 cm from the proximal end. The flow at this point was calculated from the flowmeter readings through inviscid wave propagation theory.

THEORETICAL METHODS

A simple theoretical model was developed to simulate the experiments. It assumes a straight tube, Newtonian fluid, negligible convective acceleration (long wavelength) and specifies both pressure gradient and diameter variation waveforms with a variable phase relationship. These assumptions lead to the following equation of fluid motion

$$\frac{\partial w}{\partial t} = \nu\left[\frac{\partial^2 w}{\partial r^2} + \frac{1}{r}\frac{\partial w}{\partial r}\right] - \frac{1}{\rho}\frac{\partial P(t)}{\partial z}$$

and boundary conditions

$$\frac{\partial w}{\partial r} = 0 \quad \text{at} \quad r = 0$$

$$w = 0 \quad \text{at} \quad r = R(t)$$

where w is the axial velocity, r and z are the radial and axial coordinates, respectively, $\partial p/\partial z$ is the pressure gradient, and R is the tube radius. The pressure gradient and radius are specified as time varying input waveforms

$$\partial p/\partial z = K(1 + k\cos\omega t)$$

$$R = \bar{R}(1 + k_r\cos(\omega t - \phi))$$

Before solving the equations, a radial coordinate transformation is introduced

$$\xi = \frac{r}{R(t)}$$

which has the effect of immobilizing the tube wall in the transformed coordinate (ξ). The transformed equations are then solved by a standard finite difference algorithm based on the method of lines.

It is difficult to simulate the experimental conditions precisely with the theoretical model because it requires pressure gradient as an input, whereas flow, not pressure gradient, was measured in the experiments. In the simulations, a sinusoidal pressure gradient waveform was specified which for a rigid tube produced nearly the same flow waveform and unsteadiness as the experiments described above except that the flow amplitude was somewhat higher (approximately 100% of mean flow). A sinusoidal diameter variation waveform with a constant peak-to-peak variation of 10% was imposed. The parameter varied in the simulations was the phase angle between the imposed pressure gradient and diameter variation waveforms.

RESULTS

The experimental peak WSS and reversal of WSS (as determined by the magnitude of secondary hot-film anemometer peaks) showed a strong positive correlation with the phase angle between WSS and diameter (WSS-D) and a relatively weak correlation with diameter variation. Figure 1 displays the peak WSS normalized by the Poiseuille flow WSS at the mean flow rate and mean diameter (Zp) for the curved tube (inside and outside wall) and the straight tube. Zp was nearly constant and close to its rigid tube value (3.0-curved tube outside

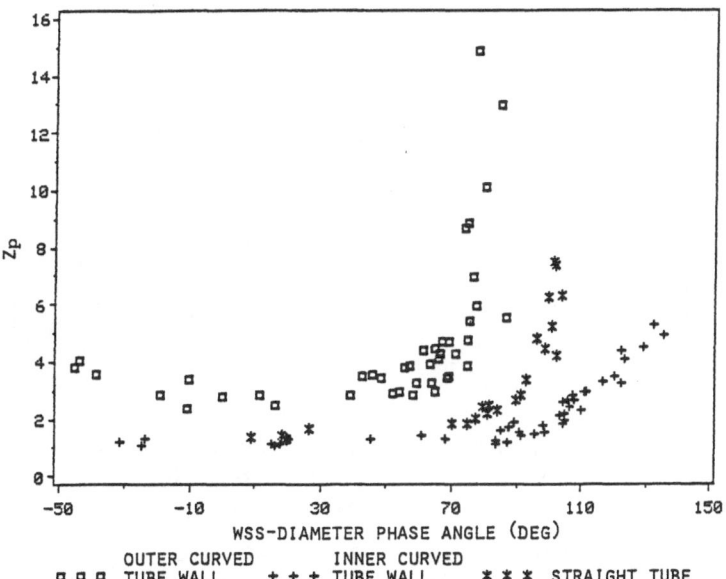

Figure 1. Normalized peak wall shear stress versus phase angle between wall shear stress and diameter variation.

wall, 2.1-curved tube inside wall, and 2.1-straight tube as computed by Chang and Tarbell [7]) for WSS-D between -50 and +70 deg. As WSS-D was increased above +70 deg there was a dramatic increase in Zp at all locations, by as much as a factor of 5. Evidence of significant flow reversal at the inside (but not the outside) wall of the curved tube and in the straight tube was observed in the secondary peaks of the anemometer bridge voltage signal. Figure 2 shows the normalized reversal peak WSS (Zrp) as a function of the WSS-D phase angle. There was little flow reversal until WSS-D reached about +80 deg, but a dramatic increase in Zrp for WSS-D greater than +80 deg. The magnitude of Zrp reached levels comparable to those observed for Zp in the sensitive range of WSS-D indicating a very intense flow reversal.

    Results of the simulations are shown in Figure 3. The left hand ordinate is the peak WSS normalized by the time-averaged WSS (Zp). This is a different normalization than was used in presenting the experimental results. A different normalization was required because the mean flow, which was held constant in the experiments, varied significantly in the simulations in which pressure gradient was held constant. The right hand ordinate of Figure 3 is the oscillatory shear index (OSI) defined by Ku et al. [8] to characterize wall shear stress reversal, and the abscissa is the phase angle between WSS and diameter (WSS-D). Dramatic increases in both Zp and OSI are observed for WSS-D above +70 deg. Zp reaches a maximum value of 24 which is about 8 times higher than the rigid tube value. OSI attains a maximum value 0.48 which is only slightly less than the value obtained when the reverse and forward WSS are equal (OSI = 0.5). The sensitive phase angle range is the same as observed in the experiments (compare Fig. 3 to Figs. 1 and 2).

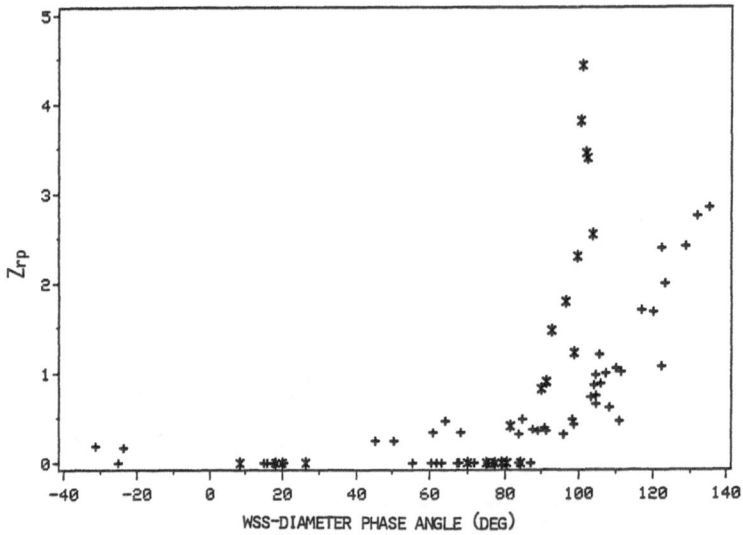

+ + + INNER CURVED TUBE WALL   * * * STRAIGHT TUBE

Figure 2. Normalized reversal peak wall shear stress versus phase angle between wall shear stress and diameter variation.

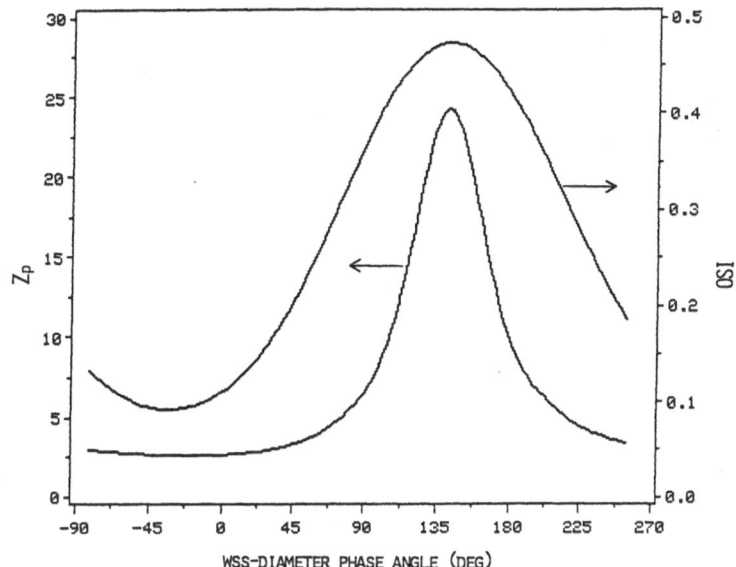

.Figure 3.   Normalized peak wall shear stress (left) and oscillatory
             shear index (right) versus phase angle between wall shear
             stress and diameter variation.

DISCUSSION

     WSS magnitude and WSS reversal may be important in atherogenesis
[6,8].   The present study indicates that vessel wall motion may
dramatically affect WSS magnitude and WSS reversal and that the phase
relationships among flow, diameter, and WSS are of critical
importance.   Since WSS-D phase angle relationships for in-vivo flow
states are not know, it remains to be seen if the phenomena we have
observed are important physiologically.

     Since WSS has not been measured in relation to flow and diameter
in vivo, we will make a case for the physiological relevance of our
results by considering pressure-flow (P-Q) relationships.   If the
rubber tube used in our experiments is taken to be purely elastic,
then the diameter and pressure waveforms are in phase.   In this case,
P-Q and D-Q phase angles are equivalent.   In our experiments, D-Q
phase angles varied between +8 and -64 deg as the distal impedance
was increased.   Aortic input impedance data is typically
characterized by P-Q phase angles in the range 0 to -60 deg for the
first four harmonics of the waveforms [1,2]. Thus, our experiments
appear to be in a physiological range of P-Q phase angles, and the
phenomena we have observed may be relevant to physiological flow
states.   Our results also suggest that subtle changes in arterial
impedance may significantly alter wall shear stress characteristics.
Such changes are known to occur in hypertension [9] and in response
to vasoactive drugs [10].

     The physical mechanism underlying the phenomena we have reported
may not be immediately obvious.   If one considers Poiseuille flow, in
which wall shear stress is directly proportional to mean velocity and
inversely proportional radius, then one expects 10% radius variations
to produce 10% variations in wall shear stress.   This would be the

situation at low values of the unsteadiness parameter ($\alpha < 1$). However, at high values of α ($\alpha > 10$), the wall shear stress in a rigid tube is directly proportional to the mean velocity and inversely proportional to the thickness of the Stokes boundary layer on the wall ($\delta = \sqrt{\nu/\omega} \equiv$ Stokes layer thickness). Since $\delta = a/\alpha$, it is clear that at high values of α, the Stokes layer thickness (δ) may be reduced to the order of magnitude of the radius variations in our rubber tubes. Under these circumstances it is plausible that seemingly small radius variations could have a significant influence on wall shear stress. This suggests that the considerable effects we have observed in our experiments and calculations at $\alpha = 12.5$ (characteristic of the thoracic aorta) would be diminished at lower α (distal vessels) and perhaps further amplified at higher α (proximal aorta).

Acknowledgment: This work was supported by USPHS Grant R01-H135549.

REFERENCES

[1]McDonald WA (1974) Blood Flow in Arteries. Williams and Wilkins Co
[2]Patel DJ, Vaishnav RN (1980) Basic Hemodynamics and Its Role in Disease Processes. University Park Press
[3]Chang LJ, Tarbell JM (1986) Proceedings of the 39th ACEMB, p 304.
[4]Chang LJ (1985) A Numerical and Experimental Study of Unsteady Flow in Rigid and Elastic Curved Tubes. Ph.D. Thesis, Penn State Univ
[5]Liepsch D, Moravec S (1984) Biorheology 21: 5
[6]Mark FF, Deters OJ, Bargeron CB, Friedman MH (1985) Proceedings of the ASME Winter Annual Meeting, p 59
[7]Chang LJ, Tarbell JM (1985) J Fluid Mech 161: 175
[8]Ku DN, Giddens DP, Zarins CK, Glagov, S (1985) Arteriosclerosis 5: 29
[9]Merillon JP, Fontenier GJ, Lerallut JF, Jaffrin MY, Motte GA, Genain CP, Gourgon RR (1982) Cardiovasc Res 16: 646-56
[10]Caro CG, Fish PJ, Goss DE, Halls J, Lever MJ, Parker KH, Stacey-Clear A (1985) Proc Physiol Soc 98P, 28-29 March

Wall Shear Stress Distribution Patterns in Arterial Stenosis Models Measured with an Electrochemical Technique

T. YAMAGUCHI and S. HANAI

Vascular Pathophysiology Laboratory, Department of Vascular Physiology, National Cardiovascular Center Research Institute, Suita, 565 Japan

ABSTRACT

An electrochemical surface shear stress measurement was applied to a model of unilateral arterial stenosis. The unilateral stenosis model consisted of a removable stenosis plug which was placed inside an electrochemical shear stress measurement test section containing 100 electrodes. Three dimensional wall shear stress distribution was measured under conditions of steady flow. We found a characteristic high and low wall shear stress distribution pattern beginning immediately downstream of the unilateral stenosis plug. Furthermore, we observed remarkable high shear stress regions on the opposite wall both up- and downstream of the stenosis; as well as on both side walls upstream of the stenosis.

INTRODUCTION

A variety of physical and physico-chemical factors have been suggested to be responsible for the localization of early atherosclerotic lesions, and thus, to influence the whole initiation process of atherosclerosis. Of these factors, wall shear stress has been suggested to play an important role in atherogenesis, since it has an inherent non-uniformity in space[1,2]. Recent human studies[3-5] have indicated that the earliest atherosclerotic changes occur preferentially at regions where average wall shear stress is expected to be low. Such a region has often been referred to as a "low shear region", a term which refers to specific locations in an artery, such as the lateral walls of symmetrical branchings, the proximal or upstream walls of asymmetrical branchings, and the distal or downstream regions of stenoses. As we discussed previously[6], the term "low shear region" can be misleading, since these regions are places where we would expect an average low shear stress from an analogy of the two dimensional steady flow field.

In fact, recent three dimensional flow visualization studies on both branching flow and stenosis flow have indicated that the blood flow in these vessel regions is far more complicated than we would expect from an analysis of two dimensional flows. Even in cases where branching is symmetric or the stenosis is smooth, complex vortices have been observed[7-8]. Also, as we have previously reported[9], remarkable alterations in wall shear stress distribution patterns have been observed in these regions. Although it has been suggested that such flows would consequently produce complex patterns of wall shear stress distribution, very little is known about the quantitative nature of the wall shear stress. In this paper, we describe an electrochemical method used to measure wall shear stress distribution patterns in a unilateral stenosis model, and compare our results with those others have obtained from flow visualization studies.

EXPERIMENTAL METHOD

(1) Electrochemical wall shear stress measurement.

The principle and outline for the application of the electro
chemical method used to determine wall shear stress distribution wa
previously reported[6], and extensively reviewed by Mizushina[10]
Thus, only a brief description of the method is outlined here.

Imagine a small cathode placed flush with the surface of a mode
flow tract. A solution of equimolar ferricyanide and ferrocyanid
flows through the model. When an electrical potential is imposed o
the cathode, the following oxidation-reduction reaction proceed
toward equilibrium at the cathode surface,

$$Fe(CN)_6{}^{3-} + e^- \rightleftharpoons Fe(CN)_6{}^{4-}. \qquad \qquad ....(1)$$

When the cathode potential is kept between -0.2 and -0.8V, the ferri
cyanide ion is completely consumed at the cathode surface. Under thes
conditions, convective transport and the diffusion govern the exten
of the reaction. Thus, the cathode current becomes a function o
convection and diffusion. Since ion transport by diffusion is though
to be negligible as compared with the convective transport of ions
the electrical or so called limiting current I_{lim}, becomes a functio
of the velocity gradient (or shear rate, S) when it is very close t
the cathode surface. This problem is able to be solve
analytically[10], and the solution is determined by using th
following equation,

$$S \propto I_{lim}{}^3 . \qquad \qquad ....(2)$$

In the present study, we performed careful electrode calibratio
measurements both before adding the stenosis plug, and once agai
after its removal in order to obtain the coefficient and power fo
solving Eq.(2). These parameters, however, differed from one electrod
to another in an unpredictable manner. We were unable to find an
systematic deviation. For example, we found that the average measure
power for Eq.(2) was 3.0, as the theory predicts, although it range
from 2.0 to 5.0. Thus, in order to obtain more reproducibl
measurements, we recalibrated each electrodes using known shear stres
values produced by Poiseuille flow. These calibration measurement
were also made both before and after making measurements using
stenosis. We used the following exponential calibration expression,

$$I_{lim} = I_0 + B \cdot S^A, \qquad \qquad ....(3)$$

where, I_0 is the current corresponding to 0 shear rate. Estimates fo
coefficient B and the power of A were determined by a least squar
fitting method using the calibration measurement data. After obtainin
the values for these parameters, wall shear rate values wer
determined by solving Eq.(3).

(2) The unilateral stenosis model

The model test section used was similar to a previously reporte
model[6]. Electrodes were made of 0.5 mm nickel wire. Four rows of 2
electrodes were implanted to a depth of 7-8mm along the length of a 3
mm diameter acrylic rod. Rows of electrodes were positioned at 90°
angles from each other, and individual electrodes were separated b
5mm. Once the electrodes were glued into place, a 20mm diameter hol
was bored through the center of the rod. In this way, we were assure

that the electrode surface was as flush as possible with the model wall. The surface of the inner wall was polished before and after each experiment in order to prevent any contaminating substances from causing non-specific chemical reactions at the electrode surface.

The acrylic test section was placed in an artificial flow system consisting of up- and downstream overflow tanks, up- and downstream flow settling chambers, a heat exchanger, filters, and a pump[6]. Flow rate was measured with a rotameter-type flow meter, and an electronic counter. The flowmeter had been precalibrated using a stopwatch and a measuring cylinder. The test fluid was a solution of 0.01 mol/l potassium ferricyanide and potassium ferrocyanide, with 1.0 mol/l sodium hydroxide added to prevent electrophoresis. The temperature of the test fluid was kept constant at 25.0°C with a heat exchanger and a precision water bath which had an error of ± 0.01 °C. A quartz thermometer was used to monitor the test fluid temperature.

Stenosis plugs of three different sizes were manufactured and tested in this study. The length of each stenosis (along the direction of flow) was equivalent to the diameter of the test section. The height of each stenosis plug varied, and was a half, a quarter, or an eighth of the diameter of the test section. The half height stenosis plug was made of paraffin, and was easily fixed to the inner wall of the test section by manufacturing it slightly wider than the pipe diameter. The quarter- and eighth height paraffin stenoses could not be easily fixed to the inner wall in the same way. This problem was solved by making the smaller stenoses from lathed steel and fixing them into place with a strong magnet attached to the outside wall of the test section. In this paper, we present results obtained using the large (half diameter) stenosis.

In calibration of measurements, we removed the stenosis plugs from the test section. Also, since the flow through our system was unidirectional, it was necessary for us to move a stenosis plug to the downstream end of a row of electrodes when making upstream flow measurements, and vice versa for our downstream measurements.

(3) The measuring system

For each set of measurements, 100 electrodes were scanned using a specially designed GP-IB controlled selector. A special set of low resistance relays were used to switch the very small cathode current, which was usually on the order of magnitude of microamperes. The cathode current, the flow rate and the temperature of the test fluid were measured simultaneously and recorded by using a 16-bit microcomputer. The test fluid viscosity was measured both before and after the experiments using a cone-plate-type viscometer. The viscosity measurement was always 1.2×10^{-3} Pa s (1.2 cP). This value was used to calculate the shear stress from the measured shear rate.

Each electrode was scanned for three different potentials (-0.4, -0.5, and -0.6 V). For each potential, we made 10 measurements which were later averaged. Each set of measurements took approximately ten minutes to complete. The data were recorded on floppy disks for subsequent analysis using the Apollo DN330 32 bits engineering work station.

RESULTS

Shear stress distribution patterns measured at three different Reynolds numbers for the half height (10mm) stenosis are shown in FIGs.1-3. A detailed discussion of the relationship between stenosis

height and wall shear stress distribution has been presented
elsewhere[9]. Reynolds numbers were calculated using the values for
the mean flow rate, the diameter of the test section (not the size of
the stenosis), and the test fluid viscosity. Reynolds numbers, 270,
660, and 1330 correspond flow rates of 5.0, 12.5 and 25.0 ml/s respectively.

In all cases, shear stress measurements made at points far upstream of the stenosis were approximately equal to the Poiseuille flow
value. If we assume a fully developed Poiseuille flow, then the wall
shear stresses should be, 7.6 x10^{-3}Pa, 1.9 x10^{-2}Pa, and 3.8 x10^{-2}Pa
for the flow rates of 5.0, 12.5 and 25.0 ml/s, respectively. At the
low Reynolds number (270), we found characteristic wall shear stress
distribution patterns up- and downstream of the stenosis. On both
side walls, there was an increase of the shear stress which was
detectable beginning about 2 diameters upstream of the stenosis. This
increase in side wall shear stress upstream of the stenosis was
usually detected before there was any observable increase in shear
stress at the wall opposite of the stenosis. The increase in shear
stress at the opposite wall is likely to be due to the effective
reduction of cross sectional area; and is considered to be analogous
with the results obtained previous two dimensional stenosis studies.
As expected, we also observed a characteristic small low shear stress
region upstream of the stenosis which was probably induced by the
presence of a horse shoe vortex[7].

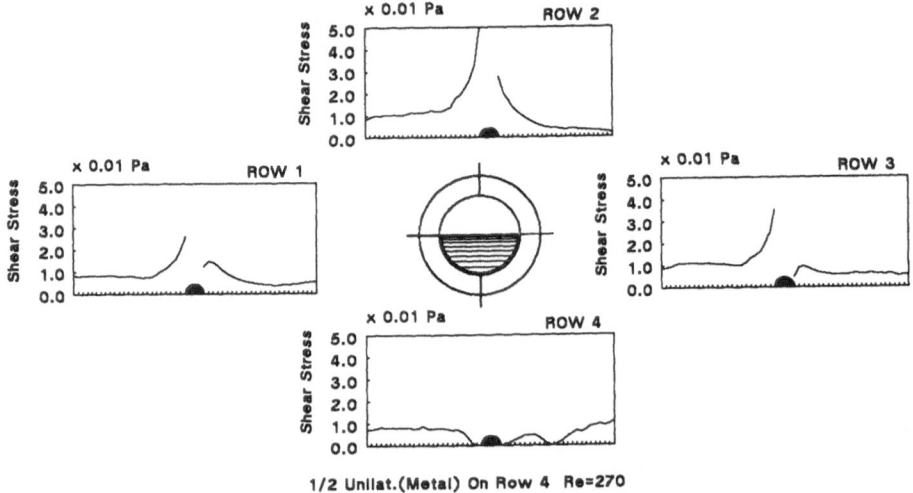

1/2 Unilat.(Metal) On Row 4 Re=270

FIG.1 Wall shear stress distribution patterns obtained using a half
height unilateral stenosis at Reynolds number 270. Each panel
corresponds to a set of measurements carried out along the direction
of flow. The position of the stenosis is indicated (●) in each
panel. Ticks on the x-axis indicate electrodes. A scheme of the
cross-sectional area of the test section, with the 4 rows of
electrodes placed at 90 angles from each other is shown.

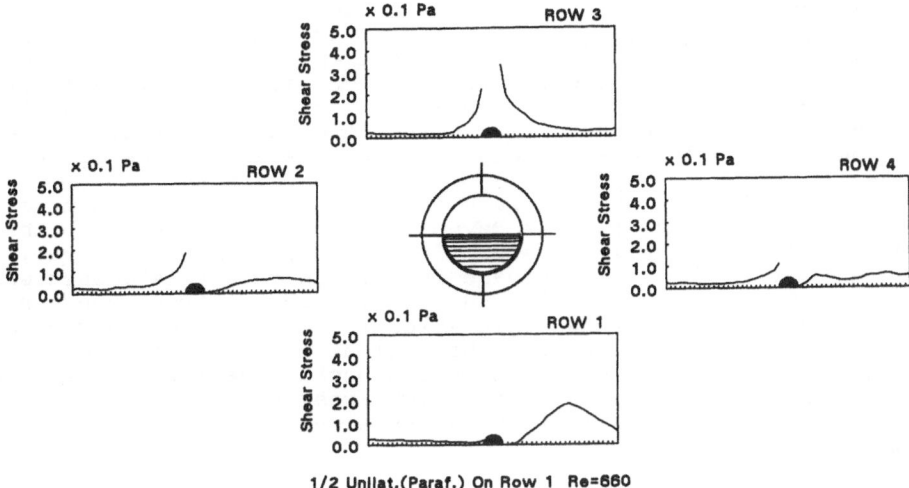

FIG.2 Wall shear stress distribution pattern obtained using a half height unilateral stenosis at Reynolds number 660. See FIG.1 caption for details.

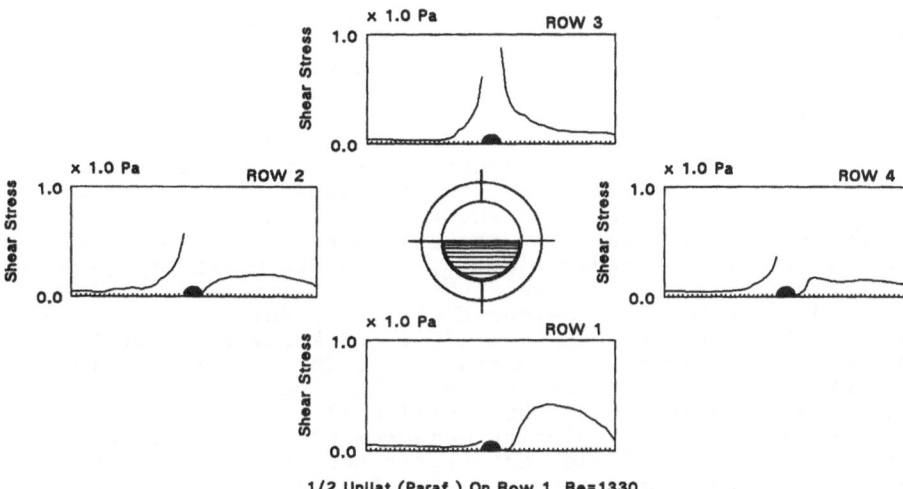

FIG.3 Wall shear stress distribution patterns obtained using a half height unilateral stenosis at Reynolds number 1330. See FIG.1 caption for details.

Another characteristic feature of our stenosis model was the presence of a marked low wall shear region about 3 diameters downstream of the stenosis. Also, on the wall opposite the stenosis, we found a very high shear stress region just downstream of the stenosis plug. However, the shear stress values taken further downstream began to decrease to a value lower than that of Poiseuille flow; and they remained low along the more distal regions of our test section.

The increase in shear stress on the side walls upstream of the stenosis which we observed at Reynolds number 270, was also observed at the two larger Reynolds number (660 and 1370) flows. However, with larger Reynolds numbers a decrease in wall shear stress downstream of the stenosis was not observed, and the wall shear stress continued to remain higher than the Poiseuille value in this region. In general, as the Reynolds number increased, the regions of low wall shear stress both up- and downstream of the stenosis became smaller, and the shear stress values at the opposite wall downstream of the stenosis remained higher than the Poiseuille flow values along the more distal regions of our test section.

DISCUSSION AND CONCLUDING REMARKS

The electrochemical method of measuring wall shear stress is widely used in chemical engineering field as a way of measuring wall shear stress in various flow tracts. Recently, this method has been applied to bio-fluid dynamics[11-14]. This method has been shown to be very sensitive to the velocity gradient in wall regions, and is thus an appropriate method for obtaining estimates of wall shear stress distribution patterns in arterial models with respect to atherogenesis[9].

Two other methods which are commonly used for measuring wall shear stress are the hot-film method and the laser Doppler technique. The hot-film method, like the electrochemical method, is based on convective transport. However, the hot-film anemometer is based on heat transfer, whereas the electrochemical method is based on mass transport. In transport theory, the thickness of the thermal or mass boundary layer plays an important role in this convective transport. The Schmidt number, a ratio of the thickness of the velocity boundary layer to the mass boundary layer, is on the order of magnitude of 10^3. This value is approximately two orders of magnitude larger than the Prandtl number, an analogous parameter for heat transfer. This indicates that the mass boundary layer thickness is about 1/100 of the thickness of the thermal boundary layer. The electrochemical method is, therefore, more suitable than the hot-film method for the measuring shear stress near the vessel wall.

The laser Doppler velocity measurement, which has become a very popular technique in fluid mechanics research, has a spatial sample volume limit of approximately 10^{-4}m. In order to estimate the wall shear rate, the velocity gradient value must be known. One drawback of the laser Doppler method is that the shear rate of a wall layer thinner than 10^{-4}m can not be measured directly due to this limitation. When the flow is fully developed, so that the velocity boundary layer thickness becomes on the order of magnitude of 10^{-2}m, as in the present study, the thickness of the mass boundary layer, on which the electrochemical method based, would be on the order of magnitude of 10^{-5}m. Thus, for this study, the electrochemical method also seems to be more suitable than the laser Doppler method for determining wall shear rate.

The electrochemical method has both a relatively high frequency response and good spatial resolution; the latter depending on the size of the electrodes relative to the size of flow field. In previous casting model studies, a large number of electrodes were placed in a casting model of the entire aorta[13]. When examining particular wall geometries, there were too few electrodes present in the region of interest to perform an analysis with good spatial resolution. In the present study, we used a more simplified model which allowed us to measure the entire flow region of interest with a relatively high spatial resolution.

Our discussion to this point has focused on experimental conditions of steady flow. This is mainly due to the complexity of measurements and thus, of data reduction in experiments performed under conditions of unsteady flow. Accurate measurements of wall shear stress in fields with rather complex geometries have been hindered by our lack of efficient methods for electrode calibration. In the present study, however, the simple Poiseuille flow could be employed for electrode calibration. By using the Poiseuille values, we were able to calibrate each of the 100 electrodes. However, there was still a considerable variability in calibration parameters from one electrode to another, even when care was taken to machine the test section and the electrodes. This technical problem should be taken into consideration when the electrochemical method is utilized to measure flow fields of complex geometry. Even a tendency of wall shear stress distribution pattern changes may not be reflected under some circumstances, especially when the power and the coefficient of Eq.(2) vary from one electrode to another.

Flow patterns have previously been demonstrated in arterial systems using the flow visualization technique. Recently, transparent arteries have been used for such flow visualization studies[8]. In these studies, complicated vortex patterns with a three dimensional nature have been demonstrated. Unfortunately, flow visualization studies usually cannot provide quantitative results about wall shear stress distribution. The results obtained in the present study provide a foundation for subsequent flow visualization studies on a quantitative basis. Our observation suggest that the horse shoe vortex which was observed in the previous studies[7-8] may be one of the fundamental flow structure occurring at sites of stenosis, branching or similar three dimensional wall irregularity. The presence of a horse shoe vortex apparently creates complex wall shear stress distribution patterns like those observed in the present study.

There are two reasons why we performed our study using a rather simple arterial stenosis model. Firstly, due to the technical difficulties described in the foregoing, it was necessary to calibrate each electrode both before and after shear stress measurements were made. In order to make these calibration measurements, it was necessary to use a circular pipe and thus, we could not use flow tracts of complex geometries. Secondly, from a pathophysiological point of view, the unilateral stenosis model is comparable to the situation found in early atherosclerotic lesions. It is well known that the earliest lesions of atherosclerosis appear unilaterally in the intima of arteries, and develop very slowly over a period of decades as localized atheromatous elevated lesions. Thus it seems likely that the entire blood flow pattern could change upon the formation of even a small atherosclerotic plaque.

The three dimensional fluid mechanical structure of blood flow, especially in regions very close to the wall, remains to be precisely described with respect to the localization of atherosclerosis. Most fluid mechanical theories of atherosclerosis do not, unfortunately, seem to be based on firm experimental findings. Thus, in order to correlate pathological and cell biological findings to fluid mechanical theories, it is necessary to perform more detailed study of flow fields in known geometrical conditions in arterial systems.

Acknowledgment: This work was supported by a Research Grant for Cardiovascular Diseases (60C-2) from the Ministry of Health and Welfare.

REFERENCES

[1]Caro CG, Fitz-Gerald JM, Schroter RC (1971) Proc Roy Soc Lond B 177:109-159
[2]Fry DL (1972) Localizing factors in arteriosclerosis. In: Likoff W, Segal BL, Insull W Jr(eds) Atherosclerosis and Coronary Heart Disease. Grune and Stratton, New York, pp 85-104
[3]Kjaernes M, Svindland A, Walloe L, Wille O (1981) Acta Path Micro-biol Scand Sect.A. 89:35-40
[4]Zarins CK, Giddens DP, Bharadvaj BK, Sottiurai VS, Mabon RF, Glagov S (1983) Circ Res 53:502-514
[5]Sakata N, Joshita T, Ooneda G (1985) Heart and Vessels 1:70-73
[6]Yamaguchi T, Hanai S (1987) Biorheology 24:753-762
[7]Fukushima T, Azuma T (1982) Biorheology 19:143-154
[8]Fukushima T, Karino T, Goldsmith HL (1985) Heart and Vessels 1:24-28
[9]Yamaguchi T, Hanai S (1988) Biorheology, in the press.
[10]Mizushina T (1971) Adv.in Heat Transfer 7:87-161
[11]Lutz RJ, Cannon JN, Bischoff KB, Dedrick RL, Stiles RK, FRY DL (1977) Circ Res 41:391-399
[12]Lutz RJ, Hsu L, Menawat A, Zrubek J, Edwards L (1983) J Biomech 16:753-766
[13]Pei ZH, Xi BS, Hwang NHC (1985) J Biomech. 18:645-656
[14]Choi US, Talbot L, Cornet I (1979) J Fluid Mech 93:465-48

Intraoperative Evaluation of Blood Velocity Waveforms in Different Coronary Artery Bypass Graft

Sequential Saphenous Vein Graft and Internal Mammary Artery Graft

F. Kajiya[1], S. Kanazawa[2], S. Matsuoka[1], Y. Ogasawara[1], K. Tsujioka[1], and T. Fujiwara[1]

Department of Medical Engineering and Systems Cardiology[1], Department of Thoracic Surgery[2], Kawasaki Medical School, Kurashiki, 701-01 Japan

ABSTRACT

We investigated the characteristics of blood velocities in different types of coronary bypass grafts, i.e., the saphenous vein graft (SVG; 6 cases) vs the internal mammary artery graft (IMAG; 6 cases) and for different positioning of the sequential saphenous vein bypass graft (SSVG), i.e., the side-to-side anastomosis (SSA) vs the end-to-side anastomosis (ESA), the life span of which are known to be different. The blood velocities were measured by the dual mode (zerocross and FFT), multichannel, high frequency ultrasound Doppler method during bypass graft surgery. Comparing the blood velocities in the SVG with those in the IMAG (longer life span), the velocity profile was much more parabolic and the velocity spectrum was narrower in the IMAG. Regarding the velocities in the SSVG (the SSA has longer life span), the skew of the velocity profile and the reverse flow at the position just proximal to the SSA were always recognized near the probe-side wall (the opposite side of the SSA), indicating the existence of flow separation and recirculation in this region. The direction of skew changed between the SSA and the ESA in almost all cases. These patterns of blood flow seem to be a contributory factor in determining the fate of the graft.

INTRODUCTION

Coronary bypass surgery has been a very frequently performed operation in order to provide adequate perfusion to an ischemic myocardium. Despite the symptomatic alleviation of angina pectoris afforded by the procedure, the problem has been the development of graft occlusion after operation. Long-term follow-up studies have now established the relatively shorter life span of the saphenous vein graft (SVG) and the better viability of the internal mammary artery graft (IMAG). One variation in the surgical procedure of the SVG is a sequential saphenous vein graft (SSVG) in which a side-to-side anastomosis (SSA) of the vein graft into a coronary artery is performed in addition to the end-to-side anastomosis (ESA). In the cases of SVBG, the patency rates of side-to-side anastomoses were reported to be better than those of end-to-side anastomoses. Several factors, some technical, determine the early fate of coronary bypass grafts. However, atherosclerosis is emerging as the major determinant of long-term vein graft viability (1). It is suggested that the local blood-flow pattern influences its development in addition to global factors such as abnormal lipoprotein levels. The possibility that differences in blood velocity waveform and velocity profile across the graft are implicated in the fate of the graft has encouraged us to conduct studies of blood velocities in different types of grafts (SVG vs IMAG) and for different positioning of the graft (SSA vs ESA). We applied the 20 MHz 80 channel pulsed Doppler velocimeter, which was developed in our laboratory, to the blood velocity measurements (2-4).

SUBJECTS AND METHODS

A total of 12 patients (9 men, 3 women) were studied. The SSVG was anastomosed to the major diagonal branch (DIAG) by SSA and to the left anterior descending coronary artery (LAD) by ESA in 6 patients (aged 39-76 years) who had 75-100% and 75-90% stenoses in the LAD and the DIAG, respectively. The IMAG anastomoses were performed to the LAD in 6 patients (aged 61-73 years) with 75-100% stenoses of the artery. The blood velocity in the SSVG was measured at three positions, i.e., 2-3 cm distal to the aorto-graft anastomosis, just proximal to the graft-DIAG anastomosis (SSA) and the bridge region between Graft-DIAG and Graft-LAD (ESA) anastomoses (Fig. 1). For the IMAG, the blood velocity was measured at two positions, i.e., several cm proximal and just proximal to the Graft-LAD anastomosis. The pulsed Doppler system used in this study detects Doppler signals from 80 channels by a zero-crossing method and analyzes Doppler signals from one optional channel by a fast Fourier transform method, both in real time (Fig. 2). The sampling volume for each sampling point is $\pi x 0.5^2 x 0.2$ mm^3. We used a cuff-type probe for the measurements of graft flow velocities.

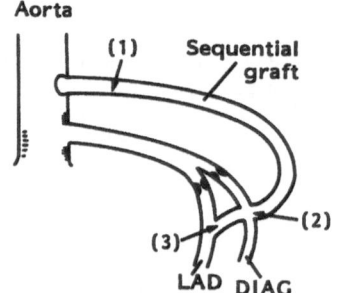

(1) portion 2-3 cm distal to the aorta-coroanry anastomosis

(2) portion just proximal to the graft-DIAG anastomosis

(3) bridge portion between graft-DIAG and graft-LAD anastomoses

Fig.1 Three positions of blood velocity measurements in the sequential saphenous vein graft (SSVG).

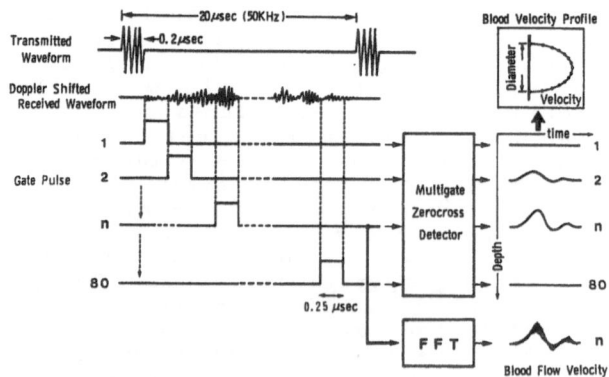

Fig.2 Principle of the 80 channel 20MHz pulsed Doppler velocimeter(3).

RESULTS

A typical recording of the SSVG waveform near the central axial region processed by FFT for three different positions is shown in Fig. 3. The velocity waveform at 2–3 cm distal to the aorto–graft anastomosis was relatively rich in systolic forward flow component and the velocity spectrum was broader compared with those in the other two positions.

The velocity profile across the vessel near the aorto–graft

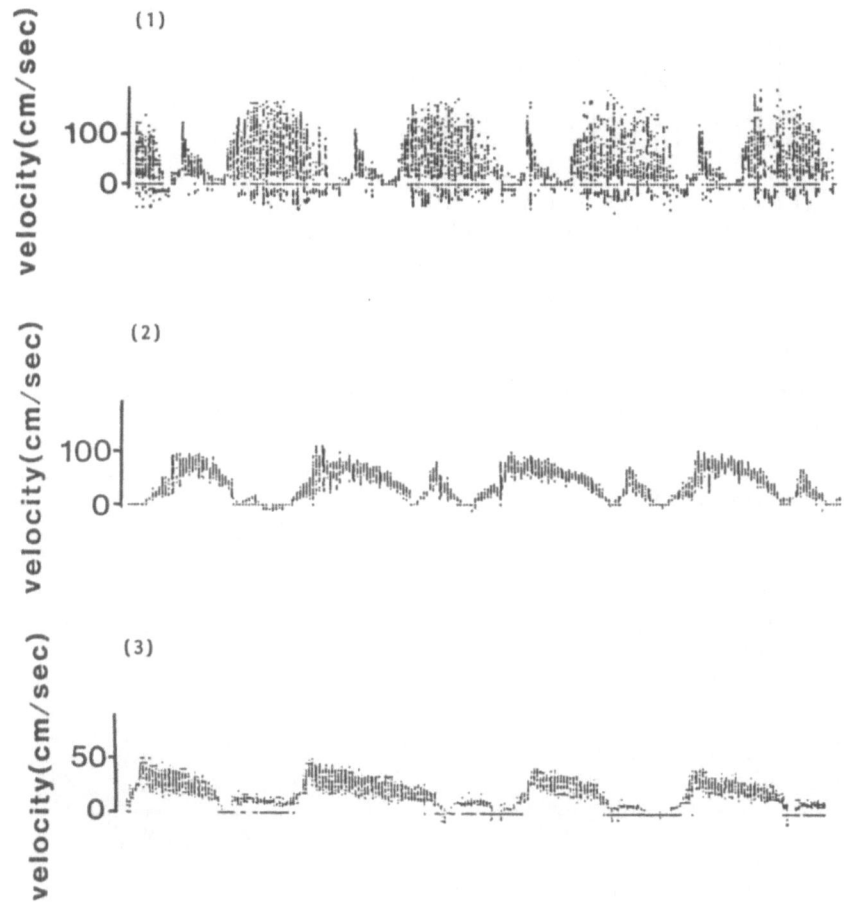

Fig.3 Blood velocity patterns at three different portions in the SSVG. (1), (2) and (3) indicate the location of measurements:see Fig.1.

anastomosis showed a relatively irregular and blunt pattern (Fig. 4). Figure 5 is a three dimensional display of the velocity profiles at the positions just proximal to the SSA and at the bridge position between the SSA and the ESA. The waveform just proximal to SSA had less of a systolic flow component. The velocity profile was skewed toward the SSA side wall, but the velocity spectrum was narrower in this area. The flow velocity near the probe side wall was reversed in most cases (dark shading) or flattened around the zero velocity line. At the bridge position, the shape of the profile showed at times a non-skewed and at other times a skewed pattern toward the probe-side wall.

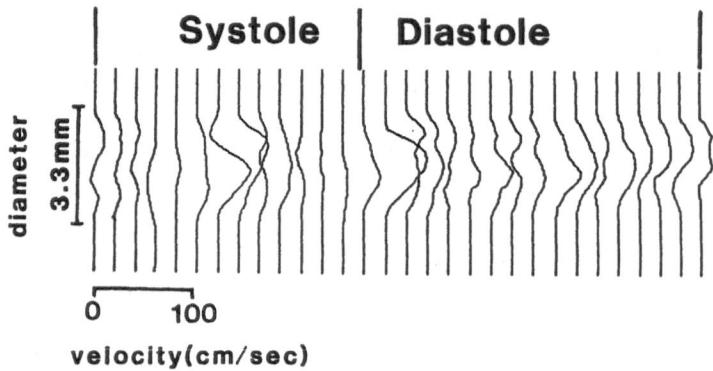

Fig.4 Blood flow velocity profile at the position 2-3 cm distal to the aorto-graft anastomosis in the SSVG.

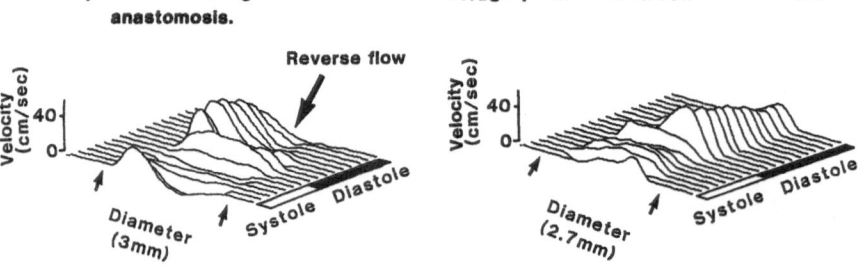

Fig.5 Three dimensional displays of the velocity profiles at the positions just proximal to the SSA and at the bridge position between the SSA and the ESA. The velocity profiles in the three dimensional display and represented by the coordinates of velocity, radial position and cardiac cycle.

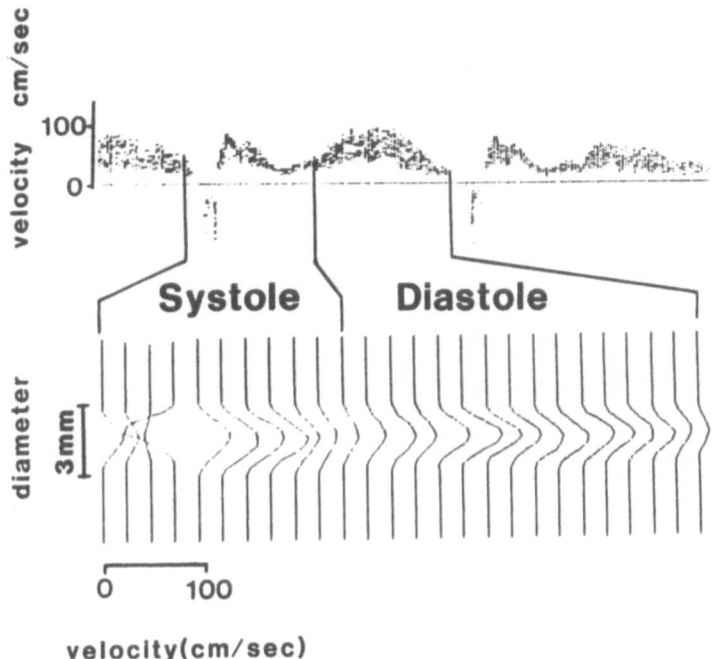

Fig.6 Blood velocity patterns in the IMAG. Top, velocity waveform at the central axial region of the vessel by FFT. Bottom, velocity profile across the vessel by zero-crossing method.

Figure 6 shows a representative recording of the IMA flow velocity just proximal to the Graft-LAD anastomosis. The velocity waveform showed a normal coronary artery flow pattern, i.e., diastolic-predominant. The velocity profile across the graft was parabolic with a narrow spectrum. The velocity configuration at the position several cm proximal to the Graft-LAD anastomosis was almost the same as that at the immediate proximal position.

DISCUSSION

The superior late patency of the IMAG compared with the SVG has been well documented by carefully designed follow-up studies. Lytle et al (5) and Campeau et al (6) noted the susceptibility of SVG to late atherosclerotic changes in 50 to 60% of grafts implanted 10 to 12 years. The long-term follow-up study of SSVG by Kieser et al (7) reported that the SSA of a double graft had a much better patency rate than the ESA.

The major contribution of our studies is a detailed description of the characteristics of the SSVG and the IMAG blood velocities which is suggested to relate to the development of atherosclerosis. For this study, we employed the 80 channel 20 MHz dual-mode (zero-crossing and fast Fourier transform FFT) pulsed Doppler velocimeter. Eighty channels were used to allow evaluation of the detailed blood flow velocity profile across the graft and the use of fast Fourier transforms was indispensable to the analysis of flow disturbances. Freed et al (8) have also shown the usefulness of 20 MHz pulsed

Doppler velocimeter for graft velocity measurements, although in their studies, the Doppler shift frequency was detected by a zero-crossing method and the number of channels of measurement was limited.

One of the prominent features of the velocity profile just proximal to the SSA in the SSVG was the skewing of the profile toward the SSA, indicating that blood is diverted down into the DIAG. In spite of the skewing, the configuration of the velocity profile was smooth and the spectrum was narrow. These flow characteristics may relate to the better patency rate of the SSA. The reverse flow near the probe-side wall implies the existence of flow separation and recirculation in this region, which dissipate energy. The change in the shape of the velocity profile between the SSA and the ESA also suggests a complex flow field. Such alterations of the velocity patterns may contribute to the poor patency rate of the ESA. The broadening of the velocity spectrum near the aorto-graft anastomosis and the relatively blunt configuration of the velocity profile may be mainly due to the entrance effect of the blood into the graft. In contrast with the SSVG, the parabolic and regular pattern of the velocity profile was observed with a narrow velocity spectrum. This non-disturbed, well-ordered velocity configuration may help to explain why the patency of the IMAG is higher than the SVG, along with its relative immunity to the atherosclerosis and the more physiological nature (intact vascular smooth muscle, the intact vasa vasorum and the matured internal elastic lamina) of the IMAG.

REFERENCES

(1) FitzGibbon GM, Leach AJ, Keon WG, Burton JR, Kafka HP (1986) J Thorac Cardiovasc Surg 91: 773-778
(2) Ogasawara O, Hiramatsu O, Kagiyama M et al (1984) IEEE Computers in Cardiol: 447-450
(3) Kajiya F, Ogasawara Y, Tsujioka K et al (1986) Circulation 74 (Suppl III): 53-60
(4) Kajiya F, Tsujioka K, Ogasawara Y et al (1987) Circulation 76: 1092-1100
(5) Lytle BW, Loop FD, Cosgrove DM, Ratliff NB, Easley K, Taylor PC (1985) J Thorac Cardiovasc Surg 89: 248-258
(6) Campeau L, Enjalbert M, Lesperance J, Vaislic C, Grondin CM, Bourassa MG (1983) Circulation 68 (Suppl II): 1-7
(7) Kieser TM, FitzGibbon GM, Keon WG (1986) J Thorac Cardiovasc Surg 91: 767-772
(8) Freed DB, Hartley CJ, Noon GP, Short D (1984) Circulation 70 (part-II): II-384 (abstr)

The Role of Flow Separation and Its Prediction in Arterial Flows

L. Fuchs[1], U. Erikson[2], and O. Smedby[2]

[1]Department of Gasdynamics, The Royal Institute of Technology, S-100 44 Stockholm, Sweden
[2]Department of Diagnostic Radiology, Uppsala University, S-751 85 Uppsala, Sweden

ABSTRACT

A new model to explain a possible mechanism for atherogenesis is presented. The model is based upon the fact that when the flow is separated there is a increase in pressure in the separated region. Further, if the separation is three-dimensional, there are spiral vortices, with axes parallel to the axis of the artery. Both these factors cause an increase in the arterial wall tension near the separated regions. The increase in the azimuthal wall tension results in axially oriented lesions. Numerical methods are used to compute the flow in systems of channels and in a three-dimensional flow past an atheroma. Such theoretical flow computations can be useful in quantifying different factors in atherogenesis.

INTRODUCTION

The role of fluid mechanics in atherogenesis has been considered extensively in the past years by different approaches. Basically, there are several hypothetical causes and processes that lead to the final formation of atheroma. The different theories, and their background, are described in some details in the review article of Nerem and Cornhill [1] and the book of Caro et al. [2] and the references therein.

Atherosclerotic lesions are primarily localized to bends and bifurcations of (medium and larger) arteries [1-2]. The intuitive suggestion that large wall shear-stresses cause endothelial erosion cannot be supported by evidence, since the largest wall shear-stresses occur at other locations than the observed lesions and secondly, the required shear-stresses (of over 40 N/m^2 [4]) are not achieved in-vivo. In contrast, the lesions do appear at 'low shear-stress' regions at the above mentioned sites. Furthermore, that model would imply a uniformly distributed endothelial damage and not in form of axially oriented streaks. Other hypothetical theories explain atherogenesis on the basis of increased transport through the endothelial layer at elevated shear-stress, and/or increased pinocytosis in such situations (see [1] and the references therein). The fact is that there is no single theory that can relate fluid mechanical features of the flow field to the findings that promote the latter theories [1].

Here, we propose a new model that may explain many of the observed phenomena associated with atherogenesis. As a complement to the new model we also present some numerical techniques that can be applied for calculation of the flow in relevant (though simplified) geometries:

two-dimensional flows in systems of channels with multiple branchings
and also certain three-dimensional calculations to simulate flows past
an asymmetric obstruction in a tube.

FLUID-DYNAMICAL BACKGROUND

In the following we shall discuss possible factors that seem to
contribute to atherogenesis. The existence of these factors in the
flow field is then verified by numerical computations. In the
discussion below, we distinguish between two different contributing
factors: one is locally increased pressure (based in inviscid
arguments) and the other is the presence of spiral, axially oriented,
vortices (due to viscosity) and the resulting shear stress that gives
rise to a distending force.

The model that we propose is based on the observation that lesions
occur in the vicinity of separated flow regions. The flow in such
separation bubbles is slow and hence there is an increase in the
pressure in such regions (Bernouli's law). Furthermore, the separation
bubble causes an increase in the mean flow velocity at the unseparated
portion of the arterial cross-section, and hence the pressure
decreases. Thus, there is a change in balance in internal pressure;
near stagnation regions (coinciding with relatively low wall shear-
stress regions) the pressure increases while at other potions of the
wall (the high wall shear-stress region) the pressure decreases. This
change in pressure has to be balanced by a change in the artery wall:
Initially, by increasing and decreasing the 'hoop' stress (and hence
the local distension of the arterial wall) at the high and the low
pressure sides, respectively. A quantitative estimate (based upon
Bernouli's principle for steady flows), indicates a total pressure
change of several percents (but less than about 10%). Such a change
would cause (using the data given in Fig. 7.5 (a) p. 94 in ref.   2),
a change in shape (of the order of some few percents). Such a
change might seem to be small, if it would be not be associated with a
possible deformation of the artery. (The arterial deformation can be
estimated using Laplace's and Hook's laws). However, the seemingly
small change in the shape of the artery, is not uniformly distributed,
and it is mainly concentrated to the higher pressure side of the
arterial wall. The distension can possibly cause axially oriented gaps
in (or at least weakening of) the endothelial cell layer. Such gaps
would, by themselves, facilitate increased transport into the arterial
wall (due to passive or active processes). The observable results of
the process would be 'fatty streaks' with an axial orientation. A
second possibility of Laplace law, is that the wall tension is not
increased, but rather the wall thickness increases by a similar
proportion. This could be a long term response to the imbalance in the
pressure and the initial increase in the distending pressure. This
second stage, is also in agreement with observation of initial intimal
thickening before atherosclerosis is established [1]. The natural self
adaptiveness to elevated distending pressure would be the deposition of
collagen fibers which, due to their high Young's modulus, can resist
shape changes in response to elevated pressure. The mechanism that is
described above, can also explain the close relationship between
hypertension and stiffening of the wall of the arterial system.

A contributing factor to the imbalance in arterial wall tension
can be related to viscous effects. Viscosity causes separation and
vorticity leading to a component of shear stress that does not exist in
the case of simple axial flows in tubes. In the presence of axially

oriented vortices, there exists a non-vanishing wall shear stress
component that gives rise to a distending force on the arterial wall.
This component of the wall shear stress is proportional to the normal
partial derivative of the azimuthal velocity component. These type of
vortices can be observed in bifurcating arteries as well as down-stream
of obstacles (such as atheroma). The distending shear stress acts in
synergy with the pressure imbalance that is discussed above. One
should observe that the component of the shear stress that we refer to
here, is not identical to the 'shear stress' that is often quoted in
the literature. In the literature one usually talks about the
component that is proportional to the normal partial derivative of the
axial velocity component. This component of the shear stress acts on
the wall in the axial direction!

NUMERICAL RESULTS AND DISCUSSION

     To quantify the different components in the model discussed above,
we have used several computer codes for simulating the flow of
incompressible fluids in certain geometries.

     First, consider the flow in a system of two-dimensional channels.
The number, the relative locations, the angles of inclination of the
different branches as well as the flow distribution in the system of
channels can be varied easily. This is achieved by using a system of
overlapping grids, that are defined independently of each other. Each
sub-channel has its own grid system, and information is transferred
among the different grids so that at convergence all the physical
parameters are independent of the grid that they are represented on.
The main difficulty with such methods is the slow convergence of the
iterative process. This difficulty has been resolved by using a Multi-
Grid method for solving the discrete problem. Details of the numerical
method can be found in [5-6]. A typical case is given in Figure 1. The
low shear-stress regions (and the separation bubbles) are found in two
main locations around bifurcations: the lateral walls, somewhat
downstream to the point of bifurcation. The extent and the location of
the stagnation points (limiting the separation bubble) depends on the
Reynolds number, the angle of inclination, the area ratio of the
daughter channels, relation to other nearby branchings and the flow
distribution into the daughter branches. The sensitivity of the flow
to changes in parameters is demonstrated in Fig. 2, where two, almost
symmetrical branches leave the main channel. The figure illustrates a
limiting case with equally distributed flow rate in both branches and
no flow in the main channel after the branchings. The small asymmetry
in geometry leads to a rather marked asymmetry in the flow field: In
one branch one can observe two separation bubbles, one with an unusual
location (at the proximal wall).

     A three-dimensional computer code has been used to simulate the
flow past an asymmetric stenosis in a tube. The stenosis is simulated
as an inner cylindrical object connected to the outer wall via two
radial walls. The unblocked cross section area can be varied by
changing either the opening angle of the two radial walls (see Figures
3) or by changing the radius of the tube. In the current computations,
we considered mainly the variation in the wall pressure in the
different geometries. Figures 3, show the pressure forces on the
boundaries for different lumen area (between 0.5 and 0.75; i.e. 50% to
25% blockage). Figures 4 show three cases with a given opening angle
but different tube diameters. One can observe again that the small
changes in the lumen area may cause clear changes in the pressure along

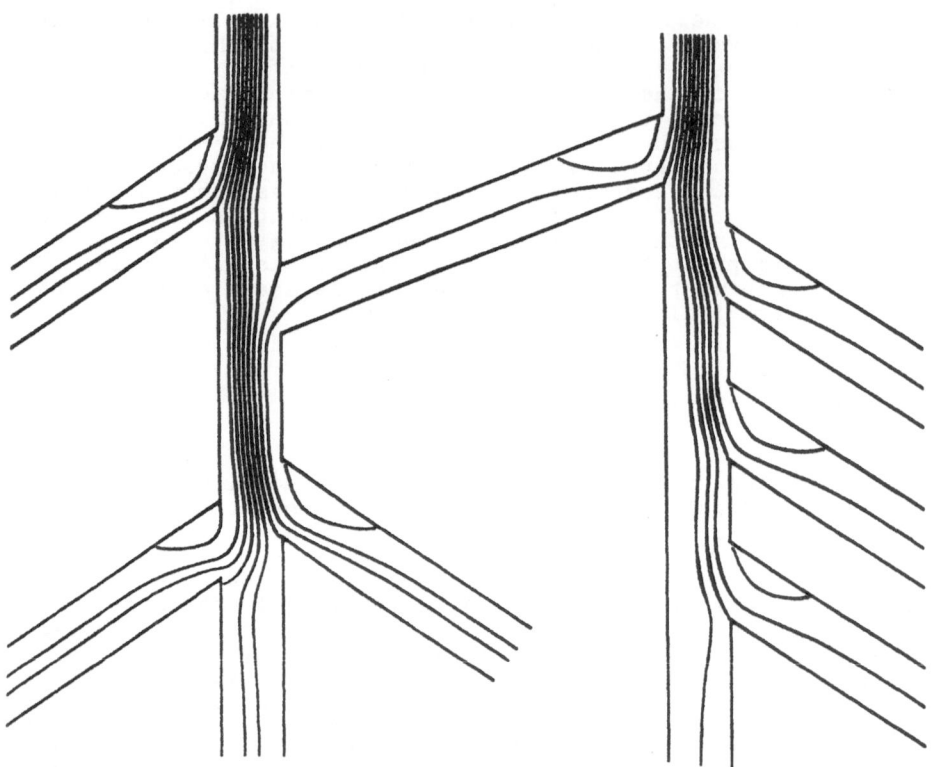

Figure 1: Flow in a system of channels. Re=200.
Right channel: Branching angles of 55° and -68°.
Left channel: Branching angles of 112° and 55°,respectively.
Mass flow: 20% of inflow value in each branch.

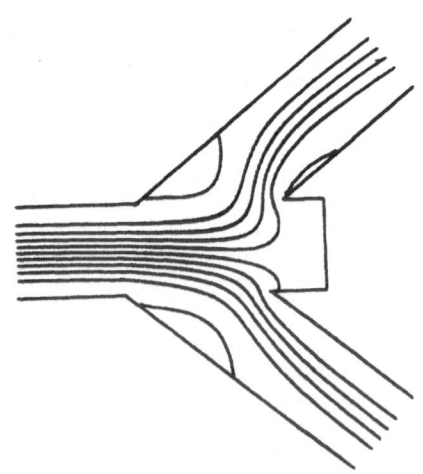

Figure 2: Streamline patter in an almost symmetric branching.
Branching angles 55° and -55°, respectively.
Equal mass flow through both branches.

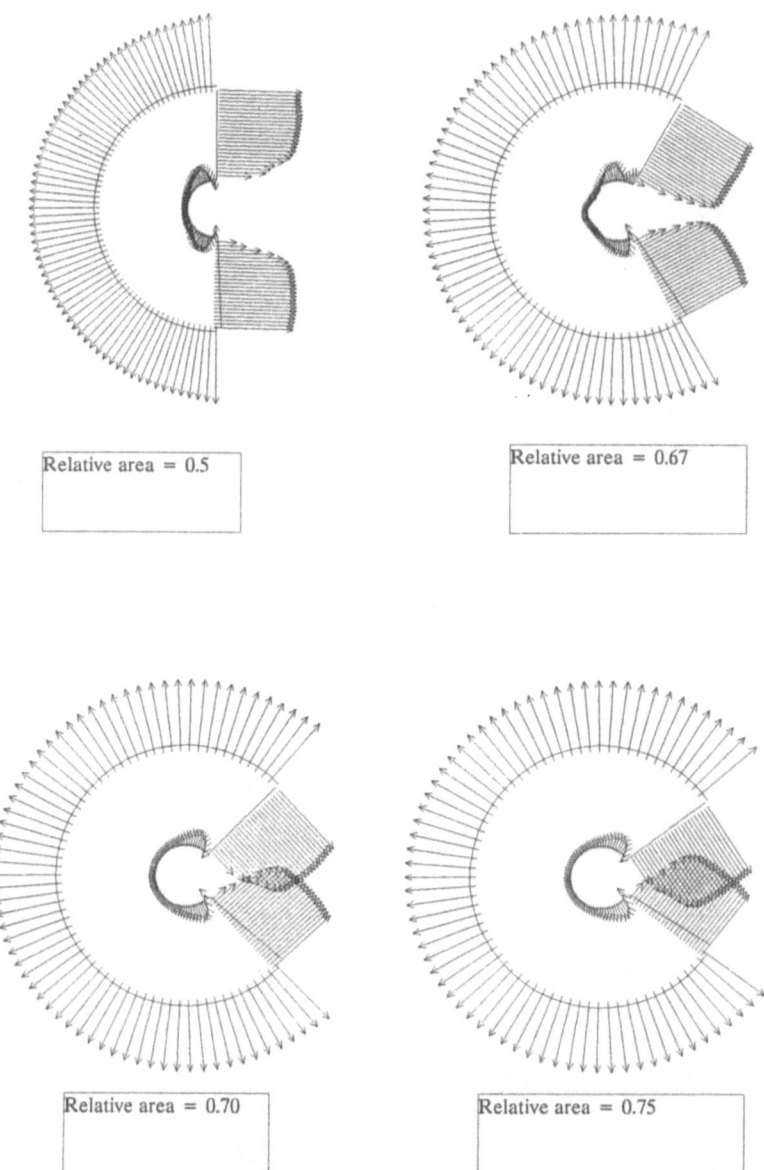

Relative area = 0.5

Relative area = 0.67

Relative area = 0.70

Relative area = 0.75

Figures 3: The pressure distribution along the inner surface
of the blocked tube. The relative area is defined as the
ratio of the free lumen to the tube cross section area.
Note the larger forces on the stenosed portions of the
wall and the constant pressure on the unblocked part.

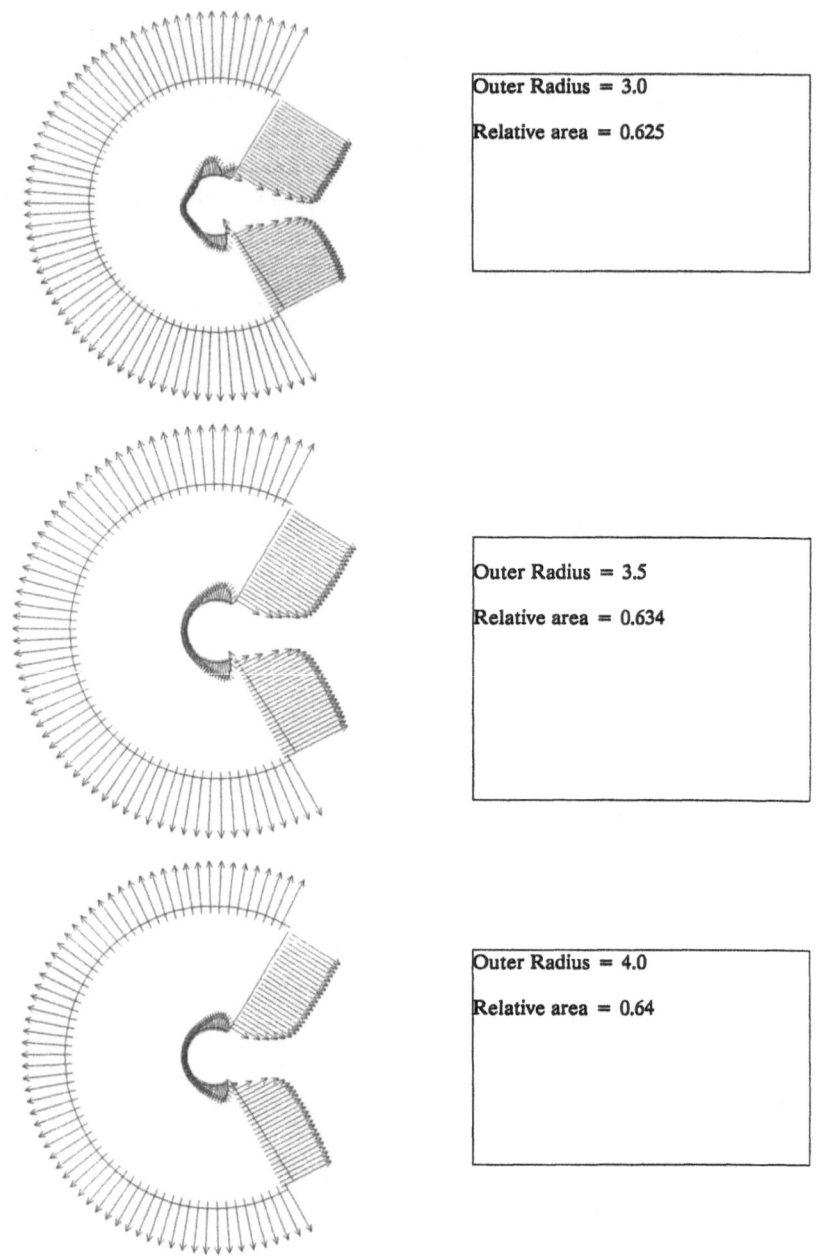

Outer Radius = 3.0
Relative area = 0.625

Outer Radius = 3.5
Relative area = 0.634

Outer Radius = 4.0
Relative area = 0.64

Figures 4: The pressure distribution on the inner surface of blocked tubes. The opening angle is fixed but tube radius is varied.

the side (radial) walls of the stenosis. In all cases, one can note
that the pressure is practically constant along the wall of the tube
with the exception of the neighborhood of the stenosis, where there is
an increase in pressure (as predicted by Bernouli's principle based on
inviscid theory). One can also note that the force acting on the wall
near the site of the stenosis is larger than at other portion of the
wall. Thus, the wall tension is largest near the edges of the
stenosis. This fact is in accordance with the model that we described
above.

The computed examples that are given here show that the multi-
parameter dependence and the sensitivity of flow to small changes,
makes a complete experimental study of such flows very difficult (if
not impractical), whereas by numerical methods the parameters can be
varied easily, and computing sequences of solution makes each solution
even cheaper (in terms of CPU time).

CONCLUSIONS

A model for atherogenesis, based on fluid-dynamical arguments has
been presented. Numerical computations done so far give qualitative
support for this theory. A quantitative study of flows in different
geometries, including the effect of the flow on the wall deformation
should be the next step of the future work.

REFERENCES

1. Nerem, R.M. and Cornhill, J.F., "The role of Fluid Mechanics
   in Atherogenesis". J. Biomech. Eng. vol 102, pp 181-189, 1980.
2. Caro, C.G., Pedley, T.J., Schroter, R.C. and Seed, W.A.,
   "The Mechanics of the Circulation". Oxford University Press,
   Oxford, 1978.
3. Zarins, C.K., Giddens, D.P. Bharadvaj, B.K., Sottiurai, V.S,
   Mabon, R.F. and Glagov, S., "Carotid Bifurcation Atherosclerosis: Quantitative Correlation of Plaque Localization
   with Flow Velocity Profiles and Wall Shear-Stress". Circ. Res.
   vol 53, pp 502-514, 1983.
4. Fry, D.L., "Certain Histological and Chemical Responses
   of the Vascular Interface to Acutely Induced Mechanical Stress
   in the Aorta of the Dog". Circ. Res. vol 24, p. 93, 1969.
5. Fuchs, L., "Computation of Viscous Flows using a Zonal-
   Multi-Grid Method". Submitted to J. Comp. Phys. 1987.
6. Fuchs, L., "Numerical Computation of Viscous Incompressible
   Flows in Systems of Channels". AIAA P-87-0367, 1987.

Numerical Simulation of a Blood Flow in a Stenosed Tube

H. Kawai[1], T. Sawada[2], and T. Tanahashi[2]

[1]Engineering Research Laboratory, Kanegafuchi Chemical Industry Co., Ltd., Takasago, 676 Japan
[2]Department of Mechanical Engineering, Keio University, Yokohama, 223 Japan

ABSTRACT

A new finite element technique which is based on the multiplier method[1] is presented to analyze incompressible flow problems. We apply this method to the flow analysis in a stenosed tube which is modeled by a cosine curve. Calculations are carried out for the flow whose Reynolds number is less than 1000. These results are compared with those obtained by a finite difference method. Separation and reattachment points agree with experimental results.

INTRODUCTION

The investigation of the flow in a stenosed tube may play an important role in making clear the mechanism of the disease which is characterized by a growing thrombus. Many studies have been performed for flow in a stenosis, both theoretically and numerically. Deshpande et al.[2] carried out the numerical analysis for a steady flow in a stenosed rigid pipe. Their results are in good agreement with experimental results. On the other hand, pulsatile flow problems in a stenosed tube have been studied by Daly[3], Clark[4] and Young and Tsai[5]. Mehrotra et al.[6] considered flow in a geometry whose cross-section is elliptic.

These investigations have treated low Reynolds number flow. Recent rapid progress of digital computers makes it possible to analyze more complicated flows, using numerical techniques. The purpose of the present investigation is to analyze a high Reynolds number steady flow in a stenosed tube which is modeled as a cosine curve. We arrange the multiplier method in either Cartesian or cylindrical coordinates and calculated steady flow patterns in two different geometries. One is flow in a rectangular channel with a step in order to test the algorithm by comparing with experimental results. The other is flow in a tube with a stenosis whose Reynolds number is less than 1000.

SYMBOLS

Typical symbols are listed as follows:

n_r, n_z: components of an outer-normal vector on a boundary
p: pressure
R: radius of the tube outside the stenotic region
r: radial coordinate

Re: Reynolds number $=\rho UR/\mu$
U: maximum velocity at the inlet
u,v: velocity components in cylindrical coordinates
z: longitudinal coordinate
α: penalty parameter $=(\lambda+\mu)/\mu$
Γ: boundary of a numerical cell
Γ_2: boundary where the Neumann's boundary condition is satisfied
δ: maximum height of a stenosis
λ: second viscosity
μ: viscosity
ν: kinetic viscosity
ρ: density
Ω: area of a numerical cell

Variables are nondimensionalized such that

$$r^*=\frac{r}{R} \qquad z^*=\frac{z}{R} \qquad u^*=\frac{u}{U} \qquad v^*=\frac{v}{U} \qquad p^*=\frac{p}{\rho U^2}$$

For simplification, the asterisk which shows a dimensionless quantity is omitted.

ANALYTICAL MODEL AND BASIC EQUATIONS

Steady laminar flow in an axi-symmetrical stenosed tube is considered as shown in Fig.1(a). Figure 1(b) indicates a numerical model which is divided into mesh elements. In the upper figure, grid lines of the z-direction are abbreviated. Basic equations in cylindrical coordinates are written as

$$u\frac{\partial u}{\partial z}+v\frac{\partial u}{\partial r}+\frac{\partial p}{\partial z}-\frac{\alpha}{Re}\frac{\partial \Theta}{\partial z}-\frac{1}{Re}\left(\frac{\partial^2 u}{\partial r^2}+\frac{1}{r}\frac{\partial u}{\partial r}+\frac{\partial^2 u}{\partial z^2}\right)=0 \qquad (1)$$

$$u\frac{\partial v}{\partial r}+v\frac{\partial u}{\partial r}+\frac{\partial p}{\partial z}-\frac{\alpha}{Re}\frac{\partial \Theta}{\partial r}-\frac{1}{Re}\left(\frac{\partial^2 v}{\partial r^2}+\frac{1}{r}\frac{\partial v}{\partial r}-\frac{v}{r^2}+\frac{\partial^2 v}{\partial z^2}\right)=0 \qquad (2)$$

$$\Theta\equiv\frac{\partial u}{\partial z}+\frac{\partial v}{\partial r}+\frac{v}{r}=0 \qquad (3)$$

The specific shape of the stenosis is given by

$$r(z)=\begin{cases} 1-\frac{\delta}{2}\{\cos(\frac{\pi z}{4})+1\} & (\,|z|\leqq 4) \\ 1 & (\,|z|> 4) \end{cases} \qquad (4)$$

Boundary conditions are given by

$$u(r)=1-r^2, \quad v=0 \qquad \text{at the inlet}$$

$$\frac{\partial u}{\partial r}=0, \quad v=0 \qquad \text{at the center line}$$

$$\frac{\partial u}{\partial z}=\frac{\partial v}{\partial r}=0 \qquad \text{at the exit}$$

$$u=v=0 \qquad \text{on the wall}$$

$$(5)$$

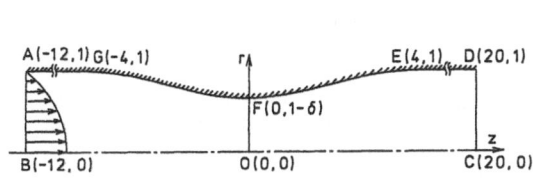

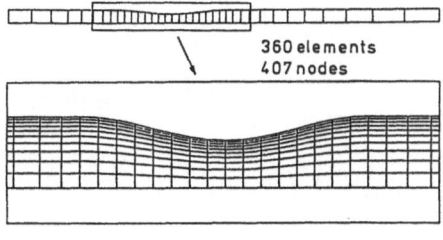

(a) Geometry for a stenosed tube   (b) Mesh system

Fig.1 Analytical model

NUMERICAL METHOD

The multiplier method, which is a version of the penalty function method[7], is applied to Eqs.(1), (2) and (3) under the boundary conditions (4) and (5). Integrating Eqs.(1) to (3) by the Galerkin method yields

$$f = \int_\Omega \left\{ \delta u^* \left(u\frac{\partial u}{\partial z} + v\frac{\partial u}{\partial r} \right) + \frac{\partial \delta u^*}{\partial z}(-p + \frac{\alpha}{Re}\Theta) + \frac{1}{Re}\left(\frac{\partial \delta u^*}{\partial z}\frac{\partial u}{\partial z} + \frac{\partial \delta u^*}{\partial r}\frac{\partial u}{\partial r} \right) \right\} r d\Omega$$

$$- \int_{\Gamma_2} \delta u^* \left\{ (-p + \frac{\alpha}{Re}\Theta)n_z + \frac{1}{Re}\left(\frac{\partial u}{\partial z}n_z + \frac{\partial u}{\partial r}n_r \right) \right\} r d\Gamma = 0 \qquad (6)$$

$$g = \int_\Omega \left\{ \delta v^* \left(ur\frac{\partial v}{\partial z} + vr\frac{\partial v}{\partial r} + \frac{1}{Re}\frac{v}{r} \right) + \frac{\partial \delta v^*}{\partial r}r(-p + \frac{\alpha}{Re}\Theta) + \frac{r}{Re}\left(\frac{\partial \delta v^*}{\partial z}\frac{\partial v}{\partial z} + \frac{\partial \delta v^*}{\partial r}\frac{\partial v}{\partial r} \right) \right.$$

$$\left. + \delta v^*(-p + \frac{\alpha}{Re}\Theta) \right\} d\Omega - \int_{\Gamma_2} \delta v^* \left\{ (-p + \frac{\alpha}{Re}\Theta)n_r + \frac{1}{Re}\left(\frac{\partial v}{\partial z}n_z + \frac{\partial v}{\partial r}n_r \right) \right\} r d\Gamma = 0 \qquad (7)$$

$$\Theta \equiv \int_\Omega \left\{ \frac{\partial u}{\partial z} + \frac{\partial v}{\partial r} + \frac{v}{r} \right\} r d\Omega = 0 \qquad (8)$$

where δu^* and δv^* are arbitrary weighting functions which are zero on the boundary, except Γ_2 and α the penalty parameter. Here the following interpolating functions are defined for a linear isoparametric quadratic element

$$\begin{cases} N_1 = (1-\xi)(1-\eta)/4 \\ N_2 = (1+\xi)(1-\eta)/4 \\ N_3 = (1+\xi)(1+\eta)/4 \\ N_4 = (1-\xi)(1+\eta)/4 \end{cases} \qquad (9)$$

Velocity components and weighting functions are written as

$$\begin{cases} u = u_i \cdot N_i \\ v = v_i \cdot N_i \\ \delta u^* = \delta u_i^* \cdot N_i \\ \delta v^* = \delta v_i^* \cdot N_i \end{cases} \qquad (10)$$

where δu_i^* and δv_i^* are arbitrary weighting functions on each local node. Substituting Eq.(10) into Eqs.(6) and (7) yields

$$\int_{\Omega_E}\left\{N_i\left(N_j u_j\frac{\partial N_k}{\partial z}u_k+N_j v_j\frac{\partial N_k}{\partial r}u_k\right)+\frac{\partial N_i}{\partial z}\left(-p_E+\frac{\alpha}{Re}\Theta\right)+\frac{1}{Re}\left(\frac{\partial N_i}{\partial z}\frac{\partial N_j}{\partial z}+\frac{\partial N_i}{\partial r}\frac{\partial N_i}{\partial r}\right)u_j\right\}d\Omega_E$$

$$=\int_{\Gamma_E}N_i\left\{\left(-p_E+\frac{\alpha}{Re}\Theta\right)n_z+\frac{1}{Re}\left(\frac{\partial u}{\partial z}n_z+\frac{\partial u}{\partial r}n_r\right)\right\}rd\Gamma_E \tag{11}$$

$$\int_{\Omega_E}\left\{rN_i\left(N_j u_j\frac{\partial N_k}{\partial z}v_k+N_j v_j\frac{\partial N_k}{\partial r}v_k\right)+\frac{\partial rN_i}{\partial r}\left(-p_E+\frac{\alpha}{Re}\Theta\right)+\frac{r}{Re}\left(\frac{\partial N_i}{\partial z}\frac{\partial N_j}{\partial z}+\frac{\partial N_i}{\partial r}\frac{\partial N_i}{\partial r}\right)v_j\right\}d\Omega_E$$

$$=\int_{\Gamma_E}N_i\left\{\left(-p_E+\frac{\alpha}{Re}\Theta\right)n_r+\frac{1}{Re}\left(\frac{\partial v}{\partial z}n_z+\frac{\partial v}{\partial r}n_r\right)\right\}rd\Gamma_E \tag{12}$$

where subscript E denotes a local element. u and v calculated from Eqs.(11) and (12) do not always satisfy the continuity equation (3). We correct u and v by adjusting p using the following equation:

$$p_E^{n+1}=p_E^n-\frac{\alpha}{Re}\Theta_E^{n+1},\qquad \Theta_E^{n+1}=\frac{1}{m(\Omega_E)}\int_{\Omega_E}\left(\frac{\partial N_j}{\partial z}u_j^{n+1}+\frac{\partial N_j}{\partial r}v_j^{n+1}+\frac{N_j}{r}v_j^{n+1}\right)rd\Omega_E \tag{13}$$

where $m(\Omega_E)$ is the area of the local element. Equation (13) is based on integration of Eq.(3). Using Eqs.(9) and (10), local finite element equations are rearranged in the form

$$f_i^E=A_{ijk}^E u_j u_k+B_{ijk}^E v_j v_k+\frac{1}{Re}\left(C_{ij}^E+\alpha D_{ij}^E\right)u_j+\frac{\alpha}{Re}E_{ij}^E v_j+F_i^E=0 \tag{14}$$

$$f_i^E=A_{ijk}^E u_j u_k+B_{ijk}^E v_j v_k+\frac{1}{Re}\left(C_{ij}^E+\alpha D_{ij}^E\right)u_j+\frac{\alpha}{Re}E_{ij}^E v_j+F_i^E=0 \tag{15}$$

where A, B, C, D, E, F, G and H are coefficient matrices. Then the global finite element equations are written by

$$f_\alpha=A_{\alpha\beta\gamma}u_\beta u_\gamma+B_{\alpha\beta\gamma}v_\beta v_\gamma+\frac{1}{Re}\left(C_{\alpha\beta}+\alpha D_{\alpha\beta}\right)u_\beta+\frac{\alpha}{Re}E_{\alpha\beta}v_\beta+F_\alpha=0 \tag{16}$$

$$g_\alpha=A_{\alpha\beta\gamma}u_\beta v_\gamma+B_{\alpha\beta\gamma}v_\beta v_\gamma+\frac{\alpha}{Re}E_{\alpha\beta}u_\beta+\frac{1}{Re}\left(C_{\alpha\beta}+\alpha G_{\alpha\beta}\right)v_\beta+H_\alpha=0 \tag{17}$$

where subscript α, β and γ are global node numbers in the whole region. Equations (16) and (17) are non-linear equations. The Newton-Raphson method is suitable for solving these equations numerically. The algorithm of the Newton-Raphson method is shown as follows:

Step 1: Initialize velocity u and v.
Step 2: Calculate δu and δv by the following equations:

$$\begin{bmatrix}\dfrac{\partial f_\alpha^n}{\partial u_\eta} & \dfrac{\partial f_\alpha^n}{\partial v_\eta}\\[2mm]\dfrac{\partial g_\alpha^n}{\partial u_\eta} & \dfrac{\partial g_\alpha^n}{\partial v_\eta}\end{bmatrix}\begin{bmatrix}\delta u_\eta^{n+1}\\[2mm]\delta v_\eta^{n+1}\end{bmatrix}=\begin{bmatrix}-f_\alpha^n\\[2mm]-g_\alpha^n\end{bmatrix} \tag{18}$$

Step 3: Stop calculation
if $\max(|\delta u_1|,\cdots,|\delta u_{nd}|,|\delta v_1|,\cdots,|\delta v_{nd}|)<\varepsilon_v$.
Here n_d is the number of total nodes and ε_v is a small value.
Step 4: Correct u_α and v_α by

$$u_\alpha^{n+1}=u_\alpha^n+\delta u_\alpha^{n+1},\qquad v_\alpha^{n+1}=v_\alpha^n+\delta v_\alpha^{n+1} \tag{19}$$

go back to Step 2.

Finally the algorithm for solving the global finite element equations (16) and (17) are indicated as follows:

Step 1: Initialize pressure and velocity at all points.
Step 2: Calculate δu and δv by solving Eq.(18).
Step 3: Correct u_α and v_α by Eq.(19).
Step 4: Stop calculation
if $\max(|\Theta_1|,\cdots,|\Theta_{nE}|)<\varepsilon_d$. Here n_E is the number of total elements and ε_d is a small value.
Step 5: Correct pressure by Eq.(13).
Step 6: Go back to Step 2.

RESULTS AND DISCUSSION

Calculation are carried out using the super-computer, HITAC S-810. The mesh contains 360 elements and 407 nodes as shown in Fig.1(b). Usually the penalty parameter is set as $\alpha=10^5 \sim 10^6$ in the penalty function method. For example, Bercovier and Engelman[8] adopted $\alpha=10^2 \Delta z^2$. The number of iterations increases slowly with Re; however, a large increase is seen when Reynolds number is 700 or more. At first, we examine the dependence of the penalty parameter on the number of iterations for $\alpha=10000$ and $\alpha=5000$. The number of iteration for $\alpha=10000$ is about 60% of that for $\alpha=5000$ in the range of $10<Re<1000$. In the present calculation, we use $\alpha=10000$.

Figure 2 shows flow patterns in a rectangular channel with a step where the Reynolds number is 125. Velocity profiles are compared with experimental results which were obtained by Denham and Patrick[9]. Since close agreement between calculated and experimental results is obtained, the scheme can be considered acceptable.

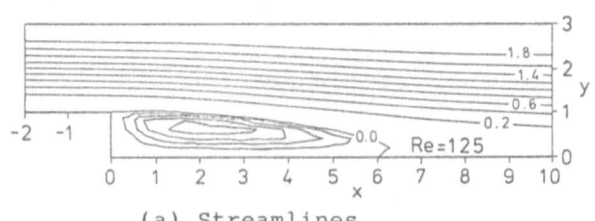

(a) Streamlines

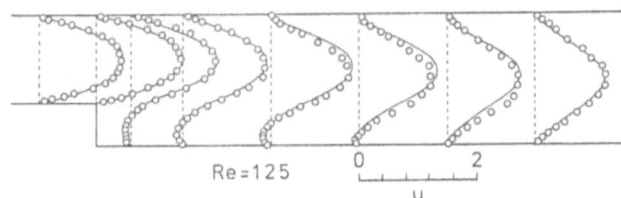

(b) Velocity profiles

Fig.2 Flow patterns in a rectangular channel

Figures 3, 4 and 5 show streamlines for Re=400, 600 and 1000, respectively. In these figures, streamlines and equi-vorticity contours are shown in upper and lower planes, respectively. It is clear that the separation region develops according to the increase in Reynolds number. Particularly at Re=1000, the separated flow region is observed downstream. Figure 6 shows the movement of the separation and reattachment points with Reynolds number. These are compared with another result obtained by the finite difference method[2] and by experiment[5]. Separation begins when Re=200 and the separated region increases with an increase of Reynolds number. Behavior of the separation point conforms to the experimental result. In contrast, some disagreement is observed for the trajectory of the reattachment point. These difference may be caused by the choice of mesh division. In addition, it may be that the reattachment point is difficult to measure as reported by Young and Tsai. Figure 7 shows the distribution of the wall shear stress for various Reynolds numbers less than 1000. A maximum shear stress is seen just before the throat. As Reynolds number increases, the peak shear stress shifts upstream slightly. A separated flow in the range from Re=400 to Re=1000 as evidenced by negative values of shear stress on the surface. This is also reported by Parvathamma and Devanathan[10].

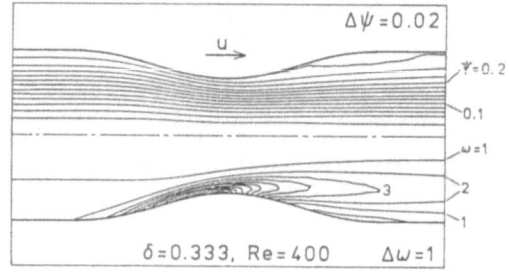

Fig.3 Flow patter in a stenosis

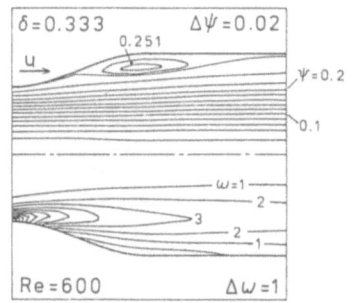

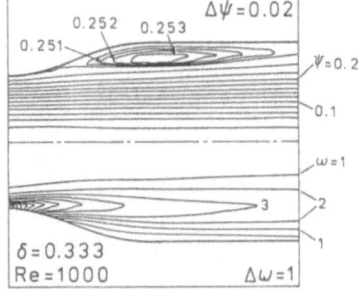

Fig.4 Flow pattern in a stenosis   Fig.5 Flow pattern in a stenosis

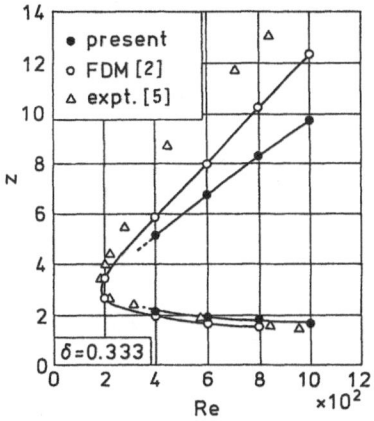

Fig.6 Movement of separation
and reattachment points
with Re

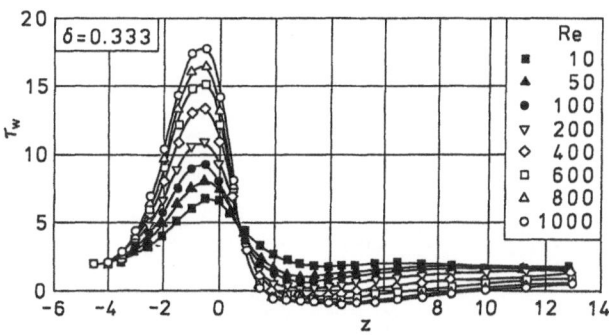

Fig.7 Distribution of shear stress

REMARKS

In the present paper we proposed a modified algorithm for the multiplier method. The present calculation adopt a model which is far from a complicated artery. The model falls short of providing the flow analysis for an arterial flow which includes unsteady, unstable and non-Newtonian flow. But it is clear that steady flow in a stenosed tube is simulated for Re<1000 by using the present method as well as by a finite difference method. Since the multiplier method is a kind of a finite element method, more complicated flow problems can be analyzed easily by the present method.

REFERENCES

[1] Mizukami A (1983) 4th Symposium on Finite Element Method in Flow Problems JUSE 49-56
[2] Deshpande MD, Giddens DP, Mabon RF (1976) J Biomech 9:165-174
[3] Daly BJ (1976) J Biomech 9:465-475
[4] Clark C (1976) J Biomech 9:567-578
[5] Young DF, Tsai TY (1973) J Biomech 6:395-410
[6] Mehrotra R, Jawaraman G, Padmanabham N (1985) Med Biol Eng Comput 23:55-62
[7] Hughes TJR, Liu WT, Brooks A (1979) J Comput Phys 30:1-60
[8] Bercovier M, Engelman M (1979) J Comput Phys 30:181-201
[9] Denham MK, Patrick MA (1974) Trans Instn Chem Eng 52:361-367
[10] Parvathamma S, Devanathan R (1983) Physiological Fluid Dynamics 1:69-73

Sinusoidal Oscillatory Flow in a Strongly Curved Tube

T. NARUSE, M. ASAI, K. NAKAZATO, and K. TANISHITA

Department of Mechanical Engineering, Faculty of Science and Technology, Keio University, Yokohama, 223 Japan

ABSTRACT

The feature of sinusoidal oscillatory flow in a strongly curved tube, which appeares frequently in the arterial vascular system, is evaluated in terms of the axial and secondary velocity profiles measured by Laser Doppler Velocimeter(LDV) and wall shear rate profiles measured by the limiting current method. It should be noted that both the velocity and wall shear rate at the inner side tend to be larger than that at the outer side in a strongly curved tube, which is in contrast to the fluid flow in a loosely curved tube.

1.Introduction

It has been suggested that the pulsatility of blood flow and the large curvature of the arteries may be associated with the localization of atherogenesis in terms of the wall shear stress acting on the arterial wall.[1] The large curvature is one of the fundamental geometries of arteries, such as the arch of aorta and the internal carotid artery.[2] In order to understand the correlation between blood flow and local atherogenesis, the flow structure in a strongly curved tube must be fully recognized. However, there are very few studies about unsteady flow in a strongly curved tube; thus the primary purpose of the present study is to provide fluid mechanical information concerning the wall shear rate and the velocity profiles in a strongly curved tube. The pulsatility used in the present study was that of a sinusoidal oscillatory flow with zero mean. This is a step in the comprehension of the features of fluid flow in the arteries.

2.Description of Experiments

2-1 Measurements of wall shear rate by the electrochemical method[3]

A schematic diagram of the experimental apparatus for the measurements of the wall shear stress is shown in Fig.1. The test section for the measurements was machined out in two halves, split at the plane symmetry, after nickel electrodes with a diameter of 0.5 mm were inserted into a flat Plexiglas plate, so that electrodes were mounted flush with the wall of the test section. The straight pipes, with a length of 1 m, was attached to both the inlet and outlet of

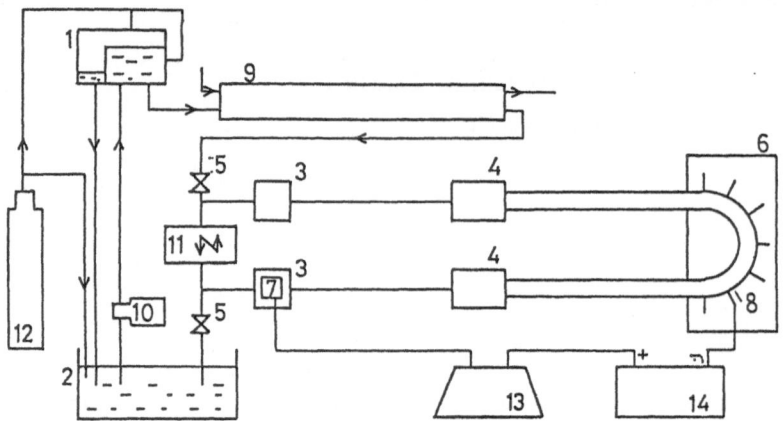

Fig.1   Schematic of experimental system (measurement of the wall
sheer stress)   1.Header tank, 2.Receiving tank, 3.Chamber, 4.Inlet
chamber, 5.Flow control valve, 6.Test section, 7.Anode, 8.Cathode,
9.Temperature control unit, 10.Pump, 11.Pulse generator, 12.N_2 gas,
13.Electro meter, 14.Voltage generator

the curved path in order to insure the same conditions at both ends
of the curved tube. The working fluid is an aqueous solution of
potassium ferricynide of 0.01 M, potassium ferrocyanide of 0.01 M,
and sodium hydroxide of 1.0 M as a supporting electrolyte. The
measurements were made at 4 streamwise stations,
θ =0° ,30° ,60° ,90° (shown in Fig.2), and 11 points at intervals of
15° from ψ =15° up to 165° (shown in Fig.2.). Oxygen dissolved in
the solution was purged with Nitrogen gas to obtain the limiting
current induced merely from the redox reaction on the electrode.

2-2 Measurements of velocity profiles using LDV

The circulating fluid used in this experiment was a 50% glycerol
aqueous solution in order to match closely the refractive index of
the Plexiglas. The measurements of velocity profiles were made in the
range of Dean number between 52 and 440, and for a Womersley
parameter between 8 and 18. The axial velocity measurements were made
in the plane of symmetry from θ =0° to 90° at 4 streamwise
stations, and the secondary velocity measurements were made at
θ =90° .

2-3 Data sampling

The analog signals from the output of the signal processor
(trucker type NIHON KANOMAX Model 1095) for the LDV and the wall
shear probes, changing periodically with time, were digitized by a
12bit A/D converter with the sampling rate 500 Hz. The number of
sampling periods was between 20 and 40 and ensemble averages were
calculated by a microcomputer (NEC PC-9801F2). Drift of the sampling
data number for different cycles was found to be within 0.1%.

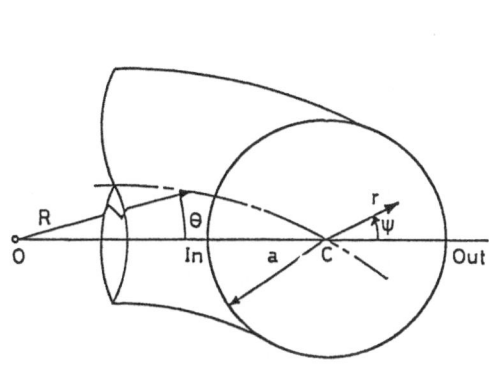

Fig.2   The system of coordinates

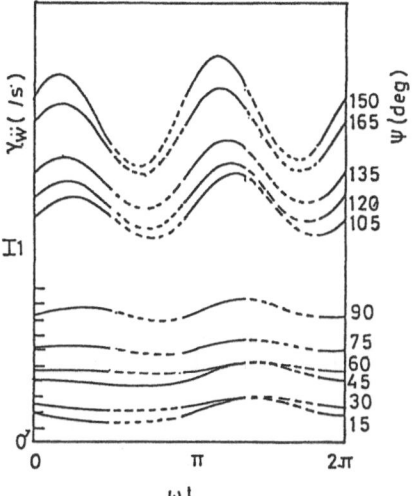

Fig.3   The traces of wall
shear rate variation at θ =90°
with De=181, α =18.0.
(De : Dean number,
α : Womersley parameter)

3.Result and discussion

     Mass and heat transfer probes measuring wall shear rate have
been widely applied for various type of fluid flow.[3] One of the
requirements to apply these methods, especially for unsteady flow, is
to correct for the frequency response of the concentration or
temperature boundary layer. The studies about frequency response of
the boundary layer to a sinusoidally varying velocity field have been
presented by Fortuna and Hanratty[4], Pedley[5], Mao and Hanratty[6],
Talbot and Steinert[7] and others. Almost all of these studies have
been carried out in an oscillatory flow field with a non-zero mean
flow. If the wall shear rate comes close to zero or reverses its
direction, the heat or mass transfer rate at the wall will maintain a
positive value well above zero regardless of the change of shear.
Therefore it is required to have careful calibration experiments for
the interpretation of the shear probe output. In this study the
reliable range of wall shear rate measured by the limiting current
method is checked by instantaneous axial and secondary velocity
profiles measured by LDV. Although LDV has also a difficulty with
measurements near the wall, it is possible to distinguish the
unreliable output of shear probe, particularly near zero shear.
  The wave forms of shear rate over the cycle at 11 points of
circumferential direction in the plane at a streamwise location of
θ =90°   are shown in Fig.3. Unreliable wall shear rates as
distinguished by velocity profiles is shown by a broken line. The
shear rates at 15° < ψ <90° tends to show similar profiles over the
cycle and remain fairly small. On the other hand, the shear rate at
105° < ψ <165° become larger and their amplitudes also increase.
The maximum shear rate appears at ψ =150° which is close to the
inner wall. The shear rate measured by the limiting current method

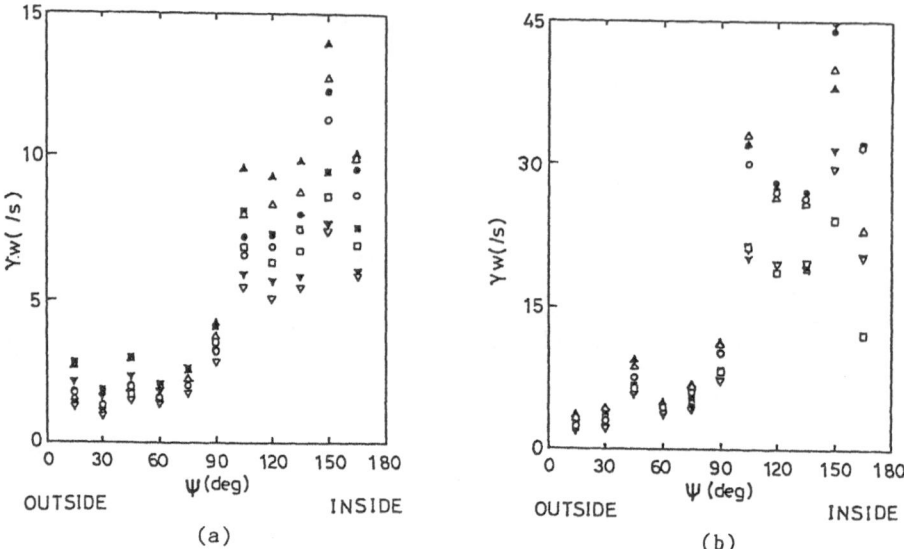

Fig.4   The distributions of wall shear rates at θ =90° with
(a) De=184,α =18.2, (b) De=459,α =18.2
(phase-symbol :0° -○,45° -△,90° -□,135° -▽,180° -●,225° -▲,
270° -◀,315° -▼)

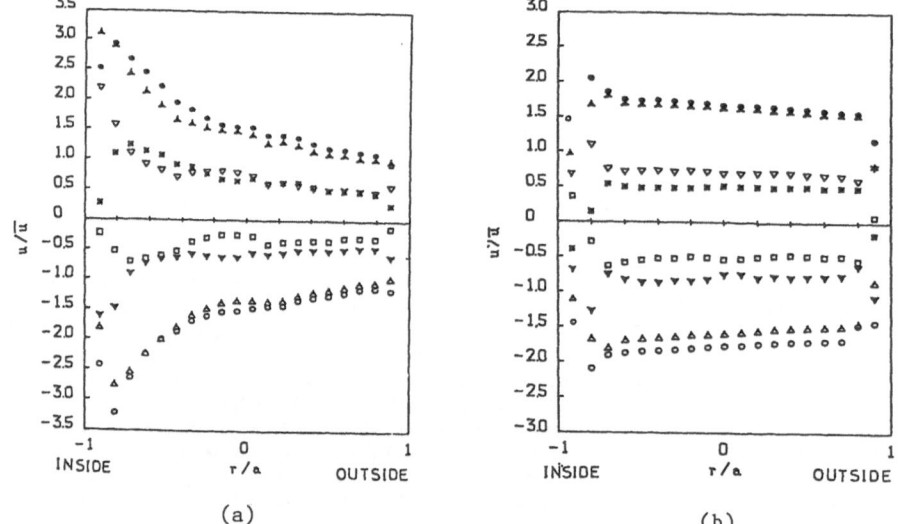

Fig.5   Axial velocity profiles at θ =90° with De = 184,α = 18.0
(a)δ =1/2, (b)δ =1/10.

can not reflect the direction of velocity, so that all of the shear
rates in Fig.3. exhibit double maximums and minimums per cycle,
appearing for both forward flow and backward flow. The wave form of
shear rate also shows a slight phase lag from the inner wall relative
to the outer wall. The wave forms of shear rates of Fig.3. are re-
plotted as a function of the circumferential angle ψ in Fig.4(a). It
is clearly seen that all of the shear rates and their amplitudes

sharply increase at ψ =90° . The effect of increasing De on the shear
rate with a fixed frequency parameter is demonstrated in Fig.4(b).
The absolute values of shear rate increase with increasing De,
although the whole profiles remain fairly constant. Wall shear stress
distributions in the entry region of a curved tube with δ =1/7 have
been measured using the electrochemical method by Choi et al.[3] in a
steady flow field with a uniform entry velocity profile. Their
experimental results have shown that the maximum shear stress occurs
at ψ =60° in the plane at a streamwise location of θ =15° , and the
circumferential angle ψ that the maximum shear stress occurs tends
to shift towards the outer side of the curvature with increasing θ .
So the fact that the maximum shear rate appears near the inner wall
obtained in this study is actually contrary to that in steady flow.
On the other hand, the wall shear stress for fully developed
sinusoidal and pulsatile flow in curved tubes was studied numerically
by Chang and Tarbell[8]. Their result demonstrate that the axial wall
shear stress at the inner wall tends to become larger as the
curvature ratio increases.
The axial velocity profiles in the plane of symmetry from ψ =0° to
180° , under the same conditions as Fig.3, are shown in Fig.5(a), and
Fig.5(b) shows the axial velocity profiles with δ =1/10. The ordinate
is the non-dimensional velocity normalized by the velocity amplitude
averaged over the cross-section. The streamwise station where θ =90°
is the center portion of the bend used in this study, so the forward
and backward flow have symmetry relative to each other.
It is shown in Fig.5(a) that the velocity near the inner wall is
nearly three times as large as that near the outer wall, which is
consistent with the shear rate profile. Fig.5(b) demonstrates a peak
velocity at the edge of the Stokes layer and almost flat profiles
throughout the cycle are observed inside the core region. The
velocity profiles are in agreement with those obtained by Sudou et
al.[9] It is evident that the effect of the curvature ratio is
important influence on the unsteady nature of fluid flow in a
strongly curved tube.

ACKNOWLEDGMENT

This work is supported in part by IBM Japan Ltd..

REFERENCES

[1] Schettler, G., Nerem, R.M., Schmid-Schonbein, H., Mori,H. &
    Diehm, C. Fluid Dynamics as a Localizing Factor for
    Atherosclerosis. 1983 Springer-Verlag
[2] Sakata, N., Machinami, M., Joshita, T. & Ooneda, G. 1985 J. Jpn.
    Coll. Angiology (in Japanese) 25-11, 1255.
[3] CHOI, U. S., TALBOT,L. & CORNET,I. 1979 J. Fluid Mech. 93, 465.
[4] FORTUNA, G., HANRATTY, T. J. 1971 Int. J. Heat Mass Transfer 14,
    1499.
[5] PEDLEY. T. J. 1976 J. Fluid Mech. 78-3, 513.
[6] MAO, Z.-X & HANRATTY, T. J. 1985 Experiments in Fluids 3, 129.
[7] TALBOT, L. & STEINERT, J. J. 1987 J. Biomech. Engrg. 109, 60.
[8] CHANG, L. J. & TARBEL, J. M. 1985 J. Fluid Mech. 161, 175.
[9] SUDOU, K., SUMIDA, M., TAKAMI, T. & YAMANE ,R. 1985 JSME (in
    Japanese) 51-463, 811.

Visualization of Velocity Profile and Measurement of Wall Shear Stress in Branched Square Tube Using Laser-Induced Fluorescence Method

K. OHBA[1], M. SATO[1,2], and S. SAKAGUCHI[1]

[1]Department of Mechanical Engineering, Kansai University, Suita, 564 Japan
[2]Kawasaki Heavy Industries, Ltd., Kobe, 650-91 Japan

ABSTRACT

Visualization and quantitative measurements of the velocity field of a laminar water flow through a branch tube of square cross section was made using a laser-induced fluorescence or phosphorescence (LIF or LIP) method. Velocity profiles in two directions across the tube were visualized in a total of 23 different cross sections located at the upstream and downstream of the branch and along the flow direction. The wall shear stress was obtained from these visualized velocity profiles and the map of the wall shear stress over the whole flow field was obtained.

INTRODUCTION

A laser-induced fluorescence or phosphorescence (LIF or LIP) method[1-3] can be used to advantage to make quantitative measurements of a complex flow field non-invasively, because it can visualize the velocity distribution directly. In the present experiments, visualization and quantitative measurements of the velocity field in a steady laminar water flow through a branching tube of square cross section with 45-deg. branch angle was made using the LIF method in order to know the detailed flow field in the branching region. Branch regions are considered to play an important role in atherogenesis. Furthermore, the distribution of a wall shear stress over the whole flow field was obtained from these velocity profiles.

APPARATUS AND PROCEDURE OF EXPERIMENT

Figure 1 shows an apparatus for the visualization and measurement of the flow velocity distribution as used in these experiments. A nitrogen pulse laser was used for exciting the fluorescence (phosphorescence) particle, thus making it fluoresce. The laser emits ultraviolet light of 5 nanosecond in pulse width, 337.1 nm in wave length and 1 MW in peak power. For the fluorescence particles, a zinc sulfide particle of about 8 μm in mean diameter and 4.1 g/cc in density was used. It was intermixed into water in a concentration of 0.1 to 0.2 % by weight. The ZnS particles, irradiated by a well collimated pulse ultraviolet laser light, emit a green fluorescence light of about 1 sec in life time. As a row of fluorescing particles moves with a flow, a

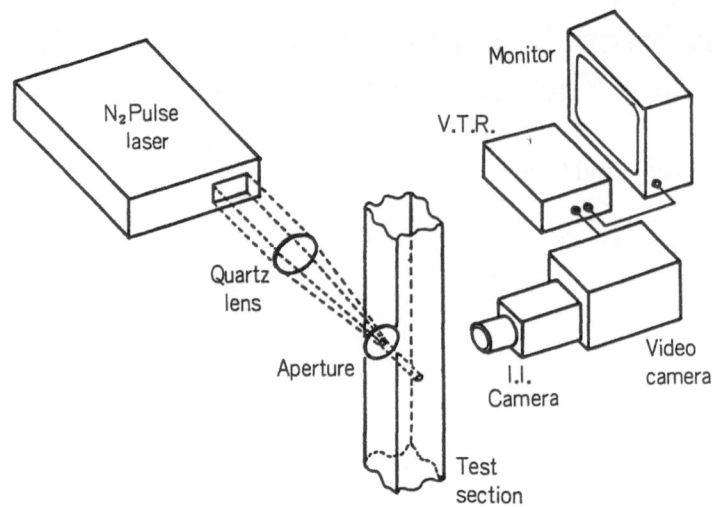

Fig.1   Schematic diagram of the apparatus for visualization and measurement of flow velocity distribution.

time line representing a velocity profile along the laser beam is
formed as shown in Fig.2.
    The motion of the time line so generated was photographed and
tracked by a high speed video camera having a time resolving power of
200 frames per second in the direction perpendicular to both the laser
beam and the flow.   The camera was equipped with an image intensifier
for amplifying the weak fluorescence light.
    Figure 3 shows co-ordinate system for the 45-deg. branch tube of
11.5 mm × 11.5 mm square cross section which was used in these experiments.   The z-axis was taken to be the flow direction, and the x- and
y- axes were taken to be perpendicular to the flow direction.   The
prime symbol (') represents the daughter tube, named as branch 2.

RESULTS AND DISCUSSIONS

    Figure 4 shows photographs of velocity profiles across the duct
visualized by the LIF method at twenty-three different cross sections
taken along the flow direction in the branch tube.   White arrow marks
represent the position of the inner walls, and furthermore, if a
straight line is drawn, connecting the vertices of the two arrow marks
which are facing each other with the time line in between, it represents the path of the laser beam.   Two kinds of profiles, i.e. distributions along the x- and y-axes, are shown at each cross section.
    It is clearly seen from Fig.4 that the first vortex appears in
each daughter tube.   It appears at the outside wall in the cross section located just after the branch point.   These vortices are considered to be generated by a flow separation due to a rapid expansion of
the duct.   A jet-like high speed flow is seen at the opposite side of
the wall at which the vortex exists.   The second vortex appears at the
inner wall in the cross section located further downstream.
    Figure 5 shows the motion of a time line representing this second
vortex.   This second vortex is also considered to be generated by a

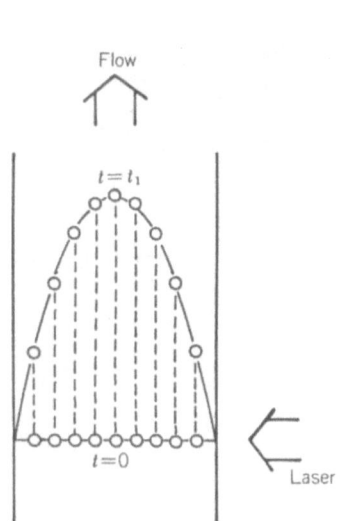

Fig.2 Time line drawn by a row of
fluorescing (phospherescing)
particles.

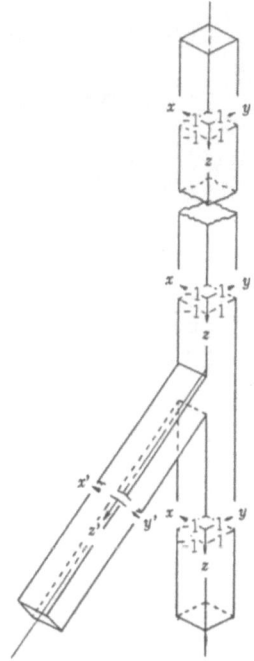

Fig.3 Co-ordinate system for the
45-deg. branch tube of
square cross section.

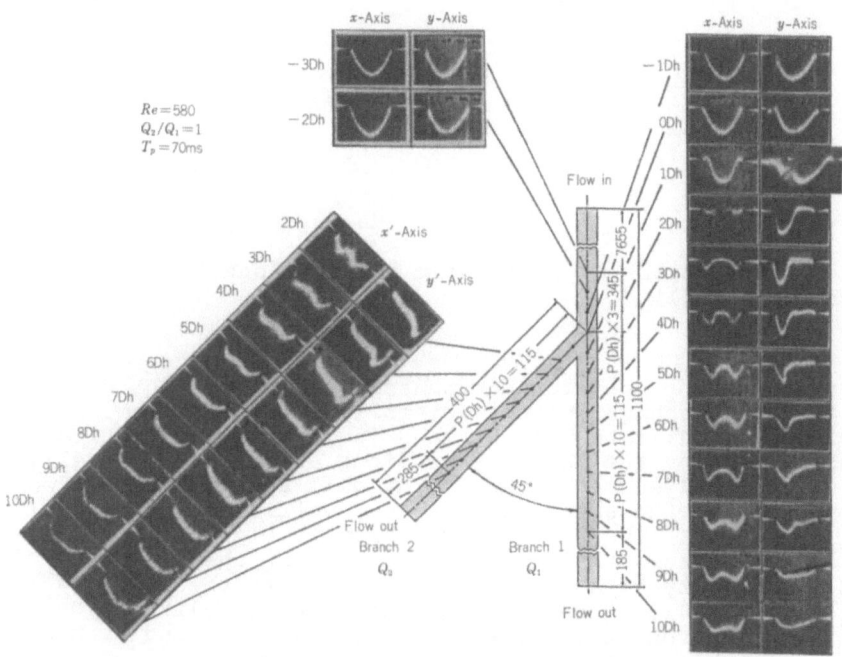

Fig.4 Velocity profiles visualized by LIF method in a branch tube.

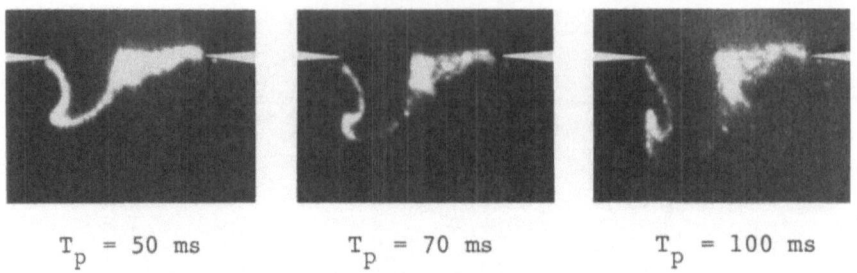

$T_p = 50$ ms $\qquad$ $T_p = 70$ ms $\qquad$ $T_p = 100$ ms

Fig.5 Photograph of time lines showing a vortex caused by flow
separation.

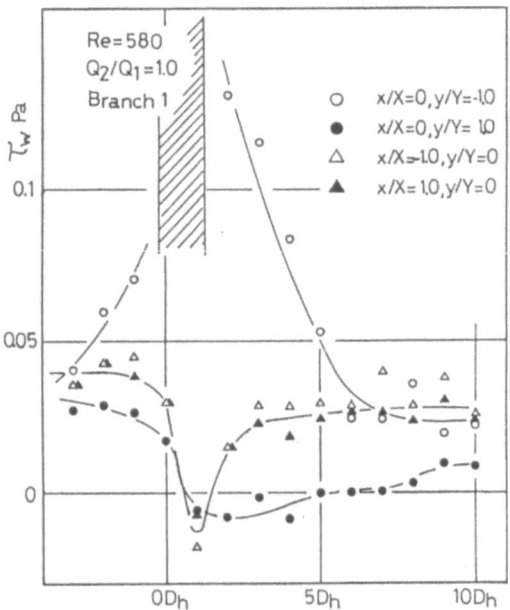

Fig.6 Distributions of wall shear stress along the flow direction
(Branch 1).

flow separation due to a rapid expansion of an apparent duct which is
caused by a reattachment of the initially separated flow.

The wall shear rate was obtained from the above-mentioned velocity
profiles by reading the velocity gradient at the wall manually or by
using picture analysis equipment. The wall shear stress τ_w was obtained by multiplying the shear rate by the coefficient of viscosity, μ,
i.e. $\tau_w = \mu(\nabla u_z)_w$. The results are shown in Figs.6 and 7. Figure 6
shows the wall shear stress distribution along the flow direction. It
is seen that a very high value of τ_w appears at the inner wall in the
branched portion, i.e. the position where the jet-like high speed flow
is seen. On the contrary, τ_w has a very low value and even has a negative value in the region of the separated flow.

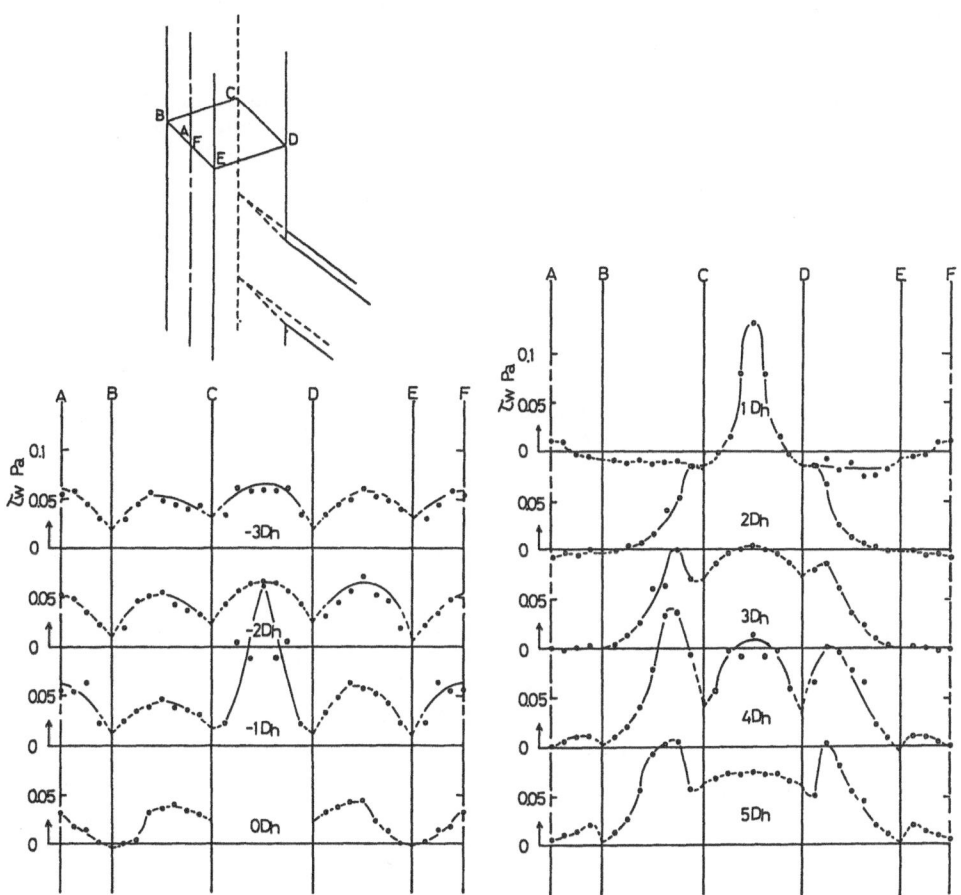

Fig.7 Map of the wall shear stress (Branch 1, -3Dh to 5Dh).

Figure 7 shows the τ_w distribution across the duct at 9 different cross sections taken along the flow direction. At the cross section 2Dh, which is located just after the branched portion, an extremely high value of τ_w is seen in the central part on the inner wall where the jet-like high speed flow appears in Fig.4. It is also seen that the τ_w takes high and low values at the center and the corner of the wall, respectively.

CONCLUSIONS

It becomes clear from the above-mentioned experiment that the detailed profile of the flow velocity and the wall shear stress can be quantitatively obtained over the entire flow field in a branch tube using the laser-induced fluorescence method. It was seen that in the region of flow separation the wall shear stress takes a very low value and takes even a negative value; while, on the contrary, it takes an an extremely high value on the wall on the opposite side in that cross section.

REFERENCES

[1] Nakatani, N. et al. (1975), J. Phs. E: Sci. Instrum. $\underline{8}$, 1042
[2] Ohba, K. and Sato, M. (1986), J. Flow Visual. Soc. Japan 6-22, 377
[3] Ohba, K. et al. (1987), J. Flow Visual. Soc. Japan $\underline{7}$-26, $\overline{3}$31

Chapter 3
Cellular or Tissue Reactions to Blood Flow

Cellular Reactions to Blood Flow

R.M. NEREM

Biomechanics Laboratory, Bioengineering Center, Georgia Institute of Technology, Atlanta, GA 30332-0405, USA

ABSTRACT

Recent investigations on mechanisms, through which a hemodynamic role in atherogenesis might be mediated, have focused on the influence of wall shear stress on vascular endothelium. Through cell culture studies, much is now known about endothelial responses to shear stress; however, a number of basic questions remain unanswered. One such question is "how does an endothelial cell recognize and then transduce a fluid mechanic signal?" Also, other cell types are also involved in the development of atherosclerosis, and it is equally important that an understanding of the influence of mechanical stresses on these cell types be achieved.

INTRODUCTION

It is now believed by many that hemodynamic factors are integral to the evolution of the disease atherosclerosis. Hemodynamics would appear to be particularly important to the determination of the spatial pattern of the disease, and in fact the primary evidence for the involvement of hemodynamics in the atherosclerotic process is the focal nature of the disease. Not only is it large, thick-walled arteries such as the aorta, the carotid, and the coronary arteries which are most commonly affected, but it appears that it is often specific regions in the vicinity of locations of arterial branching and sharp curvature which have the greatest predilection for the development of atherosclerosis.

Recent studies, which have attempted to investigate mechanisms through which any hemodynamic effect might be mediated, have emphasized the role of wall shear stress and its possible effect on the biology of the arterial wall. Of particular interest has been the influence of wall shear stress on vascular endothelium. However, other cell types, e.g. the smooth muscle cell and the monocyte/macrophage, are also important participants in the development of atherosclerosis. In these introductory comments, a brief review is provided of what is known about the reaction to blood flow of the cellular components important to the biology of the arterial wall, with the emphasis being on the endothelial cell.

ENDOTHELIAL STUDIES

From in vivo studies we know that the role of hemodynamics in the atherogenic process not only occurs in the presence of an intact endothelium, but also has a strong influence on endothelial cell shape and orientation [1-3]. Furthermore, there is evidence that regions of more rounded endothelial cells, presumably corresponding to a low shear stress environment, will exhibit enhanced permeability to plasma constituent transendothelial transport and possibly higher cell turnover rates [4]. These regions are also believed to have a higher predilection to disease [5]. Finally, it has been observed that reductions in arterial diameter produced by chronic decreases in blood flow are endothelium dependent [6].

Although such in vivo studies are informative, before any firm conclusions can be made with regard to the existence of a mechanical stimulus in the etiology of vascular disease, an evaluation of endothelial cellular responses to well-defined flow conditions is necessary. Unfortunately, vascular endothelium is not only relatively inaccessible in vivo to experimental manipulation, but also resides in a fluid mechanical environment which can only be defined qualitatively and not quantitatively. Thus, in recent years, in vitro studies of endothelial cellular dynamics have been initiated using confluent monolayers of cultured vascular endothelial cells exposed to a fluid-imposed shear stress [7-9].

There have been a number of laboratories active in this area. Our own efforts originally focused on shear stress-induced changes in endothelial cell shape and orientation [9]. However, more recently experiments have been conducted in which alterations in cytoskeletal element localization, with increases in cell stiffness [10] and an enhancement in intracellular or membrane potential [11] all have been observed. This effect is substrate dependent [9], and this suggests that the molecules of the extracellular matrix may influence the response of endothelial cells to a fluid-imposed shear stress. There have also been observed changes in endothelial cell function in response to shear stress [12-14]. In addition, in a collaborative effort with Dr. C. J. Schwartz's group in San Antonio, the influence of a steady shear stress on $125I$-LDL endocytosis by a confluent monolayer of cultured bovine aortic endothelial cells have been studied. The results indicate that shear stress increases both total and receptor-mediated LDL binding, internalization, and degradation [15].

A basic question which remains unanswered is how does an endothelial cell recognize and then transduce a hemodynamic or fluid mechanic signal? It seems reasonable to hypothesize that an endothelial cell's recognition of shear stress is a direct membrane effect. This could be due to mechano-sensitive membrane ion channels or due to some other effect on the membrane. A possible example of the latter would be an influence of shear stress on membrane phosphoinositol turnover. The intracelluar mobilization of Ca^{++} could also serve as a second messenger. This could be in place of the phosphoinositol signal transduction pathway or could occur concomitantly, with the two second messengers acting synergistically. It is well known that eukaryotic cells, when exposed to a change in chemical environment, undergo a rapid elevation in intracellular Ca^{++} concentration. The most common translator of the Ca^{++} signal is calmodulin, with many of the Ca^{++} effects being exerted through calmodulin-regulated enzymes. What is not known is whether such a response can be elicited by a change in a cell's mechanical environment.

Once possible hypothesis for the recognition and transduction of a fluid mechanic signal is that shear stress opens up mechano-sensitive ion channels, allowing for increased K^+ leakage and causing the membrane potential to become more negative, as we have observed. This further polarization of the cell membrane allows certain voltage-gated Ca^{++} channels to open with the result being an elevation in the intracellular Ca^{++} concentration. This second messenger then triggers a reorganization in cytoskeletal structure, a remodeling of extracellular matrix components, and an alteration in cell function. It is clear that experiments must be carried out in the near future to test such a hypothesis, as well as others, so that the question can be answered as to how an endothelial cell recognizes and then tranduces a fluid mechanic signal.

A CELL'S MECHANICAL ENVIRONMENT

In addition to the vascular endothelial cell, there are at least three other cell types which participate in the development of atherosclerosis. These are the monocyte/macrophage, the platelet, and the smooth muscle cell, and just as the endothelial cell is influenced by its mechanical environment, for each of these three cell types the influence of the cell's mechanical environment could be important.

In the case of the monocyte/macrophage, little is known about its response to blood flow. However, it has been reported that aortic areas demarked by Evans blue uptake (blue areas) showed preferential intimal penetration by blood monocytes [16].

This suggests the possibility of a hemodynamic effect on monocyte recruitment. Also, is it possible that the structure and function of monocytes are influenced by mechanical stresses, either while in the flow or upon invasion of the arterial wall?

For the platelet, on the other hand, it is well known the flow-related factors mediate its interaction with the arterial wall. This is true both in terms of adherence as well as aggregation [17-19]. What is not known is the influence of hydrodynamic forces on the structure and function of platelets which are adherent to the vessel wall.

With regard to the smooth muscle cell, the studies of Leung et al. [20-21], on the effect of cyclic stretching on smooth muscle cells cultured on a compliant membrane, indicate important effects of stress on cell function. This suggests that the internal stress within the arterial wall may be an important factor. It just may be that endothelial cells are more responsive to shear stress, but that vascular smooth muscle cells are significantly influenced by wall internal stresses, which in turn are dependent on intraluminal pressure, as well as the properties of the wall.

It should be noted that the exact nature of the environment imposed by blood flow may be critical to a cell's response. Existing results for the endothelial cell indicate that the influence of a pulsatile shear stress is different from that of a steady shear stress. However, if the shear stress is pulsatile, is there any difference between a reversing or a non-reversing shear stress vector? What about separated flow regions or even turbulence? A recent paper on turbulence effects on endothelial cells indicates an altered response [22]. What about pulsatile versus steady state effects on other cell types?

What about an influence of pressure on endothelial cell structure and function? If so, is there any interaction between a shear stress and a pressure effect? Although the answer to this last question is not known, in a preliminary study we have observed important effects of oscillatory pressure [23]. It may that the effect of turbulence is through pressure oscillations and not shear stress.

BLOOD FLOW AND ATHEROSCLEROSIS

Finally, one can also ask what the significance of this is to the development of atherosclerosis. A general hypothesis underlying studies of the type noted here is that mechanical signals are recognized by vascular cells such that differences in the hemodynamic environment of the different regions of the vascular system result in altered cell function and play a role in the genesis and progression of atherosclerosis. For example, differences in endothelial cell shape and cytoskeletal structure may influence cell junctions and thus endothelial permeability. Also, since cells in high versus low shear stress regions may in a sense be differentiated from one another, it would not be surprising if cell turnover rates were different. Recent unpublished results from our own laboratory indicate an important inhibitory effect of shear stress on endothelial cell proliferation in non-confluent monolayers. Whether or not this will prove to be a useful model in the study of vascular biology remains to be seen; however, the possible relationship between the observed decrease in cell proliferation and alteration in cytoskeletal structure in these non-confluent monolayer studies also may prove to be true in the in vivo case, where as noted earlier, regions of low shear appear to have higher cell turnover rates and be more prone to the development of atherosclerosis.

Also, although the emphasis here has been on shear stress and the endothelial cell, the three other cell types noted, i.e. the monocyte/macrophage, the platelet, and the smooth muscle cell, also reside in a hemodynamically-induced mechanical stress environment. As an example, Thubrikar et al. [24] have calculated the internal wall stresses in an arterial bifurcation and demonstrated regions of stress concentration, both at the flow divider and at the outer wall. This stress enhancement is found throughout the entire wall thickness and presumably would effect the structure and function of smooth muscle cells residing locally in that region. It is thus important to investigate the response of smooth muscle cells, as well as the monocyte/macrophage and the platelet, to their combined biochemical/mechanical environment.

One aspect of this is the cell-to-cell communication between different cell types. For example, if a shear stress signal is recognized by the endothelial cell as part of a vessel's vascoactive control of diameter as has recently been suggested, is this communicated to the medial smooth muscle cells and if so, how? Are smooth muscle cells in a region of stress concentration affected differently by such a signal? Is smooth muscle proliferation in the arterial wall triggered by an endothelial-derived signal? Important in all this is the recognition that cellular structure and function is dependent, not only on its biochemical environment, but also on its mechanical environment. Thus, in terms of the biology of the arterial wall, the cellular reaction to a blood flow-induced mechanical environment could be important. Only with this as a foundation can we begin to develop an understanding of the atherosclerotic disease process.

REFERENCES

[1] Silkworth, JB, Stehbens WE (1975) Angiology 26: 474-487
[2] Nerem RM, Levesque MJ, Cornhill JF (1981) ASME J Biomech Engr 103: 172-177
[3] Levesque MJ, Liepsch D, Moravec S, Nerem RM (1986) Arteriosclerosis 6: 220-229
[4] Schwartz CJ, Sprague EA, Fowler SR, Kelly JL (1983) Cellular participation in atherogenesis: selected facets of endothelium, smooth muscle, and the peripheral blood monocyte. In: Schettler G, et al. (eds) Proceedings of a Symposium on Fluid Dynamics as a Localizing Factor for Atherosclerosis. Springer Verlag, Berlin Heidelberg, pp. 200-207
[5] Repin VS, Dolgov VV, Zaikina OE, Novikov JD, Antonov AS, Nikoleva MA, Smirnov VN (1984) Atherosclerosis 50: 35-52
[6] Langille BL, O'Donnell F (1986) Science 231: 405-407
[7] Dewey CF, Jr., Bussolari SR, Gimbrone MA, Jr., Davies PF (1981) ASME J Biomech Engr 103: 177-185
[8] Eskin SF, Ives CL, McIntire LV, Navaro LT (1984) Microvasc Res 28: 87-94
[9] Levesque MJ, Nerem RM (1985) ASME J Biomech Engr 107: 341-347
[10] Sato M, Levesque MJ, Nerem RM (1987) Arteriosclerosis 7: 276-286
[11] de Souza PA, Levesque MJ, Nerem RM (1986) Federation Proc. 45: 471
[12] Davies PF, Dewey CF, Jr., Bussolari SR, Gordon EJ, Gimbrone MA, Jr., (1984) J Clin Invest 73: 1121-1129
[13] Frangos JA, McIntire LV, Eskin SF (1985) Science 227: 1477-1479
[14] Grabowski EF, Jaffe EA, Weksler BB (1985) J Lab Clin Med 105: 36-43
[15] Sprague EA, Steinbach BL, Nerem RM, Schwartz CJ (1987) Circulation (in press)
[16] Gerrity RG, Gross JA, Soby L (1985) Arteriosclerosis 5: 55-56
[17] Turitto VT, Weiss HJ (1979) Rheology 23: 735
[18] Sakariassen KS, Aarts PAMM, de Groot PG, Houdijk WPM, Sixma JJ (1983) J Lab Clin Med 102: 522-535
[19] Rhee B-G, McIntire LV (1986) Chem Eng Commun 47: 147-161
[20] Leung DYM, Glagov S, Mathews MB (1976) Science 191: 475-477
[21] Leung DYM, Glagov S. Mathews MB (1977) Experimental Cell Research 109:285-298
[22] Davies PF, Remuzzi A, Gordon EJ, Dewey CF, Jr., Gimbrone MA, Jr. (1986) Proc Natl Acad Sci 83: 2114-2117..
[23] Levesque MJ, Nerem RM (1983) Shear and pressure effects on cultured endothelial cells In: Proc. 36th Annual Conference on Engineering in Medicine and Biology, held September 11-14, 1983, Columbus, Ohio, p. 34.1
[24] Thubriker MJ, Manuel L, Eppink RL (1987) Intramural stress at arterial bifurcation in vivo. In: Proc 40th Annual Conference on Engineering in Medicine and Biology, held September 10-13, 1987, Niagara Falls, NY p. 34.1

In vivo Responses of Endothelial Cells to Hemodynamic Stress

B.L. LANGILLE, A.I. GOTLIEB, and D.W. KIM

Vascular Research Laboratory, Department of Pathology, Banting and Best Diabetes Centre, University of Toronto, and Toronto General Hospital Research Centre, Toronto, M5G 2C4, Canada

ABSTRACT

We have examined endothelial cell integrity and cytoskeleton structure at sites of flow disturbances in the vicinity of mid-abdominal aortic coarctations in rabbits. Coarctations produce high shear stresses in the inflow region and shears that fluctuate rapidly in direction immediately downstream. Both zones are characterized by elevated endothelial cell death and turnover. Furthermore, repair of endothelial injury was inhibited in both areas. Studies of cytoskeleton in the high shear regions demonstrated expression of very large and long actin microfilament bundles ("stress fibres"). We interpret this response as cellular adaptation that may limit shear-related trauma to endothelium.

INTRODUCTION

It has been proposed that abnormal hemodynamic stresses injure arterial endothelium and thereby contribute to atherogenesis. However, the nature of the injurious stress is controversial; thus, high, low and fluctuating shear all have been implicated. Furthermore, the functional significance of endothelial adaptations to altered stresses is poorly understood. We have used abdominal aortic coarctations in rabbits to manipulate in vivo shear stress, and examined endothelial cell responses to these stresses. Partial occlusion with external silk ligatures was used to produce coarctations.

FLOW CONDITIONS NEAR COARCTATIONS

We investigated how these in vivo coarctations alter local flow fields (1). An array of pulsed Doppler flowmeter crystals was used to identify variations in the magnitude of blood velocity, and also to detect regions where flow reversal occurs. In addition, we inferred direction of mean shear stress from the local orientation of endothelial cells, since it is well-established that mean shear aligns these cells. The flow patterns we defined are indicated schematically in figure 1. Three flow regimes were identified. In zone I, high shears are generated as flow funnels into the coarctation site. Shear determinations are not feasible in coarctations of this size, but a Poiseuille flow approximation implies that shear increases with the inverse cube of radius. It follows that our 60% coarctations increase shear by at least an order of magnitude. Zone II was characterized by highly complex patterns of endothelial cell orientation (figure 2). We inferred that local vortices caused by irregularities in coarctation geometry characterized this zone and produced this unusual cell alignment. In zone III, our Doppler flowmeter studies detected an annular vortex that extended approximately 6 aortic diameters downstream from the coarctation during systole. A perfectly symmetrical vortex is shown in figure 1, but this idealized situation was infrequently observed. Usually the vortex was significantly larger on the ventral side of the aorta.

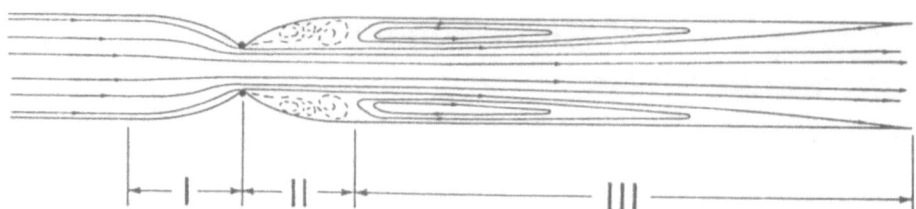

FIG.1 Steamline patterns near rabbit aortic coarctations. Streamlines were estimated by pulsed Doppler flowmetry or were inferred from endothelial cell orientation. Adapted from ref (1).

LOCAL FLOW CONDITIONS AND ENDOTHELIAL INJURY

Flow alterations caused obvious morphological changes to endothelial cells over the first 7-10 days after coarctation. Immediately upstream, cell elongation in the axial direction of the aorta increased dramatically while cells in zone II took on the pattern shown in figure 2. Over this time, cell replication, as measured by ^{3}H-thymidine autoradiography, remained below 0.1%/day. Thus morphologic changes occurred in pre-existing cells and were not a by-product of cell turnover. These morphological changes may reflect adaptations that limit cell trauma in the presence of altered shear stress; nonetheless, cell death and increased turnover rates ultimately occurred so that, by one month, turnover was two orders of magnitude higher than resting levels in both zone I and zone II.

We have concluded that both high shear stress and shear that fluctuates rapidly in direction can traumatize endothelium. It is conceivable that different arteries or different species show varying susceptibility to high versus fluctuating shear. If this is so, it may explain why anatomic correlations between shear and atherogenesis show great species variability.

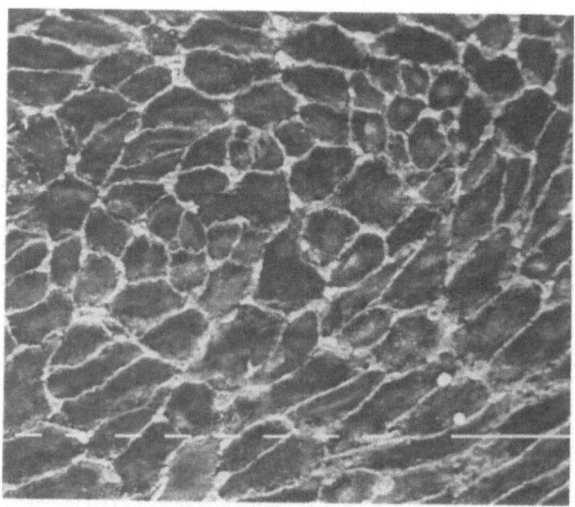

FIG 2 Endothelial cell shape and orientation seen in zone II, immediately downstream from the coarctation. Cell boundries are stained with AgNO$_3$. Short markers are 10um.

ENDOTHELIAL REPAIR

We also examined endothelial repair near coarctations. Narrow longitudinal injuries to endothelium were made by scratching the luminal surface of the abdominal aorta with a special catheter (2). Coarctations were performed immediately after injury and repair near the coarctation site was monitored. We detected complete closure of the wound through spreading of adjacent cells within 24h (figure 3A). Frequent focal regions exhibiting numerous attached white cells, probably monocytes, were observed at the junctions of spreading endothelial cells. These cells were not simply showing affinity for exposed subendothelium. Adherence to junctions occurred in preference to substrate prior to complete wound closure (figure 3B). We detected no preference for these focal regions of leukocyte attachment at different sites near coarctations, but rigorous, quantitative assessments were not attempted. Previously, leukocyte adhesion to repairing endothelium has been reported, but only in hypercholesterolemic rabbits (3).

Partial wound closure was evident after 12h; therefore, we assessed wound width at this time, to see if extent of closure was dependent on local flow conditions. We found marked inhibition of repair (up to 50% wider wounds after

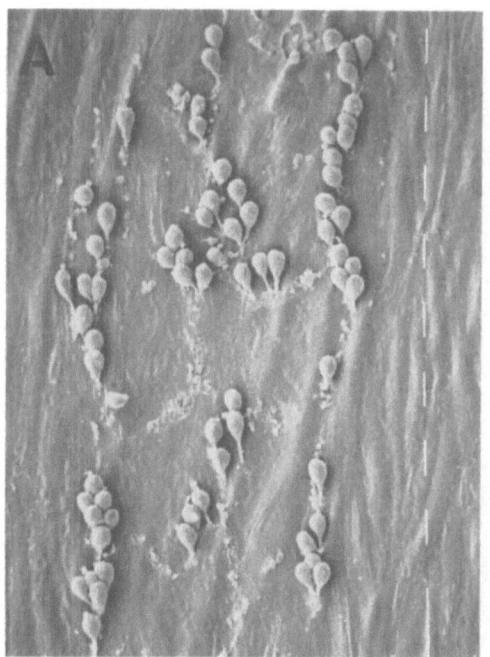 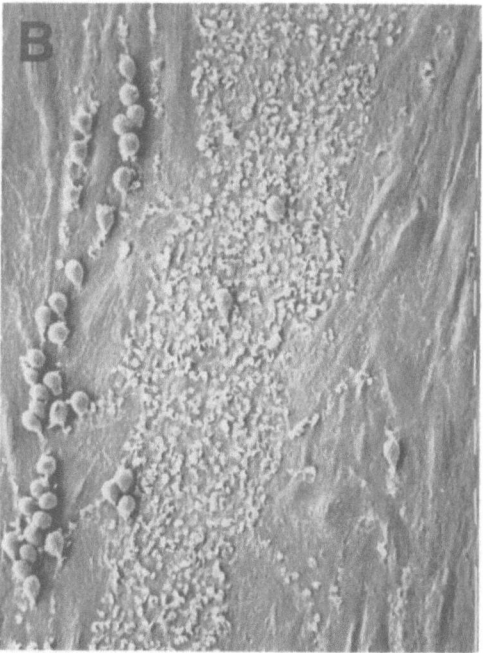

FIG 3 A. Site of longitudinal wound 24h after injury. Wound has been re-covered by spreading of adjacent endothelial cells. White cells, probably monocytes, are adherent to the junctions of the spreading cells. B. Wound site 12h after injury. Platelets are adherent to the exposed subendothelium. Leukocytes adhere to junctions of spreading endothelial cells. Short markers are 10 um.

12h) in both zone I (high shear region) and zone II (fluctuating shear region). We conclude that local flow conditions can influence endothelial integrity both by injuring the cells and by modulating repair mechanisms.

CYTOSKELETAL ADAPTATIONS TO ALTERED BLOOD FLOW

The adaptations of cell geometry to local flow conditions described above suggested that reorganization of the cell cytoskeleton has occurred. We have examined actin microfilament distribution near coarctations, because these structures are thought to be important in cell-cell and cell-substrate adhesion. In addition, microfilament reorganization plays a critical role in migration during endothelial wound healing (4).

Endothelium from control segments of abdominal aorta shows prominent actin labelling at the perimeter of the cell (figure 4A). This peripheral distribution is reminiscent of the "dense peripheral band" of actin seen in confluent endothelial cell cultures (4), although discrete filament bundles are not seen in vivo. Bundles of central microfilaments, i.e. "stress fibres", were also seen in cells from control aortic tissue. These stress fibres were relatively short and thin.

A much different actin distribution was found in the high shear region entering the coarctation. Actin staining at the periphery of cells was reduced and frequently disappeared (figure 4B & C). This peripheral actin was replaced by many long, thick stress fibres that were consistently aligned with the aortic axis. The stress fibres were not uniquely associated with cell boundaries.

The ubiquity of this pattern of actin staining in the high shear region of the coarctation suggests that it is not associated with migration secondary to death and desquamation of neighbouring cells. Cell turnover is elevated in this region but it remains below 3% per day, as measured by H-thymidine uptake (1). Furthermore, axial alignment of microfilament bundles is not consistent with patterns previously observed during wound repair (4,5). It is more likely that stress fibres are formed as part of an adaptive response that enhances the cell capacity to withstand shear-induced trauma. We are currently examining the intracellular position of these fibres, using transmission electron microscopy, to assess their association with both substrate and with cell junctions.

High shear stresses occur in unmanipulated arteries at apices of branch sites; therefore, we looked for similar stress fibre distribution at the apex of the aortic bifurcation into the iliac arteries. Again, peripheral actin staining was replaced by very long, thick stress fibres (figure 4D). This pattern of microfilament distribution was localized, as it extended only about 6 mm along the medial wall of each iliac artery. Thus, only the highest shear stresses occurring in normal rabbit arteries elicit this extreme actin redistribution. Previous studies reported microfilament redistribution near branch sites in rats and mice, but to a much lesser degree than we observe (6,7). It is not clear at this point whether species or methodological factors underly these differences, or whether the precise site at which cells were examined was critical.

Our studies have established that endothelial cells undergo marked structural and cytoskeletal alterations when exposed to changes in shear stress. The formation of very long, thick microfilament bundles under high shear suggests that these structures represent adaptations that limit shear related trauma. These bundles may be primarily load bearing structures; alternatively, they may participate in cell motility during more generalized structural modification. Ultimately, however, chronic high or fluctuating shears appear capable of injuring cells, as indicated by high cell turnover rates and impaired capacity to repair.

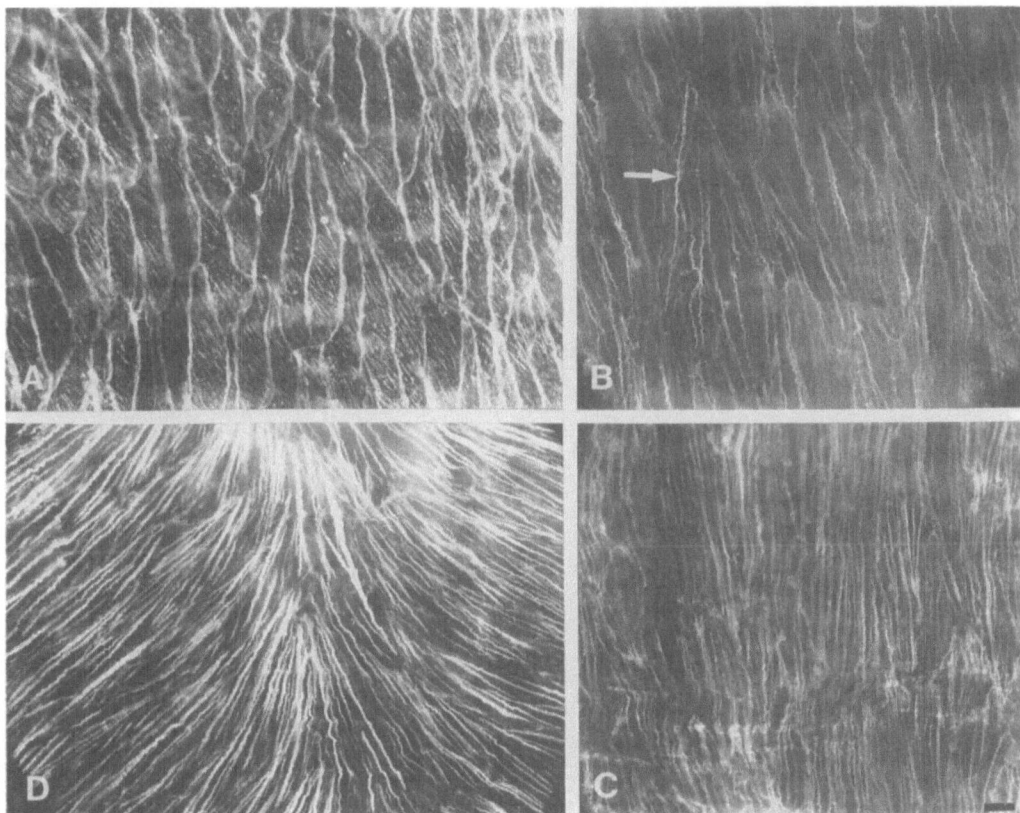

FIG 4 Endothelial cells stained for actin with rhodamine phalloidin. A. Actin
distribution in control segments showed prominent staining at the cell periphery
and short, thin central stress fibres. B. In the entry to zone I (high shear
region), well-defined peripheral staining was partially replaced by straight,
thick filament bundles. C. In the centre of zone I, actin staining is no longer
seen at the cell periphery (arrowhead). Instead, very long, thick stress fibres
are found throughout the region. D. Endothelial cell actin staining at the apex
of the aortic bifurcation, another high shear region, resembles that seen in zone
I. Marker is 10 um.

Acknowledgement: This work was supported by the Medical Research Council of
Canada, grant MA-10029.

REFERENCES

(1) Langille BL, Reidy MA, Kline RL (1986). Arteriosclerosis 6:146-154.
(2) Reidy MA, Schwartz SM (1981). Lab Invest 44:301-308.
(3) Walker LN, Bowyer DE (1984). Arteriosclerosis 1:107-161.
(4) Gotlieb AI, Spector W, Wong MKK, Lacey C (1984). Arteriosclerosis 4:91-96.
(5) Gabbiani G, Gabbiani F, Lombardi D, Schwartz SM (1983). Proc Nat Acad Sci
USA 80:2361-2364.
(6) Wong AJ, Pollard TD, Herman IM (1983). Science 219:867-869.
(7) White GE, Gimbrone Jr. MA, Fujiwari K (1983). J Cell Biol 97:416-424.

Morphological Changes in the Flow Loaded Canine Carotid Artery

H. Masuda, K. Kawamura, K. Tohda, and T. Shozawa

Second Department of Pathology, Akita University School of Medicine, Akita, 010 Japan

ABSTRACT

Morphological changes in the flow loaded canine carotid artery were studied using arterio-venous shunts. First (1 to 3 days) endothelial cells swelled. Then (7 days) they were activated with increased cytoplasmic microfilaments and thickening of the basement membrane. After 2 to 4 weeks, they proliferated with splitting and multiplication of the internal elastic lamina. In 6 to 12 months, reconstruction of the arterial wall was complete with an increase of medial elastic fibers and medial laminae. This sequence of changes in flow loaded artery may be important in considering the role of blood flow in atherogenesis.

INTRODUCTION

Thoma [1] first pointed out that the growth of the blood vessels depended on the blood flow velocity. Recently, using an arterio-venous shunt between the common carotid artery and the external jugular vein in dogs, Kamiya and Togawa [2] showed that when the blood flow rate was increased the caliber of the carotid artery enlarged over 6 months. They showed that wall shear stress regulated the growth. From the morphological point of view, the structure of an artery wall under conditions of normal blood flow rate before an arterio-venous anastomosis differs from that posed with increased blood flow 6 months after anastomosis. In this paper, we review and present our findings of the histological and ultrastructural changes in the flow loaded canine carotid artery [3,4,5,6,7,8] using the same arterio-venous shunt method as Kamiya and Togawa [2] and discuss how wall shear stress affects wall structure and may be related to the role of blood flow in atherogenesis.

MATERIALS AND METHODS

Adult dogs were used. An arterio-venous anastomosis was constructed between the right common carotid artery and the right external jugular vein following the same procedures as Kamiya and Togawa [2]. The left common carotid artery was used as a sham-operated control. Arteries were studied at 1 to 3 days (very acute stage), 7 days (acute stage), 2 to 4 weeks (subacute stage) and 6 to 12 months (chronic stage). Blood flow rates in the common carotid arteries were measured before anastomosis, just after anastomosis and at the time of sacrifice with an electromagnetic flowmeter. After the final measurement, fixation of the common carotid artery was carried out under normal pressure (about 100mmHg) using 3% glutaraldehyde solution in phosphate buffer (pH 7.4) [4]. Histological and ultrastructural observations were performed. Elastic fibers were stained by tannic acid uranyl acetate and lead citrate [9] for transmission electron microscopy (TEM). In some arteries, internal radius was measured on transversely cut histological section [8]. Morphometric studied were performed using histological sections to determine the numbers of endothelial nuclei and the medial elastic fiber content. Using TEM photographs endothelial cell number, the number of nuclei, endothelial shape and size, medial elastic fiber content [8] and volume of cytoplasmic microfilaments were determined [6]. Scanning electron microscopy (SEM) was used to determine endothelial cell density.

RESULTS

HEMODYNAMIC CHANGES: In normal and/or control common carotid arteries, the average blood flow rate was 100 to 150 ml/min. The internal radius was 0.12 to 0.15 cm. Assuming the steady flow, wall shear rate (wsr) was about 950/sec, wall shear stress (wss) was about 30 dynes/cm^2 and Reynolds number was about 370. After the shunt operation, blood flow rate was 600 to 750 ml/min. In the acute stage when the radius of the arteries is thought to be unchanged, wsr, wss and Reynolds number became 4,000 to 4,500/sec, 130 to 150 dynes/cm^2 and 1,500 to 1,900 respectively. In the subacute stage when the radius of the arteries was slightly enlarged (0.13 to 0.16 cm) and when the blood flow rate was slightly decreased (550 to 700 ml/min), wsr, wss and Reynolds number became 3,500 to 4,000, about 100 dynes/cm^2 and about 1,400 respectively. In the chronic stage when the radius of the arteries was considerably enlarged (0.15 to 0.20 cm), wsr, wss and Reynolds number were supposed to become 1,000 to 1,500/sec, 33 to 45 dynes/min and 1,000 respectively.

ENDOTHELIAL CELLS: In the shunted arteries, endothelial cells swelled in the acute stage. They were activated with protrusion, appearance of microvilli and partial disappearance of pinocytotic vesicles [3,5]. Cytoplasmic microfilament bundles [4,6], which were compatible with actin filament stress fibers increased in close correlation with the increase of blood flow rate (wall shear stress). In the subacute stage, the cells proliferated. They were compactly packed and protruded with microvilli at the surface (Fig 1 and 2), while they were flat and did not proliferate in the control arteries (Fig 3 and 4). Intercellular junctions were tall and straight, while they were low and interdigitating in the control arteries. Mitotic figures were occasionally observed by SEM. The endothelial cell density obtained by SEM was 6.15±0.68 x1,000 cells/mm^2, which was 1.84 times as many as in control arteries. They were narrow and thick, while they were rhomboid and flat in the control arteries. Their nuclei were prolate spheroid in shape, while they were flat obulate spheroid in shape in the control arteries. By morphometry on transverse TEM photographs, the endothelial cell volume in the shunted arteries was 331±53 um^3, which was 0.77 times as big as that in the control arteries. The endothelial nuclear volume was 68±8 um^3, which was the same as that in the control arteries. The cytoplasmic microfilaments were distinct and almost as abundant as in the acute stage. In the chronic stage, they were not as compactly arranged as in the subacute stage. Cytoplasmic microfilaments were distinct about the intercellular junctions, but less distinct near the abluminal plasma membrane. 10nm intermediate filaments appeared to be increased in the shunted arteries.

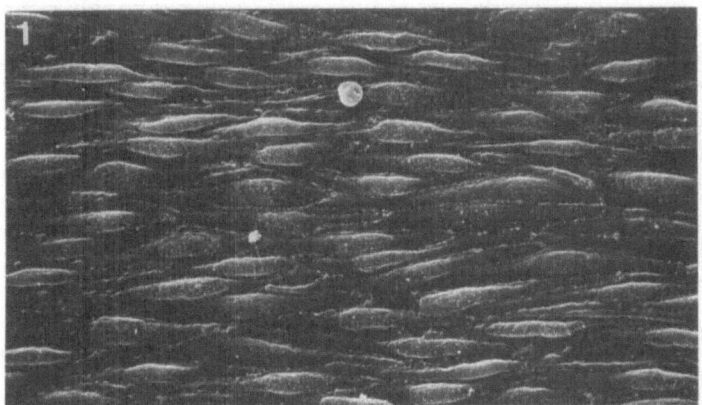

Fig 1 SEM photograph of shunted artery loaded by highly elevated blood flow rate and wall shear stress for 4 weeks (x750)

Fig 2 TEM photograph of the same artery as Fig 1 (transverse section, uranyl acetate and lead citrate, x12,000)

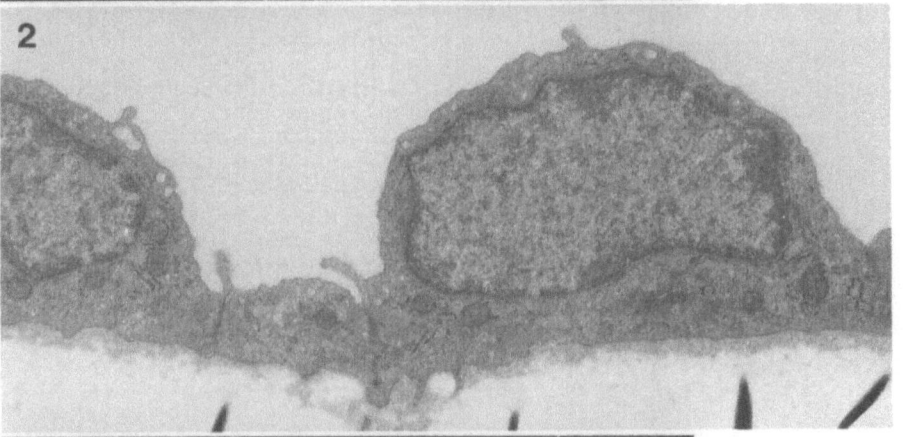

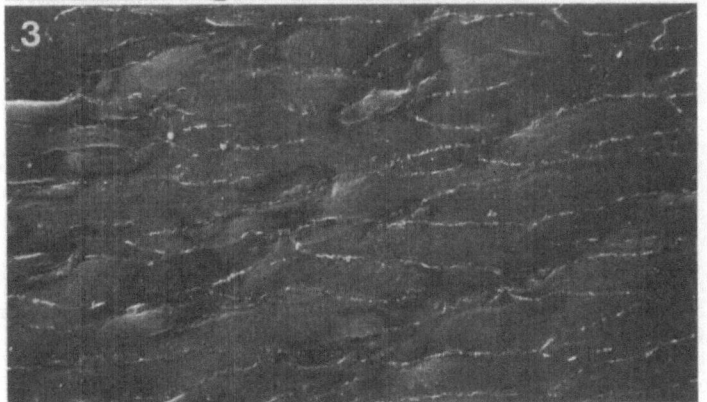

Fig 3 SEM photograph of control artery loaded by non-elevated blood flow rate and normal level of wall shear stress for 4 weeks (x750, same animal as Fig 1 & 2)

Fig 4 TEM photograph of the same artery as Fig 3 (transverse section, uranyl acetate and lead citrate, x12,000)

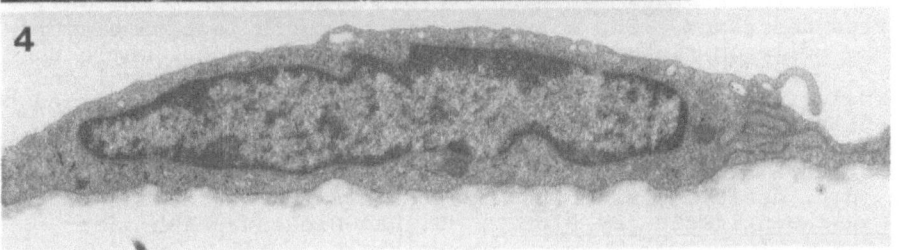

SUBENDOTHELIAL LAYER AND INTERNAL ELASTIC LAMINA: In the shunted arteries, no distinct change was observed in the very acute stage. In the acute stage, the subendothelial layer was thickened (300 to 500nm and sometimes over 500nm), while it was thin (about 50nm) in the control arteries [8]. The basement membrane was frequently multilayered. The abluminal plasma membrane of the endothelial cells sometimes showed dense bodies, which connected to the cytoplasmic microfilament bundles and subendothelial microfibrillar condensations, which formed subplasmalemmal microfilament condensations. At the luminal margin of the internal elastic lamina, there was a zone of irregular spindle to cylindrical elastic fibers. Most were arranged longitudinally with respect to the blood vessel direction. At the subacute stage, the basement membrane was still thick and irregular. The internal elastic lamina showed splitting and multiplication. Smooth muscle cells appeared in the subendothelial layer. In the chronic stage, the basement membrane was not so thick as in acute and subacute stages. The internal elastic lamina was not as split and not so layered as in the subacute stage.

MEDIA: In the shunted arteries, we could find no distinct morphological changes in the very acute stage or the acute stage. At the subacute stage, some shunted arteries with highly elevated blood flow showed an increase in elastic fibers and collagen fibers. Smooth muscle cells were activated. In the chronic stage, short elastic fibers and elastic fiber laminae were significantly increased [8] (Fig 5 and 6). The %volume of elastic fibers increased to 27% in the luminal one third of the media of the shunted arteries, while those of the control arteries were occupied 10 to 19%. Collagen fibers were increased and the smooth muscle cells appeared to be decreased in %volume.

ADVENTITIA: In the shunted arteries, collagen fibers appeared to increase in the subacute stage. Capillaries seemed distinct. In the chronic stage, collagen fibers were distinct and thick.

DISCUSSION

Morphologic changes in the flow loaded canine carotid artery are illustrated in Fig 7. Precise measurements of arterial diameter in vivo, direct evidence of cell proliferation and activation using tracers, as well as biochemical analyses of cell activity remain to be made. Evidence, such as endothelial surface changes, endothelial cytoplasmic changes and subendothelial layer changes indicate that endothelial cells are activated by elevated wall shear stress. Furthermore, as early as 7 days blood flow, i.e. wall shear stress, induces structural changes of the internal elastic lamina. In the subacute stage, we can see two dynamic changes occurring in the artery wall. Those are endothelial cell proliferation and splitting and multiplication of internal elastic lamina. At this stage, arterial growth induced by elevated wall shear stress has not been completed [2]. At the chronic stage, when the artery grows larger, the wall shear stress decreases. The structure of the media is then elastic fiber rich, collagen rich and more laminar in appearance, while the endothelial cell density decreases to the level of the control and the internal elastic lamina becomes constant and regular compaired to that noted in the subacute stage.

Thoma (1893)[1] listed three fundamental rules controlling arterial structure and the hemodynamics: 1. Das Wachsthum der Gefäss-lichtung, d.h. das Flächenwachsthum der Gefässwand ist abhängig von der Stromgeschwingigkeit des Blutes. 2. Das Dickenwachsthum der

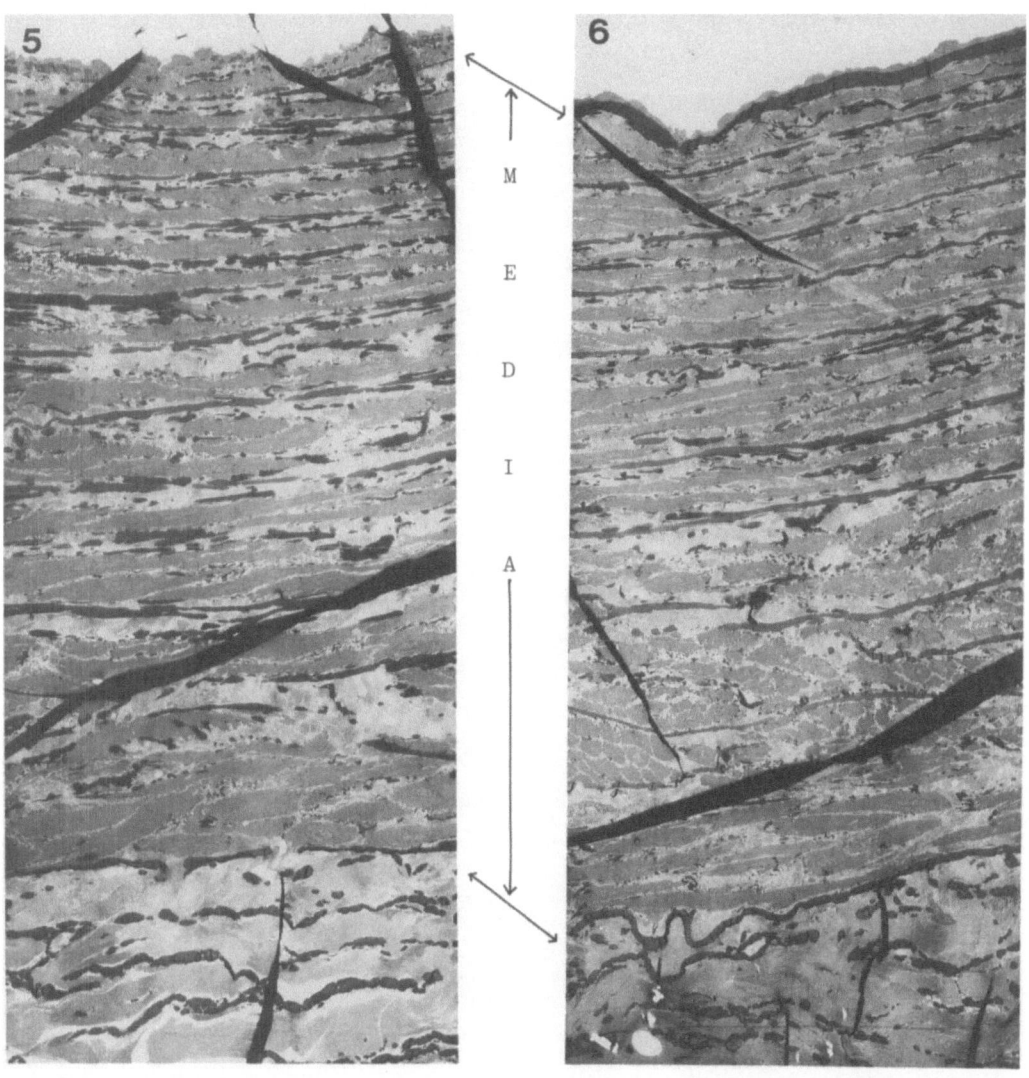

Figs 5 and 6
Transverse section of the shunted (Fig 5) & control (Fig 6) arteries
of a dog loaded by elevated blood flow for 6 months (chronic stage).
Blood flow rates were 130 ml/min (shunt) and 104 ml/min (control)
before anastomosis and were 500 ml/min (shunt) and 200 ml/min (control) at the final measurement. Low magnification TEM photograph
stained with tannic acid uranyl acetate and lead citrate (x900).
Elastic fiber was stained black. There is no intimal thickening. The
elastic fibers in the shunted artery were increased as compaired to
those in the control. The black belt-like portions across the photographs are artifacts occurred in preparing the ultrathin section. The
%volume of the elastic fibers of the shunted artery was 26.7%, 23.8%
and 14.6% in luminal 1/3, middle 1/3 and outer 1/3 layer of media as
compairing 18.8%, 16% and 8.1% of the control artery respectively.
(from Masuda et al (1987) J Jpn Soc Biorheol 1:19-26 [8])

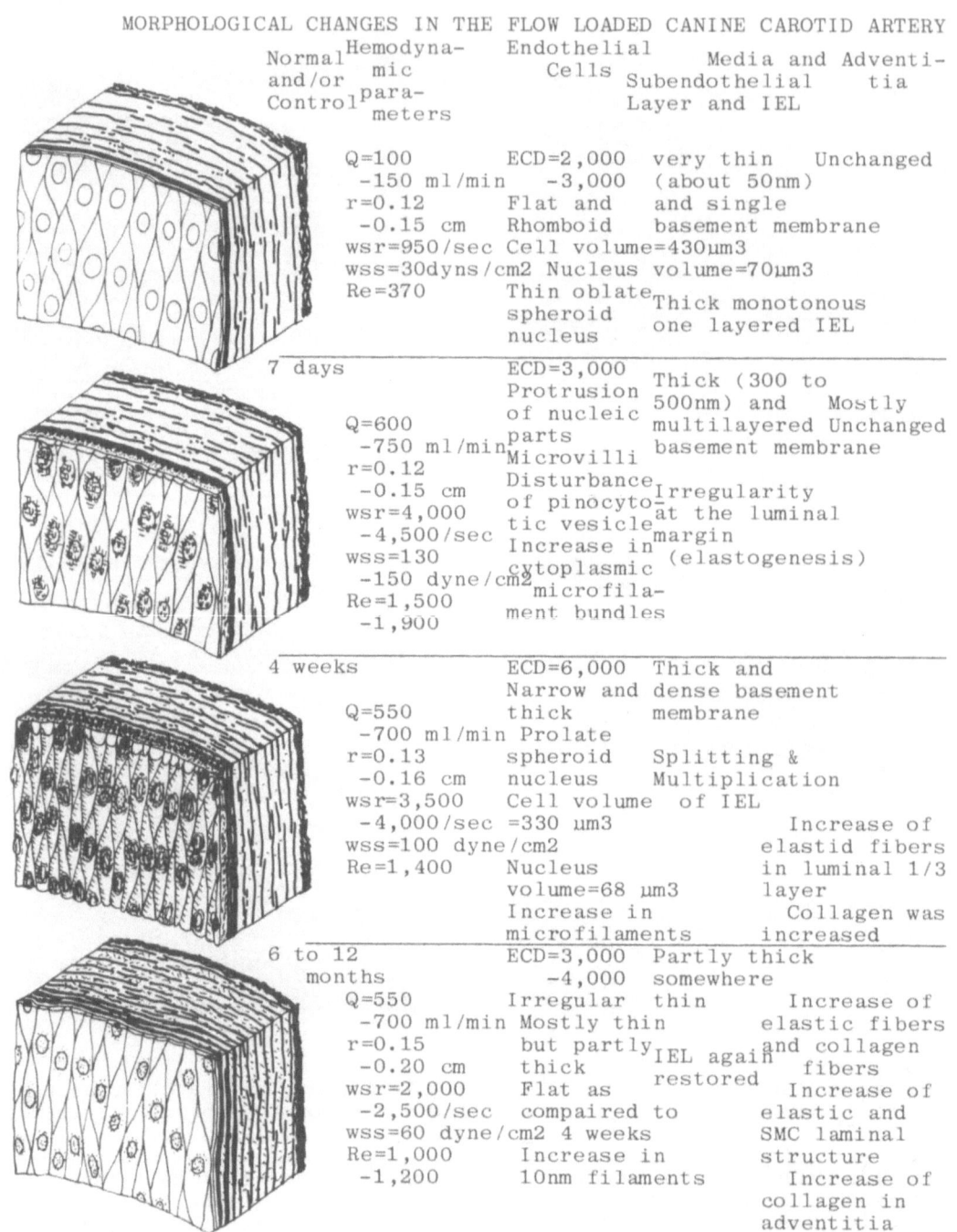

MORPHOLOGICAL CHANGES IN THE FLOW LOADED CANINE CAROTID ARTERY

Normal and/or Control	Hemodynamic parameters	Endothelial Cells	Media and Subendothelial Layer and IEL	Adventitia
	Q=100 -150 ml/min r=0.12 -0.15 cm wsr=950/sec wss=30dyns/cm2 Re=370	ECD=2,000 -3,000 Flat and Rhomboid Cell volume=430μm3 Nucleus volume=70μm3 Thin oblate spheroid nucleus	very thin (about 50nm) and single basement membrane	Unchanged
			Thick monotonous one layered IEL	
7 days	Q=600 -750 ml/min r=0.12 -0.15 cm wsr=4,000 -4,500/sec wss=130 -150 dyne/cm2 Re=1,500 -1,900	ECD=3,000 Protrusion of nucleic parts Microvilli Disturbance of pinocytotic vesicle Increase in cytoplasmic microfilament bundles	Thick (300 to 500nm) and multilayered basement membrane Irregularity at the luminal margin (elastogenesis)	Mostly Unchanged
4 weeks	Q=550 -700 ml/min r=0.13 -0.16 cm wsr=3,500 -4,000/sec wss=100 dyne/cm2 Re=1,400	ECD=6,000 Narrow and thick Prolate spheroid nucleus Cell volume =330 μm3 Nucleus volume=68 μm3 Increase in microfilaments	Thick and dense basement membrane Splitting & Multiplication of IEL	Increase of elastid fibers in luminal 1/3 layer Collagen was increased
6 to 12 months	Q=550 -700 ml/min r=0.15 -0.20 cm wsr=2,000 -2,500/sec wss=60 dyne/cm2 Re=1,000 -1,200	ECD=3,000 -4,000 Irregular thin Mostly thin but partly thick Flat as compaired to 4 weeks Increase in 10nm filaments	Partly thick somewhere IEL again restored	Increase of elastic fibers and collagen fibers Increase of elastic and SMC laminal structure Increase of collagen in adventitia

Fig.7
Q=blood flow rate of the common carotid artery, r=internal radius, wsr =wall shear rate, wss=wall shear stress, Re=Reynolds number, ECD=endo-thelial cell density (cells/mm2), IEL=internal elastic lamina, Viscos-ity=0.03 poise, specific gravity of blood=1.03, Hemodynamic parameters were mostly probable values.

Gefässwand ist abhängig von der Wandspannung, welche ihrerseits wieder
bestimmt wird von dem Durchmesser der Gefässlichtung und Blutdrucke.
3. Steigerung des Blutdruckes über eine bestimmte, vom Stoffwechsel
der umbebenden Gewebe abhängige Grenze, führt zur Neubildung von
Capillaren. However, the processes by which blood flow velocity
(rate), i.e. wall shear stress, regulates the blood vessel have not
been understood until now. From Kamiya and Togawa's experiments [2]
and our experiments, it is clear that Thoma's first rule (the growth
of the lumen of a vessel, that is the increase in surface of the wall,
depends upon the rate (velocity) of the blood flow) applies the canine
carotid arteries. Kamiya and Togawa supposed that the effects was due
to smooth muscle cell activation induced by wall shear stress dependent arterial wall permeability. It seems apparent from our studies
that the wall shear stress stimulates endothelial cells to proliferate. We think that this endothelial cell proliferation is the key
morphological event in inducing arterial growth.

Localization of atherosclerosis has been considered to be partly
due to differences in local blood flow. Atherosclerotic plaque in the
human carotid artery bifurcation was very localized forming "ring-like
lipid deposits" in the lateral wall of the sinus portion of the
orifice of the internal carotid artery [10]. This "ring-like lipid
deposits" corresponded to the marginal zone between the low-shear area
and the high-shear area. Although such analyses of human atherosclerosis is important, understanding of the reaction of blood vessels
to wall shear stress is essential for understanding atherogenesis.

Acknowledgements: This work was supported by a Research Grant for
Cardiovascular Diseases (60C-2) from the Japanese Ministry of Health
and Welfare and by a Grant-In-Aid, Scientific Research No.61570164,
from the Japanese Ministry of Education, Science and Culture.

REFERENCES

[1] Thoma R (1893) Untersuchung über die Histogenese und Histomechanik
des Gefässsystems. Verlag von Ferdinand Enke, Stuttgart.
[2] Kamiya A, Togawa T (1980) Am J Physiol 293:H14-21.
[3] Masuda H, Kikuchi Y, Nemoto T, Buchari A, Togawa T, Kamiya A
(1982) Biorheology 19:197-208.
[4] Masuda H, Shozawa T, Hosoda S, Kanda M, Kamiya A (1985) Heart and
Vessels 1:65-69.
[5] Masuda H, Shozawa T, Kanda M, Kamiya A (1985) Acta Pathol Jpn 35:
1037-1046.
[6] Masuda H, Saito N, Kawamura K, Sageshima M, Shozawa T, Kanazawa A
(1986) Acta Pathol Jpn 36:1833-1842.
[7] Masuda H, Saito N, Kawamura K, Sageshima M, Shozawa T, Kanazawa A
(1987) Acta Pathol Jpn 37:239-251.
[8] Masuda H, Kawamura K. Shozawa T (1987) J Jpn Soc Biorheol 1:19-
26.
[9] Kajikawa K, Yamaguchi T, Katsuda S, Miwa A (1975) J Electron
Microscopy 24:287-289.
[10] Masuda H, Shozawa T, Sageshima M (1987) J Jpn Atheroscler Soc
15:831-838.

Ultrastructural Changes in the Endothelial Surface of Rat Carotid Artery Induced by Blood Flow Load

A Scanning Electron Microscopical Study

K. Tohda, H. Masuda, K. Kawamura, and T. Shozawa

Second Department of Pathology, Akita University School of Medicine, Akita, 010 Japan

ABSTRACT

In order to investigate the effects of blood flow on endothelial cells, blood flow changes were produced by constructing an arterio-venous shunt between common carotid artery and external jugular vein in rats.   They were kept for 1 day, 3 days, 7 days, 2 weeks, 4 weeks and 8 weeks after operation.   Endothelial surface was examined by scanning electron microscopy (SEM).   Morphological changes, such as protrution of endothelial cells, microvilli-like projection and increase of endothelial cell density were observed in shunted artery at 2 and 4 weeks.   Decrease of endothelial cell density was observed at 8 weeks.   These results suggest that the wall shear stress induces proliferation of endothelial cells and may regurate arterial adaptive dilatation.

INTRODUCTION

Blood flow has been considered to play an important role not only in physiological responses such as growth in the vascular system [1,2,3], but also in pathological processes including athero-sclerosis [4].   The effect of the blood flow on the growth of vessel caliber was initially pointed out by Thoma [1] on the basis of observation in chick embryo.   Recently further studies of the flow-diameter relationship were reported by Kamiya & Togawa [2] and Guyton [3].   Masuda H. et al [5, 6] have studied morphological changes in flow loaded canine carotid arteries using the arterio-venous shunt system and have shown that endothelial cells show morphological changes in relation to shear stress.
In order to investigate the effect of blood flow on endothelial cells, we have chosen the rat carotid artery as the model system. The main reasons for our choice were as follows.   First to establish whether the morphological changes observed in flow loaded canine carotid artery were also present in smaller animals, and second if these changes did occure in smaller animals, such as rats and mice, how rapid the changes were.
In this report, we describes the rate and mode of the morphological changes in rat carotid artery by scanning electron microscopy (SEM) present in the form of the proliferative changes of endothelial cells in 7 days to 4 weeks and in the arterial adaptive regulatory process to the blood flow load in 8 weeks.

MATERIALS AND METHODS

54 male Sprague-Dawley (SD) rats (8 weeks-old, 250gr.) were used. They were anesthesized with sodium pentobarbital (50mg/kg) intraperitoneally. After the left common carotid artery and ipsilateral external jugular vein were exposed, a side to side anastomosis was constructed at about 2 cm from the aortic arch by following procedure. First the common carotid artery and external jugular vein were stabilized for about 1 mm using a microsurgical clamp. Then both vessels were incised about 1 mm long by surgical blade and sutured by 8 stitches, using 9-0 Nylon and micro-surgical devices under stereo-scopic microscope (first stitch at mid posterior wall, 2 stitches at both cut edges, 3 stitches at antrior wall and 2 stitches at posterior wall). The same level of right common carotid artery were used for the control in the same rats.

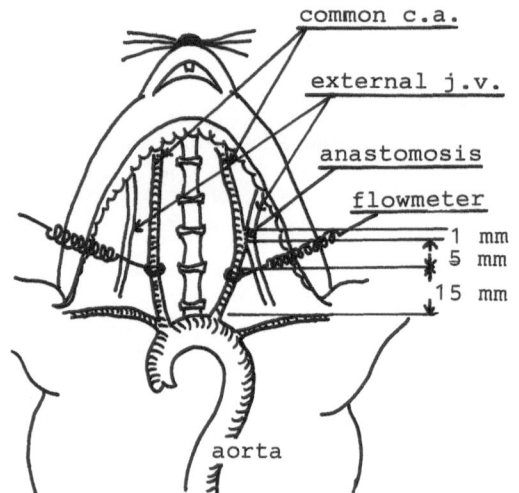

common c.a.

external j.v.

anastomosis

flowmeter

1 mm
5 mm
15 mm

aorta

Sham-operated controls were obtained by closing the anastomosis with titanium hemostatic clips before blood flowed again. They were kept for 1 day, 3 days, 1 week (3 shunted rats and one sham-operated rat in each group), 2 weeks, 4 weeks and 8 weeks (10 shunted rats and 4 sham-operated rats in each group). Blood flow rates of the common carotid arteries were measured 3 times (before anastomosis, just after anastomosis and at the final measurement) by electromagnetic flow-meter at the about 1.5 cm distal to the aortic arch and at the same level in the right control side.

At the final measurement, rats were anesthesized as before. Then fixation of the common carotid arteries was perfomed. V-5 venula was canulated in the abdominal aorta and 75 ml heparinized lactate Ringers' and sorbitol (Lactec-G injection) was injected, using the venula. Blood was drained via renal vein cut down. After the whole blood was washed out, 50 ml of 3 % glutaraldehyde solution in phosphate buffer (ph 7.4) was injected via the venula at 100 mmHg pressure. After fixation, a segment 5 mm long of the left common carotid artery at 5 mm proximal from the anastomosis was resected. A segment of the right common carotid artery at the same level was also resected for the control. Specimen were post-fixed with 1 % osmic acid solution in phosphate buffer (ph 7.4) for 1 hour at 4°C. and then dehydrated through alchohols, subjected to critical point drying and coated by evaporated gold-platinum in a high vacuum. Endothelial surface were observed by scanning electron microscopy (JEOL Co, JSMT 2001).

RESULTS

HEMODYNAMIC CHANGES: The average blood flow rate of the left
shunted common carotid artery before anastomosis was 3.1 ± 0.2 ml/
min, that after anastomosis was 17 ± 1.6 mi/min and that at the
final measurement was 22 ± 1.0 ml/min.   The blood flow rate at the
final measurement increased to about 7 times that noted before
anastomosis.   On the other hand, the average blood flow rate of the
right control side before anastomosis was 3.2 ± 0.3 ml/min, that
after anastomosis was 2.2 ± 0.2 ml/min and that at the final
measurement was 4.5 ± 0.9 ml/min.

The average blood flow rate of the left common carotid artery
of the sham-operated control rats before operation was 2.5 ± 0.2
ml/min, after operation 1.7 ± 0.3 ml/min and at the final measurement 2.1 ± 0.3 ml/min.   On the other hand, the average blood flow
rate of the right side of sham-operated control before operation
was 2.8 ± 0.3 ml/min, after operation it was 1.6 ± 0.2 ml/min and
at the final measurement flow was 2.1 ± 0.5 ml/min.

MORPHOLOGICAL CHANGES OF THE ENDOTHELIAL SURFACE: Morphological
changes such as protrusion of endothelial cells were observed as
early as 3 days (Fig. 1).   The shape of the protrusion was flat
and wide-based water-droplet like, about 11 μm in width.   A few
microvilli-like projections appeared.   In 7 days, the water-droplet
like protrusions of endothelial cells were more distinct and became
slender and tall.   Many microvilli-like projections appeared at the
tip of the protrusion.   In 2 and 4 weeks, the protrusions were
marked and tall, slender and about 4.0 μm in width (Fig. 2).
Microvilli-like projections were more distinct at the tip of the
protrusion.   A few protrusions of endothelial cells in shunted
artery of the 2 weeks group showed a cleaved appearance (Fig. 3),
suggesting an expression of mitosis.   In 8 weeks the protrusions
were still present, but were lower and their bases were wider.
Only a few protrusions showed microvilli-like projections (Fig. 4).

In the right control common carotid artery of the shunted rats,
endothelial cells were arranged like paving stones.   They were oval
rhomboid and about 12 μm in width (Fig. 5).   Protrusions were not
observed at one day, 3 days, 7 days, 2 weeks and 4 weeks, but at
8 weeks, low and small protrusions were observed (Fig. 6).   In the
sham-operated control artery, no protrusions were observed.

ENDOTHELIAL CELL DENSITY: Endothelial cell density was
determined in the 1 , 2, 4 and 8 weeks' group, using x 1000 SEM
photographs.   The endothelial cell density of the left and right
common carotid artery of the sham-operated control was about 3300
cells/mm^2.   The density of the left shunted artery in one day and
3 days was almost equal to the right control side.   In 7 days, the
endothelial cell density increased about 1.4 times as many as right
control side.   In 2 weeks, the density was about 7300 cells/mm^2,
which was two times as many as that of the right control side (about
3700 cells/mm^2).   In 4 weeks, the density still increased (about
7200 cells/mm^2).   But in 8 weeks, the endothelial cell density
decreased to the level about 3900 cells/mm^2, which was almost equal
to the right control level (about 3500 cells/mm^2).

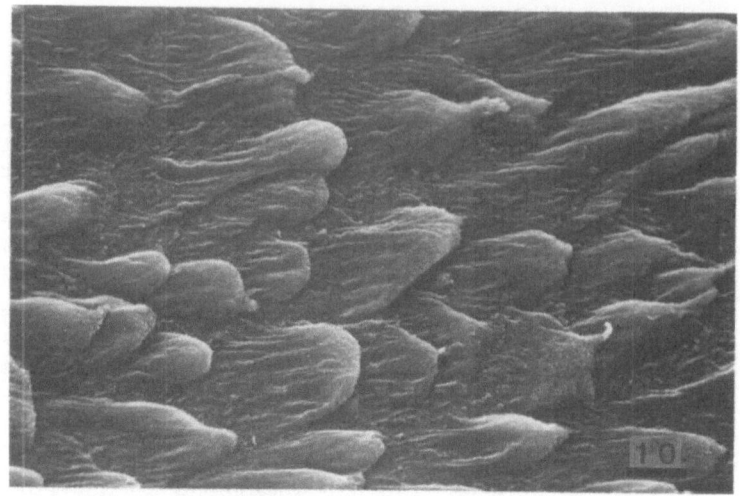

(Fig. 1) Endothelial surface of the shunted rat common carotid
artery of 3 days' group. Blood flow rate at final measurement =
19.5 ml/min (3.3 ml/min before anastomosis). Endothelial cells
start to protrude. The protrusion is flat, water-droplet like and
about 11 μm in width. The density of endothelial cell is not high.
Bar = 10 μm, scanning electron microscope (SEM).

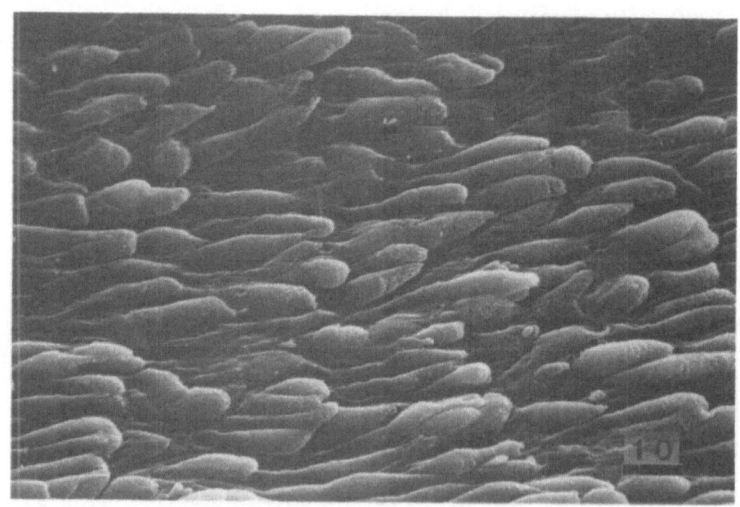

(Fig. 2) Endothelial surface of the shunted rat common carotid
artery of 4 weeks' group. Blood flow rate at final measurement =
17.5 ml/min (4.4 ml/min before anastomosis). The protrusions is
slender, tall and about 4.0 μm in width with microvilli-like
projections at its tip. The density of endothelial cell is high (
about 7200 cells/mm^2). Bar = 10 μm, (SEM).

175

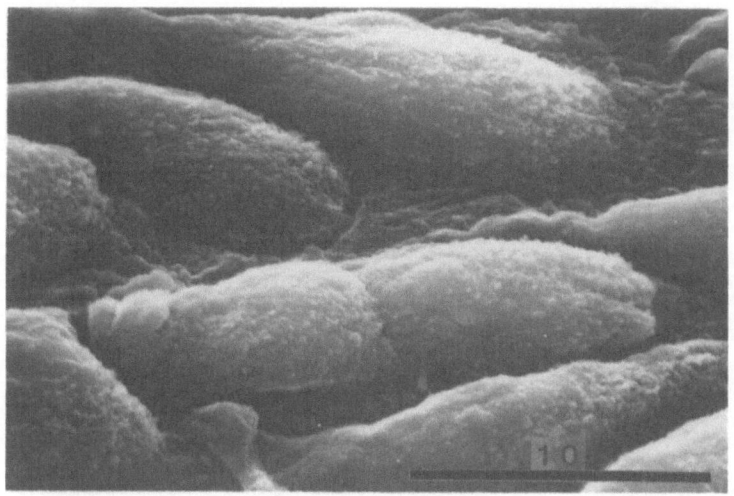

(Fig. 3) A few protrusions of endothelial cells in shunted artery of
2 weeks' group show cleaved appearance. They seem an expression of
mitosis of endothelial cells. Bar = 10 µm, (SEM).

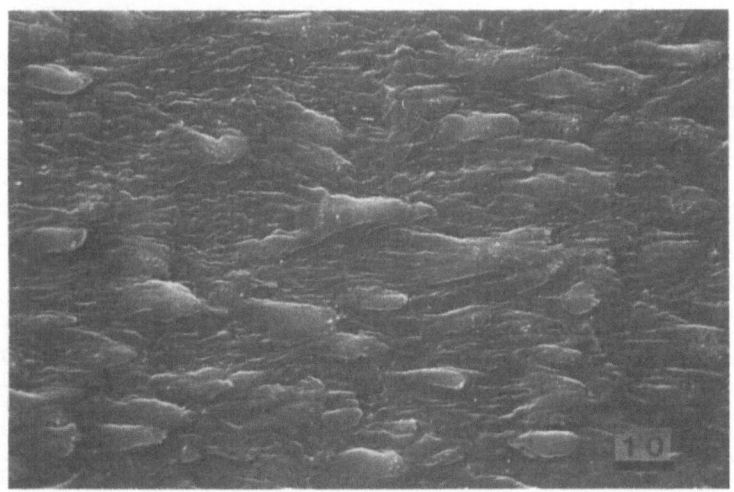

(Fig. 4) Endothelial surface of the shunted rat common carotid
artery of 8 weeks' group. Blood flow rate at final measurement =
29.9 ml/min (2.3 ml/min before anastomosis). The protrusions are
still present but its height is low and its width is short, about
5.5 um. The density of endothelial cell(about 3900 cells/mm^2) is
almost equal to the control side (about 3500 cells/mm^2).
Bar = 10 µm, (SEM).

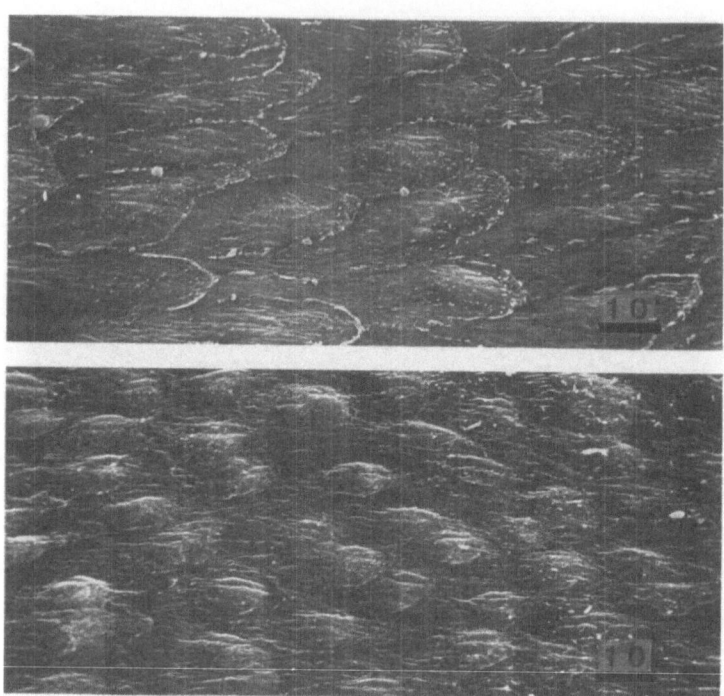

(Fig. 5) Endothelial surface of the right control side of the rat
common carotid artery of 3 days' group. Blood flow rate at final
measurement = 3.0 ml/min (2.2 ml/min before anastomosis). Protrusions are not observed. The endothelial cell is oval, rhomboid and
about 12 µm in width. Bar = 10 µm, (SEM).
(Fig. 6) Endothelial surface of the right control side of the rat
common carotid artery of 8 weeks' group. Blood flow rate at final
measurement = 6.1 ml/min (3.3 ml/min before anastomosis). The low
and small protrusions are observed. Bar = 10 µm, (SEM).

DISCUSSION

     In the present experiment, we demonstrated the blood flow
changes in the rat common carotid artery shunted to external jugular
vein, using microsurgical technique.   Small animals such as rat
were more suitable than canine to investigate the morphological and
physiological changes because of its uniformity, small specimen and
life span.   All shunted common carotid arteries consistently showed
highly elevated blood flow rate, 7 times greater than the right
control side.   We found that the morphologic changes of endothelial
cells were striking.   The protrusions and microvilli-like projections of the endothelial cells in the shunted artery appeared as
early as 3 days and changed their shapes in their course of the
experiments (3 days to 8 weeks).   Those changes were most remarkable
at 2 and 4 weeks, and at 8 weeks they were similar to the right
control side.   Moreover increased endothelial cell density (about

2 times as many as right control side) was found at 2 and 4 weeks. The density decreased again and was at nearly the control level at 8 weeks.

The findings include that endothelial cells are activated as early as 3 days after anastomosis, proliferative soon after, are compactly arranged in the non-dilated luminal surface until 4 weeks, and then cease to be activated. If they are not desquamated, the increased endothelial cells would be rearranged similarly to the control level on the dilated luminal surface by 8 weeks.
We consider that these dynamic morphological changes represent the remodeling of the artery in response to the elevated blood flow rate.

Although we intend to measure the circumferencial length of the transverse section of common carotid artery and have as yet no sufficient data on the arterial diameter, we believe that the arterial diameter would be little changed in the early stage after anastomosis (one day to 3 days), would be slightly enlarged at 7 days to 4 weeks and would be quite enlarged at 8 weeks, on the basis of the experimental data on the canine carotid artery by Kamiya & Togawa and Masuda H. et al.   Therefore the wall shear stress would be highest in 1 day to 3 days, it would slightly decrease in 7 days to 4 weeks and it would be nearly at the control level in 8 weeks. These changes of the wall shear seem to correspond to the endothelial cell morphologic and density changes.

Compared to the canine carotid artery, the protrusions of endothelial cells and microvilli-like projections were similar in rat shunted common carotid artery.   Changes in rat common carotid artery in 2 weeks corresponded to those in the canine at 4 weeks. And the changes of rat carotid in 8 weeks corresponded to those of canine at 6 months.   The endothelial surface of the rat common carotid artery showed more rapid morphological changes and more uniform hemodynamic data than that of dog.   These relationship of the arterial changes to blood flow, i.e. wall shear stress, coprresponded to those demonstrated for the canine carotid artery by Masuda H. et al.

The stimulation of endothelial cells induced by wall shear stress could be an important factor on the localization of the atherosclerosis.

Acknowledgement: This work was supported by a Research Grant for Cardiovascular Disease (60C-2) from the Japanese Ministry of Health and Welfare and by a Grant-In-Aid, Scientific Research No.61570164, from the Japanese Ministry of Education, Science and Culture.

REFERENCES

[1]Thoma R (1893) Untersuchungen uber die Histogenese und Histomechanik des Gefasssystems. Stuttgart, Verlag von Ferdinand Enke
[2]Kamiya A, Togawa T (1980) Am J Pathol 248:540-549
[3]Guyton JR, Hartly CJ (1985) Am J Pathol 248:540-549
[4]Giddens DP, Zarins CK, Glagov S, Bharadvaj BK (1983) Flow and Atherogenesis in the Human Carotid Bifurcation. In: Schettler G, Neren RM, Schmid-Schönbein H, Morl H, Diehm C(eds) Fluid Dynamics as a Localizing Factor for Atherosclerosis. Springer-Verlag, Berlin Heiderberg New York Tokyo, pp 38-45
[5]Masuda H, Kikuchi Y, Nemoto T, Bukhari A, Togawa T, Kamiya A (1982) Biorheology 19:197-208
[6]Masuda H, Shozawa T, Hosoda S, Kanda M, Kamiya A (1985) Heart and Vessels 1:65-69

Distribution of Wall Shear Stress and Microfilament Bundles in Endothelial Cells in Canine Coronary Artery *in vivo*

A. KITABATAKE[1], J. TANOUCHI[1], M. UEMATSU[1], K. ISHIHARA[1], K. FUJII[1], Y. YOSHIDA[1], H. ITO[1], M. HORI[1], N. TOMINAGA[1], H. YOSHIMURA[2], and T. KAMADA[1]

[1]The First Department of Medicine, Osaka University School of Medicine, Osaka, 553 Japan
[2]Nippon Zoki Pharmaceutical Co., Ltd., Hyogo, 673-14 Japan

ABSTRACT

The relation between wall shear stress (SS) in vivo and the micro-filament bundles (MF) in endothelial cells (EC) in the left anterior descending coronary artery (LAD) was investigated in 5 mongrel dogs. Peak shear stress was determined from the flow velocity profile at its peak velocity using a multigate 20 MHz pulsed Doppler velocimeter. Peak SS at the outer side in LAD was significantly greater than that at the cardiac side. The amount of MF in EC was evaluated in the excised vessel segments with transmission electron microscopy as the ratio of the area filled with MF to the total area of EC (F/C). F/C at the outer side was significantly greater than that at the cardiac side. These results suggested that SS increases the amount of MF in EC in canine coronary artery in vivo.

INTRODUCTION

The influence of local hemodynamics on the vascular wall has been implicated in the process of atherogenesis by many investigators. As an example, Sabbah et al reported that in human coronary artery, atherosclerotic lesions were more prevalent at the cardiac side, where the shear stress was estimated lower than the outer side [1]. In cultured endothelial cells, microfilaments, one of the major elements of cytoskeleton, have been found to increase when the cells are exposed to high shear stress [2,3]. However, the in vivo relation between local shear stress and the distribution of microfilament bundles in endothelial cells still remains speculative, mainly because of the methodological limitations to measure the fine structure of blood flow in vivo. We used a multigate high frequency pulsed Doppler technique to determine the wall shear stress in vivo and focused on the relation between local wall shear stress and the cytoskeletal structure of the endothelial cells in canine coronary artery.

METHODS

Animal preparation. We used 5 mongrel dogs (9-13 kg, average weight 12.5 kg), studied under sodium pentobarbital anesthesia (30 mg/kg body weight). The chest was opened and the proximal portion of the left anterior descending coronary artery (LAD) was carefully exposed to measure blood flow velocity. Immediately after the flow measurement, the dogs were perfused and fixed with 2% glutaraldehyde in cacodylate buffer (pH 7.3) at a constant pressure of 100 mmHg for transmission electron microscopic examination of the vascular endothelial cells.

Blood flow measurements. We used a multigate high frequency pulsed Doppler velocimeter (Fujitsu ME-110A) to obtain the blood flow velocity profile. The detailed specifications of the apparatus have been described elsewhere [4]. In brief, the carrier frequency of the apparatus was 20 MHz, with a pulse repetition rate of 50KHz. It enabled us to measure flow velocities at 80 points simultaneously along the ultrasonic beam within the depth of 15 mm with the zero-crossing method. Each sample size was 1 mm in lateral direction and 0.19 mm in depth. Thus we could obtain flow velocity profiles within a vessel in vivo without exerting any influence on the flow itself.

Blood flow velocity was measured at the proximal portion of LAD. The 20 MHz ultrasonic transducer was placed with a Doppler angle of incidence of 60 degrees against the vessel axis using a plastic cuff. Care was taken not to change the shape and direction of the vessel. The data obtained were digitized and stored in floppy disks using a 16-bit microcomputer (Fujitsu FM-11) for the calculation of shear stress.

Calculation of shear stress. We obtained flow velocity profiles in the LAD from 12 to 16 point flow velocities simultaneously measured by the Doppler velocimeter at the time when the centerline reached its peak velocity. Then the velocity gradient at each wall, where the velocity equals zero, was calculated as peak shear rate. Assuming that the blood viscosity has a constant value of 0.035 g/cm·sec, peak shear stress was determined as peak shear rate multiplied by 0.035.

Transmission electron microscopic examinations. After perfusion-fixation of the animals, the proximal portion of LAD was excised and the transmission electron photomicrographs of the endothelial cells (x17,220) were taken using a Hitachi H-600 in longitudinal as well as in transverse sections against the vessel axis. In each picture, the area of microfilament bundles (F), where more than 5 microfilaments were assembled together, and the area of a whole endothelial cell (C) were measured using a digitizer (Graphtec KD4030A). The amount of microfilament bundles was semi-quantified by calculating the F/C ratio.

RESULTS

Coronary flow characteristics in vivo. The peak flow velocity was observed in early diastole in the LAD, while in the subclavian artery (SA) or thoracic descending aorta (DA), it was observed in mid-systole. The peak flow velocity in the LAD (34±6 cm/sec) was lower than that in the SA (91±22 cm/sec, $p < 0.01$) or DA (94±17 cm/sec, $p < 0.01$). The flow velocity profile at its peak in the LAD skewed toward the outer side (Fig. 1). Therefore, the peak wall shear stress at the outer side was significantly greater than that at the cardiac side in the LAD (44.8±5.5 vs 21.2±4.3 dyne/cm^2, $p < 0.001$).

Microfilament bundles in endothelial cells. Microfilaments were observed as fine filaments of 6-7 nm in diameter in electron photomicrographs of longitudinal sections as shown in Fig. 2 and a fine dotted pattern in those of transverse sections. Thus they were considered to be oriented parallel to the vessel axis, i.e., the direction of blood flow. Comparing the amount of microfilament bundles in the endothelial cells at the outer side with that at the cardiac side in LAD (Fig. 3), F/C at the outer side was significantly greater than that at the cardiac side (18.9±9.8 % vs 12.7±6.1 %, p<0.01).

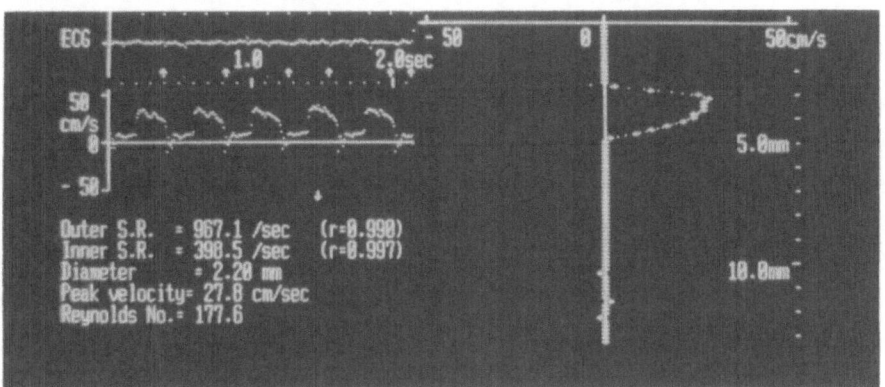

Fig. 1 Coronary flow velocity profile at its peak assessed by multigate 20 MHz pulsed Doppler velocimeter (right). The profile skewed toward the outer side in the LAD. The left panel shows the time sequential changes in the peak flow velocity (left upper) and the shear rates (left lower).

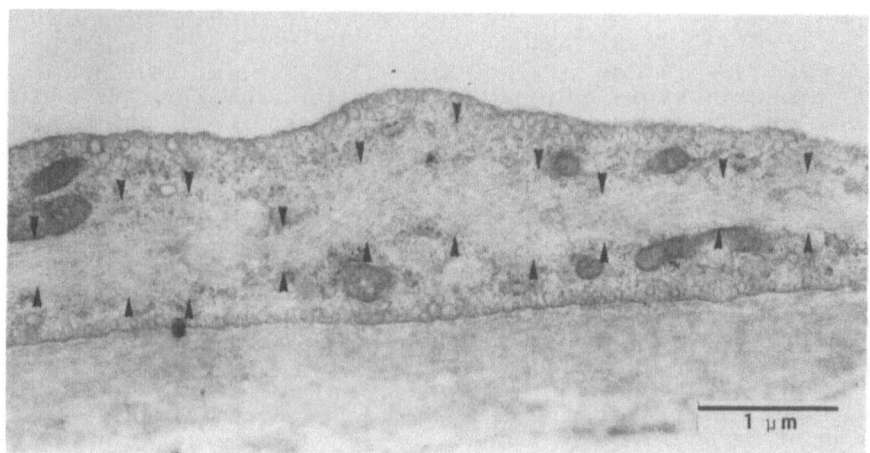

Fig. 2 Transmission electron photomicrograph of an endothelial cell in canine left anterior descending coronary artery (longitudinal section). There was a bundle of microfilaments oriented parallel to the vessel axis as indicated by the black triangles.

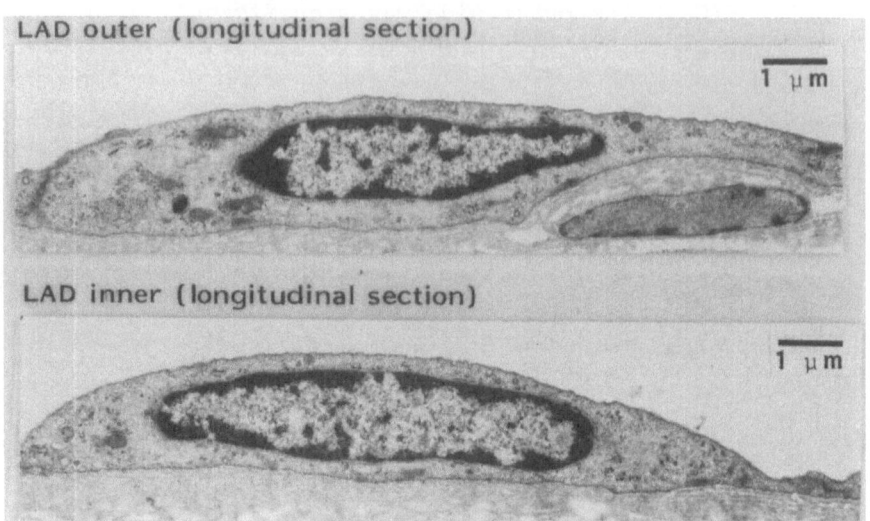

Fig. 3 Transmission electron photomicrographs of the endothelial cells at the outer side and at the cardiac side in the LAD. Microfilaments were more widely distributed in the cell from the outer wall.

DISCUSSION

In this study we determined the wall shear stress _in vivo_ in the canine coronary artery by a multigate high frequency pulsed Doppler technique, and the relation between wall shear stress and the distribution of microfilament bundles in coronary endothelial cells was assessed.

Microfilament bundles in endothelial cells, which is an important structure in the support of the membrane and in the maintenance of cell shape, were reported to increase _in vitro_ when exposed to high shear stress [2,3]. The _in vivo_ distribution of microfilament bundles has also been studied using vertebrate vascular endothelial cells [5,6]. As an example, in the thoracic descending aorta, the microfilament bundles were widely distributed and oriented parallel to the direction of flow, while in the inferior vena cava there were very few microfilaments with no preferred orientation. Furthermore, using an arterio-venous shunt method, microfilaments in endothelial cells have also been reported to increase _in vivo_ under the condition of increased blood flow [7]. Since the veins might be expected to have lower shear stresses than the arteries, and the increased flow volume might result in an increase in shear stress, these results have suggested that local hemodynamic factors, especially shear stress, may influence the abundance of microfilaments in the cytoskeletal structure. Nevertheless, this conclusion has remained speculative due to the limitation of measuring shear stress _in vivo_. In the present study, we used a high frequency multigate pulsed Doppler technique, which enabled us to obtain instantaneous blood flow velocity profiles in vivo without exerting any influence on the flow itself. Shear rate could be calculated from the velocity gradient at the wall and the shear stress was determined as shear rate multiplied by blood viscosity. The high resolution of this Doppler technique enabled us to measure the flow in small vessels like the LAD. Thus we could compare shear stresses in vivo with the distribution of microfilament bundles in endothelial cells in the canine coronary artery.

In the proximal portion of left anterior descending coronary artery, the distribution of microfilament bundles in the endothelial cells at the outer side was more prominent than that at the cardiac side, where peak shear stress at the outer side was greater than that at the cardiac side. The difference in peak shear stress between the outer side and the cardiac side might be due to the curving of the vessel along the epicardium. These findings suggest that in the canine coronary artery, microfilaments, one of the major elements of cytoskeleton, may increase under the condition of high shear stress in vivo.

It might be expected that at an early stage in atherogenesis the cytoskeleton of endothelial cells could play an important role in determining the permeability of endothelium to macromolecules and/or migrating cells such as monocytes [8,9]. In this aspect, endothelial cells exposed to high shear stress would have a more highly developed cytoskeletal structure as an adaptation to its mechanical stress environment, which could suppress transcellular and/or junctional transport. Thus, in low shear regions, the influx of macromolecules such as LDL and cellular components like macrophages would have increased, resulting in a higher predilection for the initiation of atherogenesis. We demonstrated the distribution of local wall shear stress and microfilament bundles in endothelial cells in the canine coronary artery under physiological condition. Although further analyses are needed for pathologically altered shear stresses, and the relation between the structure and the function of the endothelial cells remains to be clarified, the present study suggests a possible link between local hemodynamic forces and the initiation of atherogenesis.

Acknowledgment: This work was supported in part by a Research Grant for Cardiovascular Diseases (60C-2) from the Ministry of the Health and Welfare, Japan, and by a Grant-in-Aid for Scientific Research (61570415) from the Ministry of Education, Japan.

REFERENCES

[1] Sabbah HN, Khaja F, Hawkins ET, Brymer JF, McFarland TM, van der Bel-Kahn J, Doerger PT, Stein PD (1986) Relation of atherosclerosis to arterial wall shear in the left anterior descending coronary artery of man. Am Heart J 112: 453-458
[2] Franke RP, Graefe M, Schnittler H, Seiffge D, Mittermayer C (1984) Induction of human vascular endothelial stress fibers by fluid shear stress. Nature 307: 648-649

[3] Wechezak AR, Viggers RF, Sauvage LR (1985) Fibronectin and F-actin redistribution in cultured endothelial cells exposed to shear stress. Laboratory Investigation 53: 639-647

[4] Kajiya F, Ogasawara Y, Tsujioka K, Nakai M, Goto M, Wada Y, Tadaoka S, Matsuoka S, Mito K, Fujiwara T (1986) Evaluation of human coronary blood flow with an 80 channel 20 MHz pulsed Doppler velocimeter and zero-cross and Fourier transform methods during cardiac surgery. Circulation 74(suppl III), 53-60

[5] White GE, Gimbrone MA Jr, Fujiwara K (1983) Factors influencing the expression of stress fibers in vascular endothelial cells in vivo. J Cell Biol 97: 414-424

[6] Wong AJ, Herman IM, Pollard TD (1983) Actin filament stress fibers in vascular endothelial cells in vivo. Science 219: 867-869

[7] Masuda H, ·Shozawa T, Hosoda S, Kanda M, Kamiya A (1985) Cytoplasmic microfilaments in endothelial cells of flow loaded canine carotid arteries. Heart and Vessels 1: 65-64

[8] Shasby DM, Shasby SS, Sullivan JM, Peach MJ (1982) Role of endothelial cell cytoskeleton in control of endothelial permeability. Circ Res 51: 657-661

[9] Wysolmerski R, Lagunoff D (1985) The effect of ethchlorvynol on cultured endothelial cells: a model for the study of the mechanism of increased vascular permeability. Am J Pathol 119: 505-512

Adaptive Enlargement of Arteries in Response to Increased Flow and Increased Intimal Plaque

C.K. Zarins[1], S. Glagov[2], and D.P. Giddens[3]

[1] Department of Surgery, University of Chicago, Chicago, IL 60637, USA
[2] Dapartment of Pathology, University of Chicago, Chicago, IL 60637, USA
[3] The School of Mechanical Engineering, Georgia Institute of Technology, Atlanta, GA 30332-0405, USA

ABSTRACT

We studied adaptive changes in artery diameter in response to increased blood flow and increasing intimal plaque. Experimental increase in blood flow through an arteriovenous fistula resulted in an increase in lumen diameter such that wall shear stress was normalized. Increasing intimal plaque in human coronary arteries resulted in arterial enlargement which acted to counter or prevent lumen stenosis. Such enlargement was effective in preventing left main coronary stenosis in arteries with plaques occupying less than 40% of the internal elastic lamina. In the distal left anterior descending coronary artery, the most diseased arteries overcompensated and had enlargement of the lumen despite the presence of extensive plaques. The development of stenosis, preservation of a normal lumen caliber or lumen enlargement may depend on local differences in response and on the relative rates of plaque deposition and compensatory arterial enlargement.

INTRODUCTION

Shear stress has been implicated in the pathogenesis of atherosclerotic lesions and in the localization of plaques at certain points in the arterial tree[1]. Shear stress has also been implicated as being important in the regulation of artery size[2]. It has long been recognized that during embryologic development, arteries with high flow enlarge, while those with low flow diminish in size. We experimentally increased blood flow in monkeys by creating a right iliac arteriovenous fistula[3]. This resulted in an immediate increase in wall shear stress and served to stimulate arterial dilation. After 6 months, blood flow was increased 10-fold in the right iliac artery compared to the left iliac and flow velocity was increased more than 2-fold. However, wall shear stress in the right iliac (16 ± 4 dynes/cm^2) was the same as in the left (15 ± 2 dynes/cm^2) because of a 2-fold increase in lumen diameter[3]. Thus, the artery had enlarged sufficiently to normalize wall shear stress.

Intimal plaque deposition has the effect of decreasing arterial lumen diameter. This results in a focal lumen stenosis and a local increase in flow velocity and wall shear stress at the site of the intimal plaque. The expected adaptive response to the increase in wall shear stress would be arterial dilation at that site. Arterial enlargement has been demonstrated in response to diet-induced atherosclerosis in experimental animals[4]. To determine whether adaptive arterial enlargement in response to enlarging intimal plaques occurs in human atherosclerotic arteries, we studied sections of the left main[5] and left anterior descending coronary artery[6] in pressure perfusion-fixed adult postmortem hearts.

MATERIAL AND METHODS

Adult hearts obtained at autopsy were weighed and fixed by controlled-pressure perfusion of the coronary arteries with 10 percent formalin for 90 minutes at 100 mmHg. After fixation, the coronary tree was injected with a warm, liquid barium-gelatin mixture under controlled pressure and immersed in cold formalin to solidify the mixture and prevent collapse of the arterial tree. Sections were taken of the left main coronary artery and at 4 standard locations of the left anterior descending (LAD) coronary artery. Microscopical sections were projected onto a digitizing plate for quantitative determination of lumen area, intimal plaque area and the area encompassed by the internal elastic lamina (IEL). The IEL area was considered to be a measure of artery size or potential lumen area if no atherosclerotic plaque were present. The relationship of artery size to intimal plaque area and other variables was evaluated by regression analysis.

RESULTS

For the left main coronary artery and at each level of the left anterior descending coronary artery, there was a positive correlation between artery size (IEL area) and intimal plaque area (lesion area). The correlation was highly significant at each level (p <.001) indicating that enlargement of the artery corresponds closely to increases in intimal plaque area.

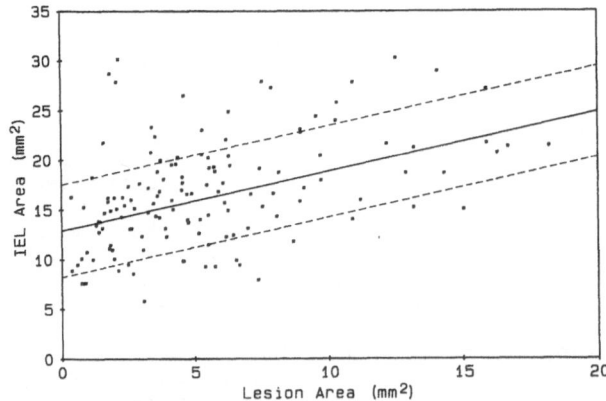

Figure 1: Graph showing positive correlation between artery size (IEL area) and intimal plaque (Lesion area) in the left main coronary artery. Reproduced with permission from Glagov et al (1987) "Compensatory Enlargement of Human Atherosclerotic Coronary Arteries" N Eng J Med. 316(22):1371-1375.

Stepwise regression analysis revealed that intimal plaque was the primary determinant of artery size at all locations in the left coronary artery. Age and heart weight were minor determinants in the left main coronary, but were an order of magnitude less than intimal plaque area in determining artery size.

When lumen area was plotted against percent stenosis, expressed as the percent of IEL area occupied by intimal plaque, the data points fell into two regions. In arteries with less than 40 percent stenosis, there was no relation between lumen area and percent stenosis indicating that arterial enlargement kept pace with increasing plaque and thus prevented the development of stenosis. Where plaque resulted in more than 40 percent stenosis, however, lumen area decreased in direct relation to the percentage of stenosis suggesting a failure of the compensatory adaptive process[5].

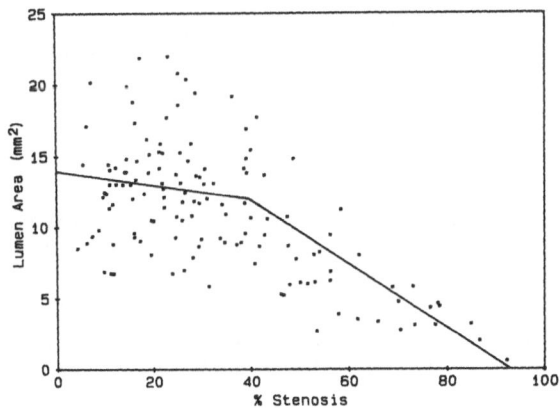

Figure 2. Lumen area plotted against percent stenosis. For stenoses less than 40 percent, there is no decrease in lumen area due to arterial enlargement. For stenoses greater than 40 percent, increased plaque results in progressive lumen stenosis. Reproduced with permission from Glagov et al (1987) "Compensatory Enlargement of Human Atherosclerotic Coronary Arteries" N Eng J Med 316(22):1371-1375.

The rate of increase in artery size relative to the increase in plaque area differed at different sites in the coronary tree. In the left main and proximal LAD, the rate of increase in artery size was less than the rate of increase in plaque area (0.60 for the left main and 0.76 for the proximal LAD). In the mid LAD, the rate of increase in artery size was the same as the increase in plaque area (1.1). However in the distal LAD, artery size increased at a greater rate (1.6) than plaque area. These differences resulted in the development of stenosis at the most diseased left main and proximal LAD levels, a normal lumen caliber in the mid LAD and an increase in lumen diameter distally in the most severely diseased LAD arteries[6]. Thus there are local differences in the adaptive response to increasing intimal plaque. Overcompensation with increasing lumen diameter as well as inadequate compensation with decreasing lumen diameter can occur. The mechanism of this response and its regulation require further study.

CONCLUSION

Local hemodynamic conditions are important in regulating artery size. Increases in blood flow and increases in intimal plaque deposition result in compensatory arterial enlargement possibly by the mechanism of restoring wall shear stress to normal. Such arterial enlargement can prevent or limit lumen stenosis in arthersclerotic arteries. Clinically, local differences in the relative rates of plaque growth and artery enlargement may determine whether clinically significant stenoses develop, whether normal lumen area is preserved or whether there is lumen enlargement.

ACKNOWLEDGEMENT

This work was supported by:

National Institutes of Health grant HL15062 and
National Science Foundation grant CME 7921551

REFERENCES

[1]. Zarins CK, Giddens DP, Bharadvaj BK, Sottiurai VS, Mabon RF, Glagov S. (1983) Carotid bifurcation atherosclerosis: Quantitative correlation of plaque localization with flow velocity profiles and wall shear stress. Circ Res 53:502-514.

[2]. Kamiya A, Togawa T. (1980) Adaptive regulation of wall shear stress to flow change in the canine carotid artery. Am J Physiol 239:H14-H21.

[3]. Zarins CK, Zatina MA, Giddens DP, Ku DN, Glagov S. (1987) Shear stress regulation of artery lumen diameter in experimental atherogenesis. J Vasc Surg 5:413-20.

[4]. Bond MG, Adams MR, Bullock BC. (1981) Complicating factors in evaluating coronary artery atherosclerosis. Artery 9:21-9.

[5]. Glagov S, Weisenberg E, Zarins CK, Stankunavicius R, Kolettis GJ. (1987) Compensatory enlargement of human atherosclerotic coronary arteries. N Engl J Med 316:1371-5.

[6]. Zarins CK, Weisenberg E, Kolettis GJ, Stankunavicius R, Glagov S. Differential enlargement of artery segments in response to enlarging atherosclerotic plaques. Submitted to the J of Vasc Surg.

The Effect of a Fluid-Imposed Shear Stress on the Mechanical Properties of Cultured Endothelial Cells

M. Sato[1], M.J. Levesque[2], and R.M. Nerem[2]

[1] Institute of Basic Medical Sciences, University of Tsukuba, Tsukuba, 305 Japan
[2] Biomechanics Laboratory and School of Mechanical Engineering, Georgia Institute of Technology, Atlanta, GA 30332-0405, USA

ABSTRACT

The mechanical properties of cultured bovine aortic endothelial cells exposed to a fluid-imposed shear stress were studied using the micropipette technique. The cells, which were attached to a Thermanox plastic substrate, were exposed to a specific steady or pulsatile shear stress. The cells exposed to shear stress demonstrated a mechanical stiffness which was significantly larger than those of control cells, being dependent both on the level of shear stress and the duration of exposure. The cells exposed to pulsatile shear stress became much stiffer in their mechanical property than those exposed to steady shear stress. This effect was particularly dramatic in the case of high shear stress.

INTRODUCTION

Although there is considerable indirect evidence that hemodynamic forces are a factor in the process of atherogenesis, the detailed mechanisms are still poorly understood and the precise role is uncertain [1,2]. Recently, hemodynamic forces have been found to affect the shape and orientation of endothelial cells studied both in vivo and in vitro [3-7]. When endothelial cells are exposed to a fluid-imposed shear stress the process of adaptation or response is expected to involve not only cell orientation and elongation, but also a change in the supporting, internal structure. Furthermore, this could be reflected in the mechanical properties of the endothelial cells, and any change in these properties could be important to the deformation a cell undergoes as part of the adaptation process. Such properties would appear to be a close correlate of cell structure and function. In this study, the mechanical properties of cultured bovine endothelial cells, exposed to either a steady or pulsatile fluid-imposed shear stress and then detached, were studied using the micropipette technique. These data demonstrate an important effect of shear stress on the mechanical properties of the endothelial cell.

METHODS

Bovine aortic endothelial cells cultured in our laboratory on Thermanox plastic coverslips were used. Fully confluent cultured endothelial cell populations from the 7th to 9th generation were studied. The age or passage time of the cultures varied from 2 to 9 days. The cells were exposed to a steady shear stress using a parallel plate flow chamber. The description of the flow chamber and the analysis of the laminar fluid flow have been reported previously [6]. Cultured endothelial cells on a coverslip with a diameter of 13 mm were positioned in the central part of the flow chamber. This flow chamber had a flow section which was 220 μm in height, 17 mm in width, and 50 mm in length. The chamber, a reservoir, and a circulation circuit were filled with culture medium (modified Dulbecco medium (MDM), containing 25 mmol/l Hepes buffer and 20 % fetal bovine serum and antibiotics). The endothelial cells in the chamber were exposed to a specific shear stress condition defined by the dimensions of the flow chamber and the pressure drop across the chamber. The MDM in the reservoir was kept at a constant temperature of 37 ± 0.5 °C. A gas mixture of 95 % air and 5 % CO_2 was provided to the MDM in the reservoir. The exposure time of cells to shear stress was in the range of 0.5 to 24 hours and the shear stress imposed on the cell population was either 10, 30, or 85 dynes/cm². In another series of experiments, pulsatile shear stress of either 7 ± 4, 30 ± 15, or 50 ± 25 dynes/cm² was applied to the cells by a roller pump using the same flow chamber.

After exposure of cells to a known shear stress and for a specified length of time, the endothelial cells were detached from their substrate by scratching the coverslip with a sterile wood stick. The sheet of cell aggregates was detached further by aspiration through a 1 ml pipette. Before measurement, endothelial cell suspensions were stirred for approximately 15 seconds on a test-tube stirrer. The prepared cells were studied at room temperature and as soon as possible after detachment, usually within 6 hours. Cell shape and the measured mechanical properties did not show any significant change with time during this period.

Micropipettes with an internal diameter ranging from 2.0 to 3.4 μm (2.7 ± 0.95 μm), were prepared from glass tubes with the use of a micropipette puller. The micropipette was filled through a 0.2 μm membrane filter with the same MDM used for the cell culture by use of a 1 ml syringe. This fluid-filled micropipette was connected to a pressure control line and was fixed to the stage of the microscope. A schematic diagram of the experimental system used is shown in Fig. 1. The details of this measuring system and the methods were already reported in previous papers [8,9]. The endothelial cell suspension was loaded into the cell chamber (1 mm in height and 10 mm in width) which was held by a manipulator. The suspended cells were observed through a long working distance objective lens (x20 or x100) under the microscope. The tip of the micropipette was made to approach the surface of a spherical endothelial cell by manipulating both the cell chamber and the stage of the microscope. To determine the zero pressure level, the height of the reservoir was changed by a slight adjustment of the micrometer so as to just maintain the cell in its initial position. First, a negative pressure of about 2 mmH_2O was set by using the micrometer, and then a portion of the endothelial cell was aspirated into the micropipette. In preliminary experiments, the aspirated part of the cell continued to deform after the application of pressure, but an almost steady state was observed to occur within 8-10 minutes. Therefore, in our experiments the negative pressure was maintained for 10 minutes at each setting and then increased in a stepwise fashion several times. In this way, the aspirated length (L) of the membrane in the micropipette was measured at several different negative pressures (ΔP) during the loading process. After the aspirated length of the cell membrane had attained a length twice the radius of the micropipette, the negative pressure was decreased and the cell was unloaded. The image of the cell shape and the deformation process was observed by a TV camera and was recorded on a video tape recorder. After each experiment, the aspirated length of the cell was measured on a TV monitor screen by replaying the recorded tape.

The data in the form of L versus ΔP represent, in effect, a stress-strain relationship. The data are presented here in the form of a mechanical stiffness parameter, $K = Rx\Delta P/(L/R)$, where $Rx\Delta P$ is the tension being exerted and L/R is the nondimensional strain imposed on the cell (R is the micropipette radius) [9]. With the use of a Minc

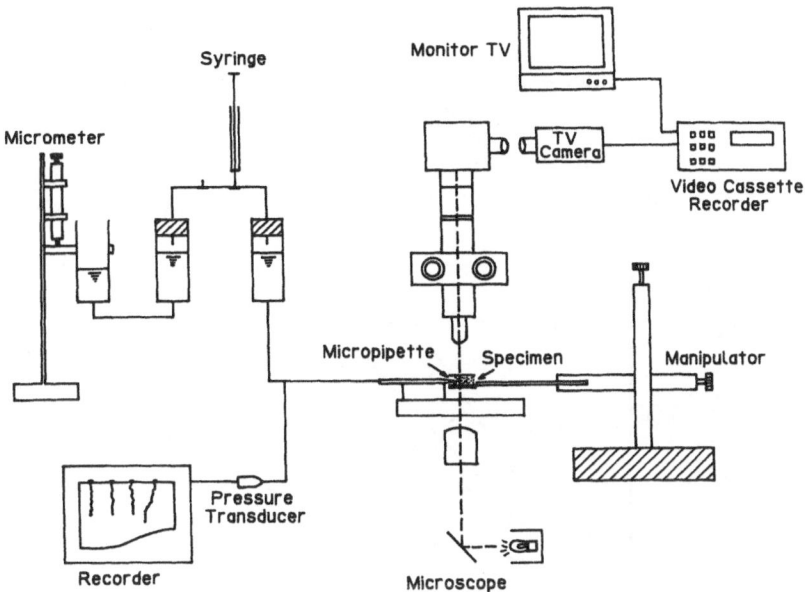

Fig. 1 Schematic diagram of the experimental setup for the micropipette technique. The left part of the diagram shows the pressure reservoirs and pressure measuring device. The center shows the micropipette and cell suspension on the microscope stage. The top shows the data acquisition system.

II microcomputer, linear regression analysis was performed on individual experiments using a least-squares curve fit. In cell experiments, it was possible to assess linearity over the full range of pressures.

RESULTS AND DISCUSSION

The characteristics of changes in the configuration of endothelial cells during or after exposure to shear have been shown previously [6,9]. During exposure to shear, the en face shape of the cells on the substrate became more elongated and their long axis became oriented to the direction of flow. This change was dependent on both the level of shear stress and the duration to exposure. After detachment, the cells exposed to shear maintained their deformed shape. This is in contrast to cells in a static, no-flow environment which became spherical in shape upon detachment. Furthermore, the degree of elongation appears to depend on the level of the shear stress to which the cell has been exposed.

The cells exposed to high shear stress were stiffer than cells exposed to a low shear or to a static, no-flow condition. This is evidenced by the fact that a larger suction pressure was needed to deform the cell to the same extent. An example of this is shown in Fig. 2 where a typical loading curve is shown for cells exposed to shear stresses of 10, 30, and 85 dynes/cm^2, respectively, as well as for a cell from a control, no-flow condition. As may be seen from Fig. 2, the relationship between the pressure difference and the aspirated length is approximately linear during the loading process [8,9]. The slope of such a relationship is used to define the stiffness parameter, K. Values of the mechanical stiffness parameter, $K = R \times \Delta P/(L/R)$, obtained from cells exposed to shear stress for different

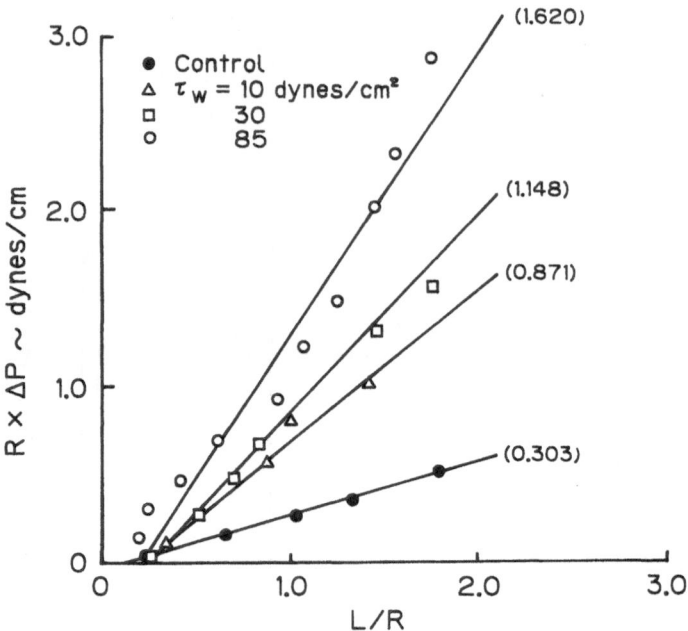

Fig. 2 Effects of shear stress on the stress-strain response
of endothelial cells. RxΔP is the tension imposed on the
cell and L/R is the nondimensional length of aspiration,
where L is the aspirated length of cell in the micropipette
and R is the radius of the micropipette. The lines represent
the computerized linear regression using a least-squares fit
analysis. The numbers in parentheses are the slopes in
dynes/cm and represent the stiffness parameter, K.

exposure times were calculated and the mean values normalized by those
for the control conditions, K_C, are shown in Fig. 3. The results for
0.5 to 1.5 hours of exposure are not presented in Fig. 3 because only
the most elongated cells were measured and they may not be a good
representation of the total population [9]. It should be noted that
the cells exposed to a shear stress of 85 dynes/cm² for only a few
hours had a value of the stiffness parameter almost four times higher
than that for control conditions. This is in contrast to a shear
stress of 30 dynes/cm², where cells exposed for approximately 4 hours
had a relatively low value of the mechanical stiffness parameter.
However, with longer exposure times, the mechanical stiffness increased to a level approximately three times higher than that for
control cells. This time-history of the mechanical stiffness parameter during the response of endothelial cells to shear stress is illustrated in Fig. 3. Data for cells exposed to a shear stress of 10
dynes/cm² are also included. These cells show a similar trend to
those at 30 dynes/cm², having a lower value of the mechanical stiffness parameter for times of 4 hours or less, but evidencing an increase for longer times. After 24 hours of exposure to shear stress,
the increase in the stiffness parameter was statistically significant
as compared to control values for all three shear stress levels
employed ($p < 0.05$).

The normalized stiffness parameter of the cells exposed to pulsatile shear stresses are also shown as solid circles in Fig. 3. For
the shear stress of 30±15 dynes/cm², the effect of exposure times

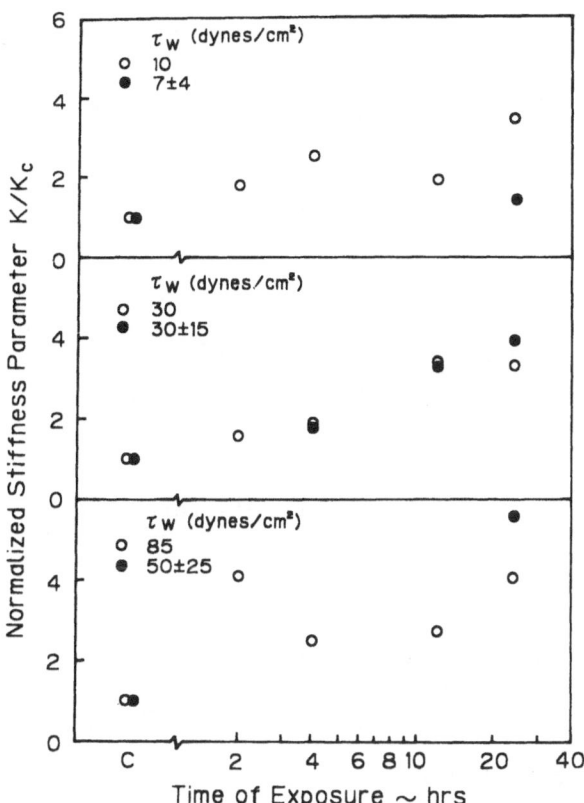

Fig. 3 Effect of exposure time on the normalized stiffness parameter for the different steady and pulsatile shear stress levels.

indicates almost the same trends as those for steady shear stress. However, in the case of longer exposure time, 24 hours, the stiffness parameter for the pulsatile shear stress has a higher value than that for steady shear stress. This effect is remarkable in the case of the highest shear stress: the mechanical property for a pulsatile shear stress of 50 ± 25 dynes/cm^2 becomes much stiffer than that for the steady shear stress of 85 dynes/cm^2. The cells exposed to the pulsatile shear stress of 7 ± 4 dynes/cm^2 do not show significant change in stiffness parameter.

Along with the change in endothelial cell shape, it has been observed that endothelial cells become stiffer in response to shear stress. The effect of shear stress on shape as a function of time was reported previously [6]. The changes with time in cell mechanical properties appear to be due to certain structural changes in the cytoskeleton which are in response to shear. It has been observed that an increased number of stress fibers aligned with the flow field in response to a fluid shear stress level of 85 dynes/cm^2 for 4-hour exposure [9]. It was also apparent that there was a widening of intercellular spaces with few connecting microfilaments. With the longer exposure time of 12 hours, the stress fibers were mostly aligned with the direction of flow, but a few intercellular spaces were still present. After a 24-hour exposure to shear stress levels of 30 and 85 dynes/cm^2, the stress fibers were aligned with the direction of flow. For the two lower shear stress levels (i.e., 10 and 30 dynes/cm^2) intercellular spaces were often seen with short microfilaments that seemed to connect adjacent cells together. For the highest shear stress level, intercellular spaces were no longer visible and there was a higher concentration of microfilament bundles at the cell periphery. It was concluded, thus, that the increase in cell stiffness may parallel the reorganization of the cytoskeleton and, in particular, the microfilament system. In an independent study, we have investigated the importance of two components of the cytoskeleton, (e.g., microfilaments and microtubles) in relation to endothelial cell mechanical properties [10]. Endothelial monolayers under no-flow conditions were incubated with cytochalasin B and colchicine to disrupt the microfilament or microtubular system respectively. We found that microfilaments contributed more to endothelial cell mechanical properties than microtubles. This suggests that, in the presence of shear stress, the microfilaments may make the greater contribution to endothelial cell mechanical properties.

CONCLUSION

Cells exposed to shear stress demonstrated a mechanical stiffness significantly greater than that of control cells, which was dependent on both the level of shear stress and the duration of exposure. The cells exposed to pulsatile shear stress became much stiffer in their mechanical property than those exposed to the steady shear stress. This effect was remarkable in the case of the highest shear stress. The present data suggest that the response of an endothelial cell to shear stress includes an alteration in both its structure and its mechanical properties. More detailed comparisons of structure and cell function between in vivo and cultured endothelial cells are needed to apply the results of in vitro observations of mechanical properties to the endothelial cells of living blood vessels.

Acknowledgement: These experiments were carried out in the Bioengineering Research Center, University of Houston, Houston, Texas. Support for this research was provided by the National Institute of Health, Grant HL-26890, and the State of Texas Advanced Technology Program.

REFERENCES

[1] Nerem RM, Cornhill JF (1980) J Biomech Eng 102:181-189
[2] Ross R (1981) Arteriosclerosis 1:293-311
[3] Flaherty JT, Pierce JE, Ferrans VJ, Patel DJ, Tucker WK, Fry DL (1972) Circ Res 31:23-33
[4] Nerem RM, Levesque MJ, Cornhill JF (1981) J Biomech Eng 103:172-176
[5] Dewey CF Jr, Bussolari SR, Gimbrone MA Jr, Davies PF (1981) J Biomech Eng 103:177-185
[6] Levesque MJ, Nerem RM (1985) J Biomech Eng 107:341-347
[7] Silkworth JB, Stehbens W (1975) Angiology 26:474-487
[8] Sato M, Levesque MJ, Nerem RM (1987) J Biomech Eng 109:27-34
[9] Sato M, Levesque MJ, Nerem RM (1987) Arteriosclerosis 7:276-286
[10] Levesque MJ, Sato M, Nerem RM (to be published)

The Effect of Fluid Shear Stress on the Growth Behavior of Vascular Endothelial Cells *in vitro*

J. ANDO, C. ISHIKAWA, T. KOMATSUDA, and A. KAMIYA

Research Institute of Applied Electricity, Hokkaido University, Sapporo, 060 Japan

ABSTRACT

Cultured monolayers of bovine aortic endothelial cells were subjected to fluid shear stress in a specially designed apparatus, in which the rotation of a disc plate in a dish forced the culture medium to flow concentrically. The effect of the shear load was evaluated from the number of regenerated cells, in a denuded area that had been created by mechanically removing some cells before rotating medium, and the changes in DNA synthesis. Cells were stained with propidium iodide after digestion in RNase and the relative DNA content per cell was determined by microspectrophotometry. The cell number observed in the denuded area after the exposure to a shear stress of 1.3-4.1 dynes/cm² for 24-48 hours was about twice as great as that of the static control. The DNA content of cells subjected to shear stress was significantly greater than that of paired, unstressed control cells. The histogram of DNA content per cell showed that the stress loaded cultures contained a relatively high proportion of cells located in the mitotic phase of the cell cycle as compared with the controls. These results indicate that fluid shear stress can stimulate the regeneration of and DNA synthesis in vascular endothelial cells.

INTRODUCTION

Endothelial cells lining the inner surface of the vessel are continuously subjected to fluid shear stress resulting from the flow of blood. Many previous studies have pointed out that such hemodynamic stresses can influence some aspects of endothelial cell biology. For example, it has been observed both in vivo [1] and in vitro [2] that the endothelial cells alter their shape and orientation in response to shear stress. Furthermore, there is increasing evidence that endothelial cells respond to changes in shear stress and consequently modulate such functions as histamine synthesis [3], prostacyclin production [4], the formation of endothelial stress fibers [5] and fluid phase endocytosis [6]. With respect to its effect on endothelial cell growth, however, only a few studies have been published, one reporting a negative result [7] while others have been positive [8].

According to the endothelial injury hypothesis [9], denuding injury is followed by platelet adhesion and aggregation, which in turn releases a growth factor able to stimulate the proliferation of smooth muscle cells. It is also accompanied by an increased endothelial permeability to lipids, and the combination of all these factors causes arteriosclerotic lesions. The ability of endothelial cells to regenerate following desquamation, therefore, appears to influence significantly the initiation and development of arteriosclerosis. Recently, it

has also been suspected that the cell turnover of the arterial endothelium is closely related to transendothelial macromolecular transport
and thereby to atherogenesis as well [10]. It would therefore be of
interest to know the effects of fluid shear stress upon endothelial
cell growth and regeneration, since this would materially help us to
understand the growth of the vascular system, as well as atherogenesis.

The present study was designed to evaluated the effects of shear
stress on the growth behavior of endothelial cells, particularly on the
migration, proliferation and DNA synthesis during the regenerative
process after mechanical denudation.

EXPERIMENTAL METHOD

Primary cultures were obtained from the descending thoracic aorta
of a fetal calf by brief collagenase digestion of the intimal lining
and were grown in Medium-199(GIBCO). Fetal bovine serum (20%), 100U/ml
penicillin, 100 μ g/ml streptmycin, and sodium bicarbonate were also
added to the medium. The cells were routinely passaged by trypsiniza-
tion in a trypsin/EDTA solution before confluence. Both primary and
passaged cultures had a homogenous monolayer configuration similar to a
cobblestone pavement, an appearance typical of the endothelial cell
layer. The purity of the cultures was also demonstrated both by the
presence of factor VIII related antigen and by positive fluorescence
after the uptake of fluorescence-labeled low density lipoprotein (Dil-
Ac-LDL, Biomedical Technologies Inc.). Cells used in the present experiments were in their fourth to tenth passages.

To impose shear stress on cultured endothelial cells, we have
developed a loading device. A flat disc of stainless steel was held on
the surface of the tissue culture medium and was rotated by a DC motor.
When the disc was rotated, the medium in the dish was forced to flow
concentrically, thus producing a fluid shear stress on the endothelial
monolayers growing at the bottom. The fluid shear stress (τ) induced by
this device is given by the equation which is shown in Fig. 1. This
device is capable of producing laminar shear stresses ranging from 0.5
to 5 dynes/cm^2. For the flow field generated in this study, the maximum
Reynolds number was less than 10. Under these conditions, it is quite
likely to assume that the effects of the radial secondary velocity are
negligible because the viscous forces are always predominantly greater
than the inertia forces. The absence of turbulence has been also confirmed with flow visualization using suspended polystyrene flakes and a
high speed video.

In these experiments, nearly equal numbers of cells were seeded
onto a pair of round polystyrene dishes. When the cells achieved con-
fluency, a denuded area was created manually in the center of the cell
layer by drawing a cell scraper (COSTAR) over them. After photographs
were taken of the area adjacent to the denuded area and of an area in
the intact monolayer, the two dishes were placed in the shear load
devices at 37°C and 5% CO_2 for 24-48 hours. In one dish, the disc was
rotated at a chosen velocity to impose the shear load of 1.3-4.1
dynes/cm^2 while the other dish was allowed to remain still as a stationary control.

Soon after the dishes were removed from the incubator, the same
areas that had been indicated by spot markers were photographed. The
borderline between the intact and the denuded areas and the spot marker
were manually traced on the photograph taken at the beginning of the
experiment. The tracings were accurately superimposed onto the same
areas in the photographs taken at the end of the experiment and the
border line was drawn on the photographs. Then the number of cells in
the denuded area was counted and expressed as cells per centimeter of

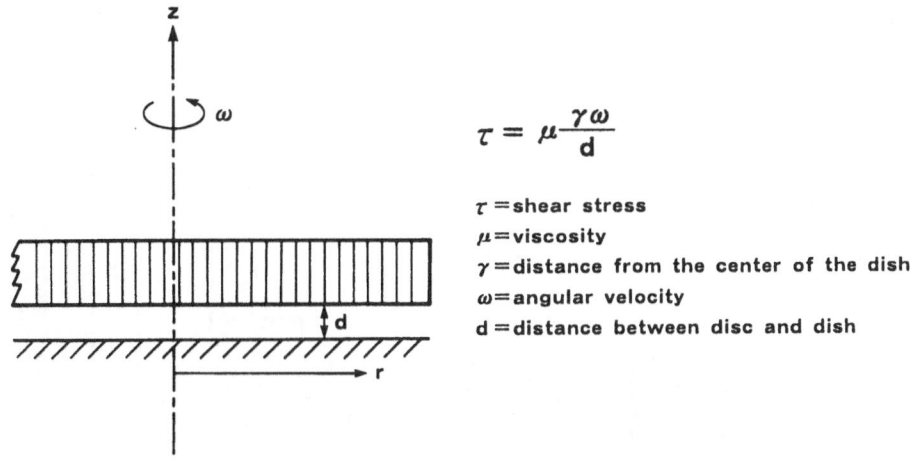

$$\tau = \mu \frac{\gamma \omega}{d}$$

τ = shear stress
μ = viscosity
γ = distance from the center of the dish
ω = angular velocity
d = distance between disc and dish

Fig.1 A cutway view of the device and the equation used for calculating shear stress.

borderline. Counts were made in specimens from the static control, as well as from the upstream and the downstream areas exposed to shear stress.

The cells were fixed in 70% ethanol for 6 hours and were treated with 0.1% RNase for 30 minutes. They were then stained with propidium iodide for microspectrophotometric measurement of the DNA content in each cell nucleus. This measurement can be carried out because the complex of propidium iodide and DNA emits a reddish-orange fluorescent light (670 nm) when excited by a green light (535-550 nm) and because the intensity of the fluorescent light is in proportion to its DNA content [11]. Three hundred cells were randomly chosen from the areas near the denuded part and in the intact monolayers, and the fluorescence intensity of each cell was measured using a NIKON MICROPHOT-FX P1 (Nihon Koagaku Co.). The resulting data were treated as the relative DNA content per cell and presented as DNA-content distribution histograms.

RESULTS

The cells in the device remained viable without any signs of degeneration, such as vacuolation of cytoplasm or desquamation, while being subjected to shear stress for 24-48 hours.

The cell number in the denuded area was compatible between the cultures subjected to shear stress and the static controls. The results, which are summarized in Fig. 2, showed that the cell number in the shear-loaded cultures was greater than that in the static controls. The difference between the downstream and the static control was statistically significant (p<0.01 to p<0.05), indicating that either cellular migration or proliferation, or both, had been stimulated by the exposure to shear stress. The cell density in the areas near the denuded parts and the intact monolayers showed a slight increase or no change during the period from 24-48 hours. In the denuded area,

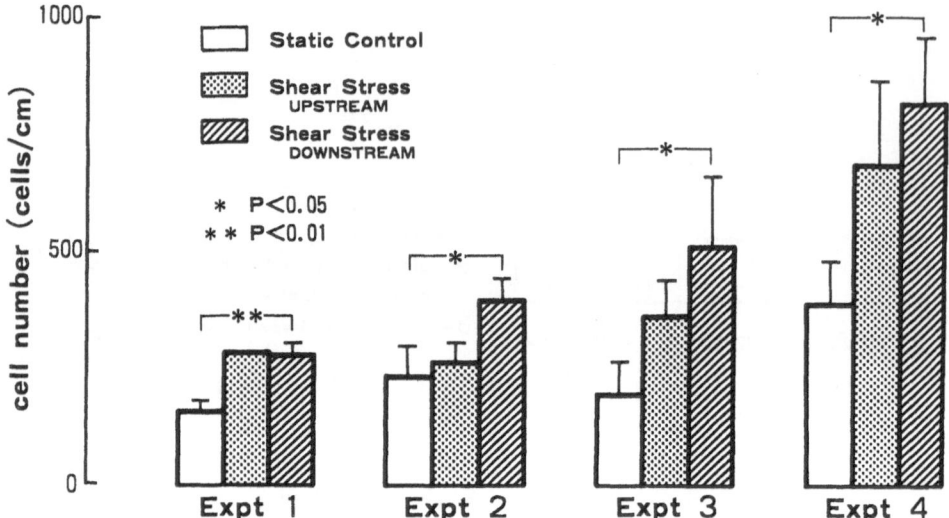

Fig.2   Number of cells counted in the denuded area.

an increase in cell number appeared to occur more prominently in the
downstream than in the upstream parts (Fig.2).
     Using the fluorescence in each nucleus of those 300 cells measured
in both the areas near the denuded part and the intact monolayers, we
calculated the mean DNA content per cell and compared the figures for
static controls and shear loaded cultures. The results are summarized
in Table 1. In all the experiments, the mean DNA content of the cells
subjected to shear stress was greater than that of the static controls.

TABLE 1

RELATIVE DNA CONTENT PER CELL[a]

| | Near denuded area | | Intact monolayer | |
Expt.	Static Control	Shear Stress	Static Control	Shear Stress
1	149.7±96.9	164.5±97.4	171.5±74.1	198.5±98.6*
2	131.1±51.1	187.4±74.6**	122.7±43.3	161.9±57.1**
3	142.2±54.7	191.8±71.4**	107.0±36.4	144.9±53.9**
4	155.1±76.1	200.5±94.4**	160.4±75.3	210.8±87.0**
5	132.4±57.8	189.0±64.2**	139.0±61.1	188.0±80.7**

a. Values are expressed as means ±SD, n=300.
* p<0.005, ** p<0.001 when compared to the static control.

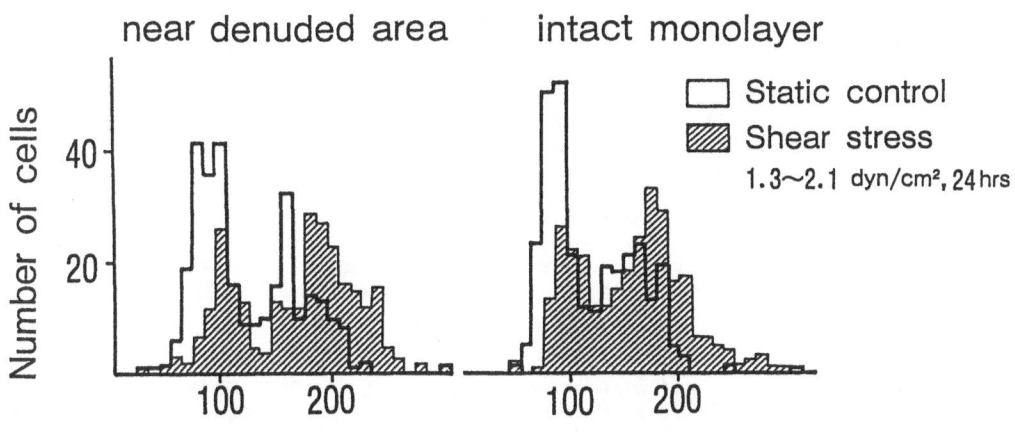

Fig.3 DNA histograms.

The difference between the two was statistically significant (p<0.005 to p<0.001), except near the denuded part in experiment 1. When the mean DNA content of the cells near the denuded area was compared with that in the intact area, there was no significant difference between the two portions.

Histograms of the DNA content per cell were also made to assess the effect of shear stress on the distribution of cells in the cell cycle. Fig.3 shows the DNA histogram obtained in the present experiment. In this figure, the left peak represents the cells of normal DNA content (1 x DNA) in the resting state (G_1/G_0 phase in the cell cycle), and the right peak shows those of the doubling content (2 x DNA) in the mitotic state (G_2/M phase), while the intermediate continuum contains cells in the S phase. The results show that the cultures subjected to shear stress for 24-48 hours contained a relatively low proportion of the cells located in the left peak and a relatively high proportion of cells in the right peak, when compared with the configuration of the stationary controls. These findings indicate that the fluid shear stress load induced the shift of the cell distribution to increase the number of the cells in the mitotic state.

CONCLUSION

In the present study, we created mechanical denudation in postconfluent endothelial cultures and examined the cell appearance in response to shear stress. Our data showed that the number of the cells counted in the denuded area after 24-48 hours of culture under fluid shear stress was significantly greater than that of the static control. The cells in the denuded area can be regarded as a mixture of migrating and proliferating cells. Because, if the greater majority of the cells in the denuded area are migrating cells, there must be a decline of cell density in the intact monolayer toward the border line, but the cell density never decreased. Our findings, therefore, indicate that endothelial cell regeneration, including migration and proliferation, is stimulated by shear stress. In order to further evaluate the effect of shear stress on endothelial cell proliferation, the change in DNA synthesis following exposure to shear stress has been examined. The data show that shear stress enhances the DNA synthesis in cultured endothelial cells. The experimental environment of our study indicated that this change in DNA synthesis is essentially elicited by laminar shear stress and has no connection with the effects of turbulence, blood pressure, pulsation, or any chemical growth factors which might act in vivo. Although further studies are needed to clarify arterio-genesis, our findings that endothelial cells respond to fluid shear stress by changing their functions may bring us closer to understanding the role of hemodynamic force in the pathogenesis of atherosclerosis.

ACKNOWLEDGEMENT: The authors wish to thank Dr. T. Shimamoto, Nissan Hospital, Mr. H. Nomura and Mr. T. Kabashima, for their aid in develop-ing the cell culture system. This work was partly supported by a grant-in-aid, for special project research no.61132008, from the Japanese Ministry of Education, Science and Culture and a research grant from the Atherosclerosis Study Association.

REFFERENCES

[1]Reidy MA, Langille BL (1980) Exp Mol Pathol 32:276-289
[2]Remuzzi A, Dewey CF, Davies PF, Gimbone A (1984) Bioreology 21:617-630
[3]Rosen LA, Hollis TM, Sharma MG (1974) Exp Mol Pathol 20:329-343
[4]Frangos JA, Eskin SG, McIntire LV, Ives CL (1985) Science 227:1477-1479
[5]Franke RP, Grafe M, Schnittler H, Seiffge D, Mittermayer M, Drenckhahn D (1984) Nature 307:648-649
[6]Davies PF (1984) Quantitative aspects of endocytosis in cultured endothelial cells. In: Jaffe EA(eds) Biology of Endothelial Cells. Martinus Nijhoff Publishers, Boston, pp 365-376
[7]Dewey CF, Bussolari ST, Gimbrone MA,Davies PF (1981) J Biomech Engr 103: 177-184
[8]Eskin SG, Sybers, HD, O'Bannon W, Navaro LT (1982) Artery 10: 159-171
[9]Ross R, Glomset JA (1976) N Engl J Med 295:369-377
[10]Weinbaum S, Tzwghai G, Ganatos P, Pfeffer T, Chien S (1987) Am J Phsiol 248:H945-H960
[11]Crissman HA, Steinkemp JA (1973) J Cell Biol 59:766-771

Turbulence, Disturbed Flow, and Vascular Endothelium[†]

C.F. Dewey, Jr.[1], P.F. Davies[2], and M.A. Gimbrone, Jr.[2]

[1]Fluid Mechanics Laboratory, Massachusetts Institute of Technology, Cambridge, MA 02139, USA
[2]Vascular Research Division, Brigham and Women's Hospital, Harvard University Medical School, Boston, MA 02115, USA

ABSTRACT

In a series of recent experiments, we have measured striking differences between cultured endothelial cells subjected to *laminar* flow and cells subjected to *turbulent* flow. In steady laminar flow, as well as laminar flow oscillated at frequencies up to 1 Hz, there is no evidence of increased cell turnover compared to static controls even though the cells undergo significant realignment in a period of 24 hours. With turbulent flow that contains a broad spectrum of higher-frequency small-scale oscillations, the most visible endothelial cell response is increased mitosis. This cell division occurs at time-average shear stresses as much as a factor of 5 smaller than the steady laminar shear stress required to cause alignment. One possible mechanism for this behavior is discussed.

INTRODUCTION

The vascular endothelial lining *in vivo* comprises the interface between flowing blood and the vessel wall, and thus is subjected to a variety of hemodynamic forces. A major component of these is *wall shear stress*, the tractive force produced by flowing blood upon the luminal endothelial cell surface. Shear stress has been implicated in the pathogenesis of atherosclerosis because a strong correlation exists between the location of developing arterial lesions and regions where large fluctuations in wall shear stress occur [6, 13, 14, 16, 17, 21]. Early studies by Fry [13] clearly established that extremely high shear stresses could *directly* injure the vascular endothelial lining. However, since frank endothelial desquamation is not typically observed microscopically in early atherosclerotic plaques [3], it is more likely that subtle functional changes are involved in lesion initiation [15].

The experiments reported here use an *in vitro* model system, based on a cone-and-plate Couette flow device, in which cultured endothelial monolayers are exposed to well-characterized shear stresses, comparable to those encountered *in vivo*, for intervals ranging from minutes to days [26]. A spectrum of shear-induced alterations in endothelial structure and function have been observed in this experimental system. In early experiments, relatively modest levels of *laminar* shear stress (<10 dynes/cm^2) were found to dynamically mold endothelial cell shape and cytoskeletal organization, enhance the rate of fluid phase endocytosis, stimulate prostaglandin production, and alter cell surface adhesivity for blood cells [4, 7-9].

RESPONSE OF CELLS TO TURBULENT FLOW

A surprising experimental discovery made in the cone-plate apparatus was a very large increase in endothelial cell division caused by turbulent flow [5]. **Figure 1** shows that flows contain-

† Research supported by The National Institutes of Health, Grant HL25536.

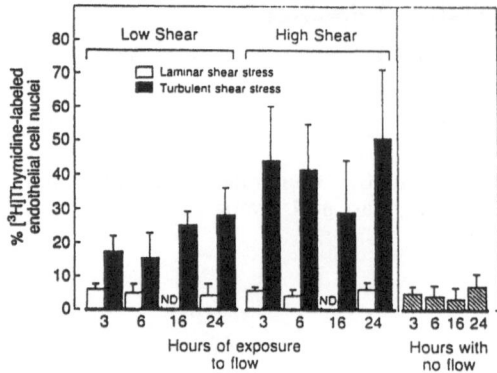

Figure 1. Endothelial growth stimulation by turbulent flow. Low shear is 1.5 dynes/cm^2 and high shear is 14 dynes/cm^2 (Davies et al. [5]).

ing turbulence can cause a sizable fraction of the cell population in confluent "quiescent" monolayers to commit to cell division even at a shear stress as low as 1.5 dynes/cm^2. This level of mean shear should be compared with the threshold of 8 dynes/cm^2 required to cause alignment in laminar flow on the same substrate. Numerous studies have provided estimates for shear stress under human arterial conditions [1, 6, 11-14, 19, 28] that provide a range of shear stress levels from 5 to 150 dynes/cm^2 at different sites in the arterial tree, again substantially larger than the turbulent threshold observed in our experiments.

In order to interpret the detailed shear stresses acting on the endothelial cells in turbulent flow, a large (2 meter diameter) cone-and-plate apparatus was built to model the conditions existing inside the small devices that are used for testing endothelial cells. We duplicated the non-dimensional flow parameters that govern turbulence and studied the turbulent eddy scales.

The turbulent flow contained a spectrum of eddy sizes very similar to the spectrum observed in turbulent boundary layers. Many of the same scaling laws were in evidence. For example, it was found that the velocity variation near the wall was linear whereas the velocity profile varied logarithmically according to the well-known 'law of the wall' at larger distances from the wall. **Figure 2** presents the turbulent spectrum in coordinates normalized to the local gap height. The fluctuation spectrum was smooth and without distinct peaks. Scaling of this result to the cone-plate turbulent flow experiments with cells provides evidence of *spatial turbulent scales that are as small as individual cell dimensions*. This has led to the possibility that *differential forces between cells* caused by turbulence can influence cell division.

POSSIBLE EFFECTS OF DIFFERENTIAL FORCES ON CELLS

Recent evidence has established that intact monolayers of endothelial cells have a well-developed network of intercellular channels. Small molecules can pass rapidly between the cells, allowing neighbors to share inorganic ions, metabolites, and small "messenger" molecules [18, 20]. Lowenstein [20] cites evidence that such channels could play a key role in controlling cell growth. Conversely, the disruption of such channels could lead to cell proliferation similar to that which we have seen with turbulent flow.

Spagnoli et al. [27] have found direct evidence that loss of junctions between endothelial cells is associated with high proliferative activity. Their experiments were performed on rabbit aortas that were injured in vivo. Cell division was assessed by sacrificing the animals at specific times after injury and measuring the correlation of nuclear uptake of ^{3}H-Thymidine with presence or absence of gap junctions. Their examination of freeze-fracture electron micrographs revealed that intercellular junctions were disrupted in endothelial cells that were migrating and proliferating to effect wound repair, whereas at two weeks, when the wound was healed and the migration and cell division had ceased, the junctional complexes had returned to their control (contact inhibited) conformation.

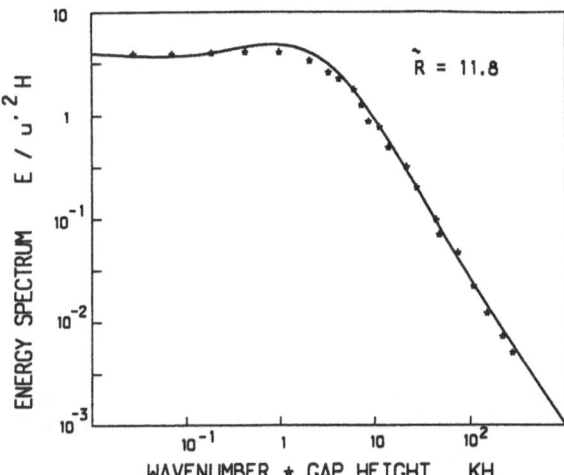

Figure 2. Spectrum of turbulence in a cone-plate flow apparatus (Einav et al.[10]).

Schwartz and his colleagues [25] have found a lack of tight intercellular junctions between endothelial cells that have migrated and proliferated to repair wounds in rat aortae. These results are consistent with previous postulates of a correlation between the absence of gap junctions and cell proliferation [23 and references in 20].

We suggest that disruption of the intercellular channels by differential turbulent forces acting on adjacent cells could be the mechanism whereby cell division is promoted in otherwise contact-inhibited endothelial cell layers. This hypothesis is based on the idea that the endothelial cell membrane is flexible and, without intracellular structural elements, lacks the rigidity to resist deformation caused by fluid shear stress. If the membrane is deformed, junctional complexes could be subjected to a tearing stress sufficient to disrupt the delicate trans-membrane junctions between the cells.

In our studies, the endothelial cells were exposed to turbulence without prior conditioning by flow. Previous laminar flow experiments [9, 29] have demonstrated that substantial intracellular structure, consisting of actin and myosin filaments oriented in the direction of flow, is polymerized in vascular endothelium subjected to modest levels of laminar shear stress. It is therefore possible that laminar flow can provide internal structure that may mitigate some of the effects of turbulence that promote cell proliferation.

In addition to direct mechanical means of affecting intercellular junctions, indirect means may also be possible. Davies [2] and Lowenstein [20] review a number of mechanisms that can regulate the opening and closing of gap junctions. It should also be noted that intercellular gap junctions can form between endothelial cells and smooth muscle cells as well as between cells of similar type. *In vivo*, therefore, the integrity of gap junctions will be subjected to a variety of complicated influences, of which shear stress is only one.

The mechanisms through which turbulence effects changes in the endothelium remain to be clarified, and the differential forces themselves are only one of the manifestations of turbulence that may be influential. Much research remains to be done on these topics.

REFERENCES

[1] Beere, P.A., Glagov, S. and Zarins, C.K. [1984] **Science, 226,** 180-182.

[2] Davies, P.F. [1986] **Laboratory Invest., 55,** 5-24.

[3] Davies, P.F., Reidy, M.A., Goode, T.B., and Bowyer, D.E. [1976] **Atherosclerosis, 25,** 125-130.

[4] Davies, P.F., Dewey, C.F.Jr., Bussolari, S.R., Gordon, E.J., and Gimbrone, M.A.Jr. [1984] **J. Clin. Invest., 73,** 1121-1129.

[5] Davies, P.F., Remuzzi, A., Gordon, E.J., Dewey, C.F.Jr., and Gimbrone, M.A.Jr. [1986] **Proc. Natl. Acad. Sciences USA, 83,** 2114-2117.

[6] Dewey, C.F., Jr. [1979] Ch. 2 of **Dynamics of Arterial Flow** [Eds. S. Wolf and N.T. Werthessen, Eds.], Plenum Press, N.Y., pp 55-103.

[7] Dewey, C.F.Jr. [1984] **J. Biomech. Eng., 106,** 31-35.

[8] Dewey, C.F., Jr., Bussolari, S.R., Gimbrone, M.A., Jr. and Davies, P.F. [1981] **J. Biomech. Eng., 103,** 177-185.

[9] Dewey, C.F., Jr., Gimbrone, M.A., Jr., Bussolari, S.R., White, G.E. and Davies, P.F. [1983] in **Fluid Dynamics as a Localizing Factor for Atherosclerosis,** (Eds. G. Schettler et al.), Springer-Verlag, pp 182-187.

[10] Einav, S., Hartenbaum, H., and Dewey, C.F.Jr. [1986] **Bull. Am. Phys. Soc., 31,** 1693.

[11] Friedman, M.H., Hutchins, G.M., Bargeron, C.B., Deters, O.J., and Mark, F.F. [1981] **Atherosclerosis, 39,** 425-436.

[12] Friedman, M.H. and Deters, O.J. [1987] **J. Biomech. Eng., 109,** 25-26.

[13] Fry, D.L. [1968] **Circ. Res., 23,** 165-197.

[14] Fry, D.L. [1976] in **Cerebrovascular Diseases** (Ed. P. Scheinberg), Raven Press, pp. 77-95.

[15] Gimbrone, M.A., Jr. [1986] in **Atherosclerosis VII, Proceedings of the 7th International Symposium on Atherosclerosis,** [Eds. Fidge,N.F. and Nestel,P.J.] Excerpta Medica, 367-369.

[16] Ku, D.N., Giddens, D.P., Zarins, C.K., and Glagov, S. [1985] **Arteriosclerosis, 5,** 293-302.

[17] Langille, B.L., Reidy, M.A., and Kline, R.L. [1986] **Arteriosclerosis, 6,** 146-154.

[18] Larson, D.M. and Sheridan, J.D. [1982] **J. Cell Biol., 92,** 183-191.

[19] Levesque M.J. and Nerem, R.M. [1985] **J. Biomech. Eng., 107,** 341-347.

[20] Lowenstein, W.R. [1987] **Cell, 48,** 725-726.

[21] Naumann, A. and Schmid-Schönbein, H. [1983] in **Fluid Dynamics as a Localizing Factor for Atherosclerosis,** (Eds. G. Schettler et al.), Springer-Verlag, pp 9-25.

[22] Nerem, R.M., and Levesque, M.J. [1983] in **Fluid Dynamics as a Localizing Factor for Atherosclerosis,** (Eds. G. Schettler et al.), Springer-Verlag, pp 26-37.

[23] Pitts, J.D. [1978] in **Intercellular Junctions and Synapses** (J.D. Feldman and N.B. Gilula, Eds.), Chapman and Hall, London, p. 63.

[24] Remuzzi, A., Dewey, C.F.Jr., Davies, P.F., and Gimbrone, M.A.Jr. [1984] **Biorheol., 21,** 617-630.

[25] Schwartz, S.M., Stemerman, M.B., and Benditt, E.P. [1975] **Am. Journal Pathology, 81,** 15-42

[26] Sdougos, H.P., Bussolari, S.R., and Dewey, C.F.Jr. [1984] **J. of Fluid Mech., 138,** 379-404.

[27] Spagnoli, L.G., Pietra, G.G., Villaschi, S., and Johns, L.W. [1982] **Laboratory Invest., 46,** 139-148.

[28] Tarbell, J.M., Chang, L.J. and Hollis, T.M. [1982] **J. Biomech. Engng, 104,** 243-245.

[29] White, G.E., Gimbrone, M.A.Jr., Fujiwara, K. [1983] **J. Cell Biol., 97,** 416-424.

Effects of Blood Flow on Development of Atheromatous Plaques at an Experimental Inter-Carotid Anastomosis (Model Carotid Bifurcation)

M. Kashihara[1], S. Ueda[2], and K. Matsumoto[2]

[1]Taoka Hospital, Tokushima, 770 Japan
[2]Department of Neurological Surgery, School of Medicine, The University of Tokushima, Tokushima, 770 Japan

ABSTRACT

Atherosclerosis often develops at the carotid bifurcation. In order to analyse blood flow in this region in vivo, we constructed a bifurcation by microsurgical anastomosis of the carotid arteries in the rabbit. In animals with hypercholesterolemia, fully developed atheromatous plaques developed in three months. The stages involved in their development were first, changes in the endothelial cells aligned in the direction of blood flow, second, adhesion of leucocytes, mainly macrophages, at the lateral wall of the bifurcation, and then formation of thick atheromatous plaques. The proximal side of the plaques was smooth and rich in collagen fibers, while the distal side was rough and contained many foam cells.

INTRODUCTION

Atherosclerosis often develops at the carotid bifurcation. Various factors are involved in the development of atherosclerosis, including flow dynamics, lipid composition and the cell components of the blood and vascular wall. There are reports of studies of each of these factors separately[1,2,3]. To examine the interactions of blood flow and the artery wall at the carotid bifurcation, we developed a model in rabbits. This paper describes sequence of changes during the development of atherosclerosis in this model and especially the interaction of leucocytes and endothelial cells.

MATERIALS AND METHODS

The right carotid artery of rabbits was cut in the mid-cervical region and the distal side was anastomosed end-to-side to the left carotid artery. The right carotid artery was analogous to the internal carotid artery(MIC), and distal part of the left carotid artery corresponded to the external carotid artery(MEC)(Fig.1).

In the first experiment, mild cholesterolemia of 50 to 100 mg/dl of serum cholesterol was induced by administration of cholesterol at 0.25g per day as a suspension in the drinking water. The animals were examined by angiography and measurements of blood flow and serum cholesterol were made. Histological examinations were made 1, 3, 6, 12 and 20 months after formation of the artificial bifurcations.

In the second experiment, 22 rabbits were given one percent cholesterol chow from the day after formation of the anastomosis. After a month, the blood cholesterol level had increased to 800 to 1000 mg/dl. Measurement of blood flow and histological examinations by light microscopy, transmission electron microscopy and scanning electron microscopy were made at weekly intervals for 12 weeks after the anastomosis.

RESULTS

The anastomosic sites healed within a month. The diameter of the proximal part of the carotid artery increased from a preoperative value of about 1.5mm to 3.0mm postoperatively. Angiography demonstrated counter-clockwise rotation of the bifurcation, i.e., the MEC shifted to the right side and the MIC to the caudal side. Light microscopic examination showed that a small pouch was formed in the flow-dividing region at the bifurcation. However, this pouch did not result in an aneurysm during the follow-up period of 20 months. Thickening of the media in the proximal portion of the bifurcation was also noted, especially at the origin of the MIC.

Atherosclerosis was evaluated by observations of the severely cholesterol-laden rabbits. In the first three weeks after the construction of the bifurcation, when hypercholesterolemia had not yet been induced, the endothelial cells changed their alignment in the direction of flow (Fig.2). Electron microscopic examination revealed mild subendothelial edema (stage 1). After one month, adhesion of leucocytes was noted at the lateral wall of the bifurcation (Fig.3). Some of these cells appeared to penetrate through the endothelial cell layer (stage 2). After six weeks, continued adhesion of leucocytes and proliferation of endothelial cells and smooth muscle cells produced an atheromatous plaque (stage 3)(Fig.4). Thickening of the plaque and/or distal extension occurred in some cases (stage 4), a change attributable to severe rheological stress at the bifurcation. Marked proliferation of collagenous fibers was produced at the proximal side of the plaque, while on the distal side, abundant adhesion of leucocytes and release of foam cells were observed (Fig.5).

CONCLUSION

A bifurcataion model was developed in rabbits. Rheological stress modified the vascular wall after the development of the bifurcation, and hypercholesterolemia induced atheromatous plaques. Both adhesion of leucocytes and rheological stress were important factors in development of atherosclerosis. The histological composition of the atheromatous plaque was also found to be affected by location in the blood stream.

REFERENCES

(1) Hrapchak BB, Bond MG, Wood LL, Hostetler JR (1980) Atherosclerosis 35:243-258
(2) Texon M, Imparato AM, Helpern M (1965)   JAMA 194:1226-1230
(3) Zarins CK, Giddens DP, Bharadvaj BK, Sottiurai VS, Mabon RF Glagov S (1983) Circ.Res 53: 02-514

Fig.1 Diagram of the carotid bifurcation model in rabbits.Anastomosis was performed with 10-0 suture under an operative microscope. MIC:model internal carotid artery MEC:model external carotid artery IC:internal carotid artery EC:external carotid artery CC:common carotid artery.

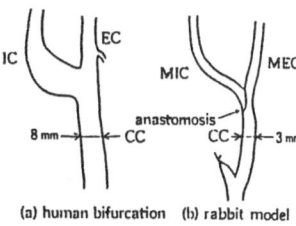

Fig.2 Scanning electron microscopic appearance of the inner surface of the bifurcation in stage 1. Endothelial cells disappeared and new endothelial cells proliferated, shown at higher magnification on the right.

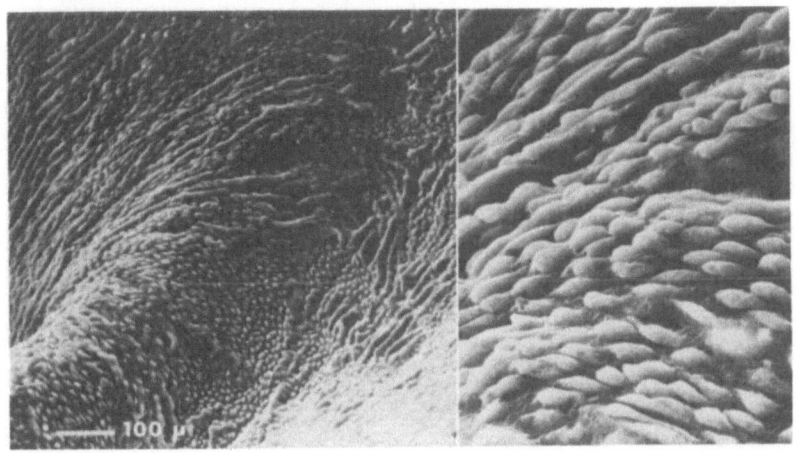

Fig.3 Adhesion of leucocytes to the lateral wall of the bifurcation in stage 2. Numerous adherent leucocytes are seen(left), and some of them penetrated through the endothelial cells(right). The area enclosed in a rectangle in the figure on the top left is shown at higher magnification on the bottom left.

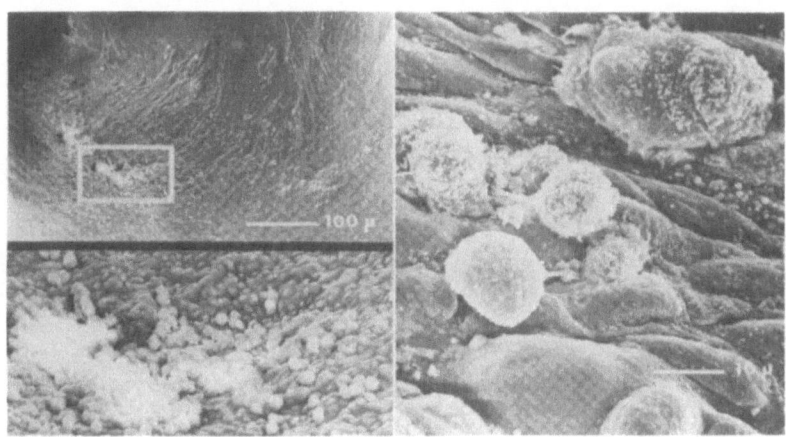

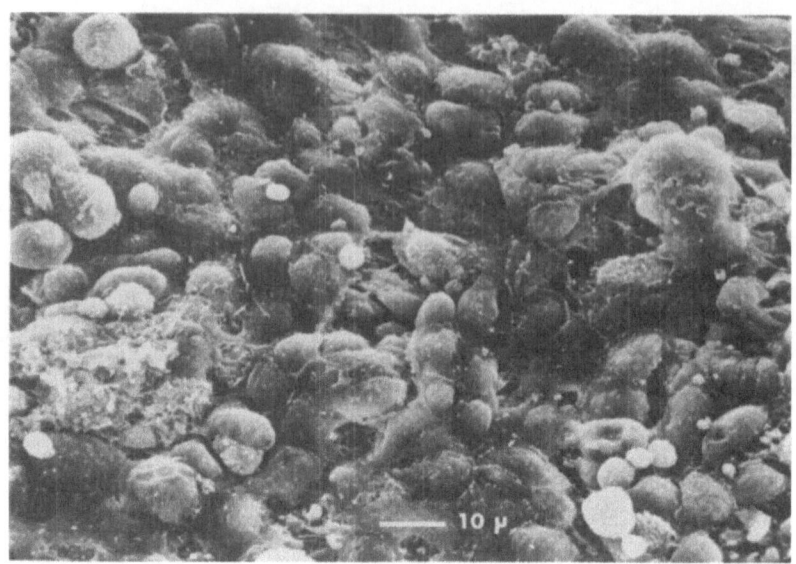

Fig.4 Surface of a thin atheromatous plaque at stage 3. Many kinds
of cells, such as monocytes, lymphocytes, platelets and endothelial
cells, are seen.

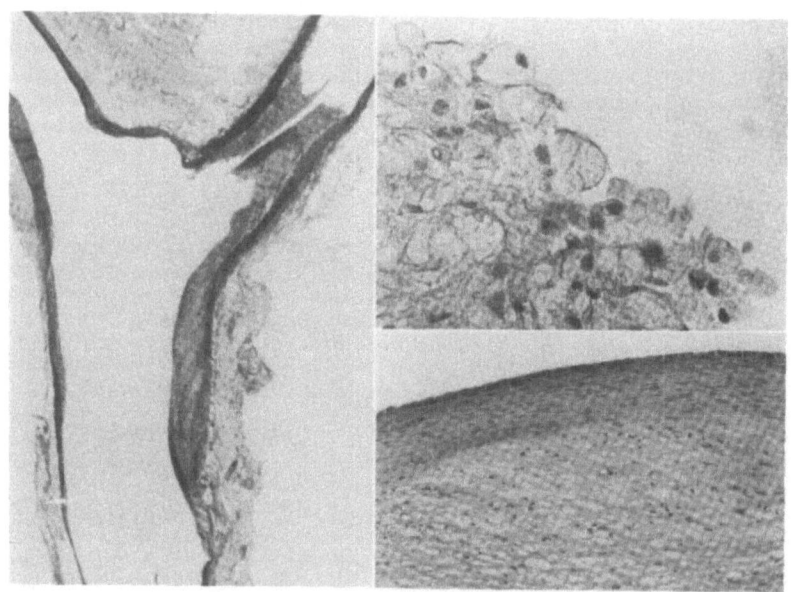

Fig.5 Light microscopic appearance of carotid bifurcation in stage 4.
A well developed atheromatous plaque is seen in the lateral wall of
the bifurcation(left). Its distal edge(top right) has a rough surface
with foam cells and its proximal surface(bottom right) is smooth with
fibrous tissue.

Arterial Tortuosity

D.L. NEWMAN and C.M. WENN

Medical Radiations Unit, Department of Applied Physics, Royal Melbourne Institute of Technology, Melbourne, Australia

ABSTRACT

The tortuosity of the abdominal aorta and common iliac arteries in man is reported. Tortuosity coefficients t_1, t_2, t_3 and t_4 were calculated from the digitisation coordinates of the midlines of the vessels as presented from aortograms of 91 patients. The results indicate an increase in tortuosity with age. The haemodynamic consequences of arterial tortuosity are discussed and the concept of tortuosity as an age dependent geometrical risk factor suggested.

INTRODUCTION

Haemodynamic theories of atherogenesis have been largely confined to the region around an arterial junction (1-3). However, the disease is frequently more generalised and widespread. It is necessary therefore, to consider haemodynamic factors which are not confined to the junction region. A geometrical, age related factor is the bending or tortuosity that is commonly observed in the abdominal aorta and iliac arteries but which have not previously been quantified.

METHODS

91 aortograms were examined, 50 males and 41 females. The age range was 12 to 89 years. The reason for the investigations was suspected trauma or renal disease. None of the patients presented with symptoms of arterial occlusive disease.
    The midline of the abdominal aorta and the midlines of the common iliac arteries were digitised to a precision of 0.1mm to obtain the x coordinates in vertical increments of 10mm. Tortuosity coefficients were obtained from the standard deviations of the successive lateral shifts, dx of the x coordinates of the vessel midlines, t_1, t_2 and t_3 being the coefficients for the abdominal aorta and right and left iliac arteries respectively and t_4, the coefficient for the whole segment.
    For a straight vessel, these coefficients would be equal to 0.00, whilst a tortuous segment would have a coefficient greater than 0.00. The magnitude of the coefficient may, therefore, be used to quantify the degree of tortuosity.

RESULTS

    Fig. 1 shows typical digitised aortograms with the corresponding values of the tortuosity coefficients. As may be seen, a straight vessel has a coefficient which lies between 0.05 and 0.10, this representing the digitisation error.

    The tortuosity coefficients were obtained for all the aortograms and their variation with age is shown in Fig. 2. It can be seen that there is an increased incidence of vessel tortuosity with age particularly above the age of 40 years. A few younger individuals did however, exhibit fairly pronounced vessel tortuosity. The iliac arteries showed a greater tendency for tortuosity than the abdominal aorta. There was no significant difference between males and females although a few male patients exhibited vessel tortuosity at a younger age.

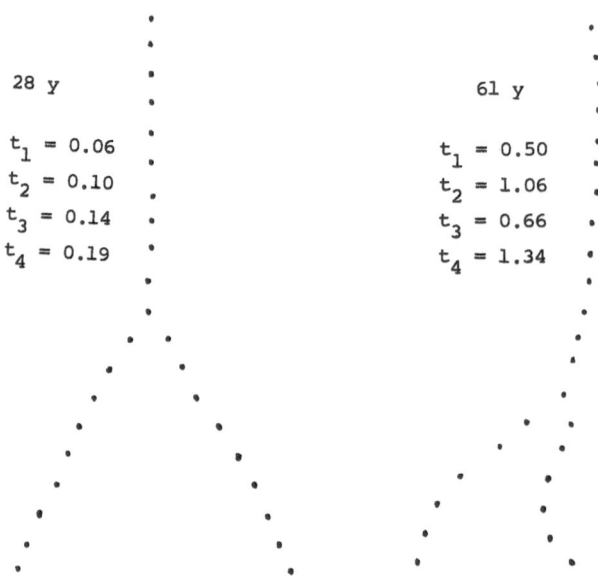

28 y

$t_1 = 0.06$
$t_2 = 0.10$
$t_3 = 0.14$
$t_4 = 0.19$

61 y

$t_1 = 0.50$
$t_2 = 1.06$
$t_3 = 0.66$
$t_4 = 1.34$

FIG. 1   Digitised appearance and tortuosity coefficients of aortograms of patients showing increasing tortuosity with age.

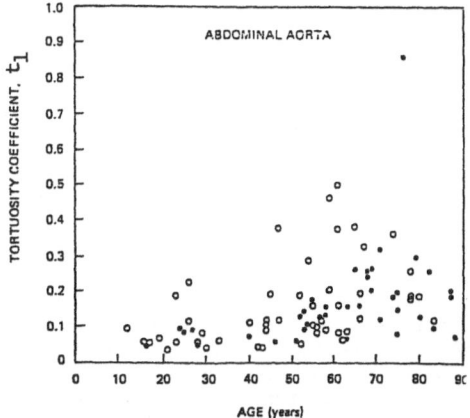

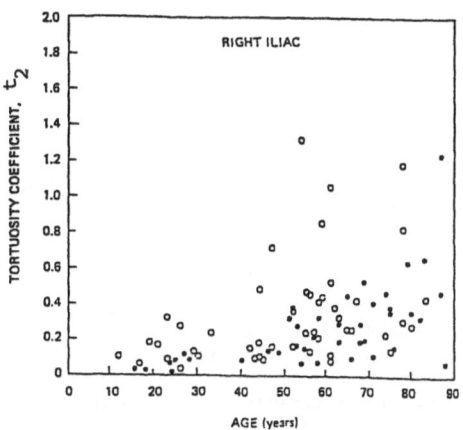

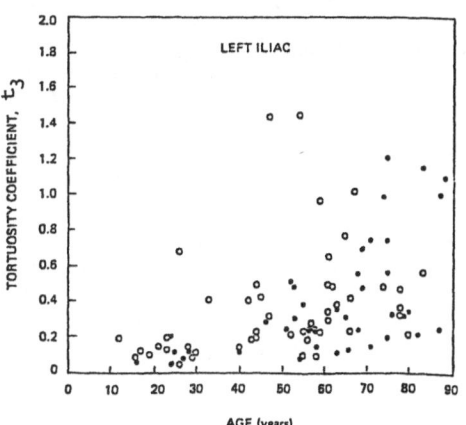

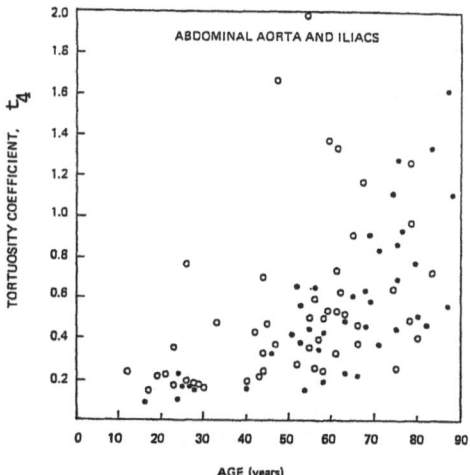

FIG. 2   The variation of the tortuosity coefficients with age for the abdominal aorta, the right and left common iliac arteries and the lumped segment (abdominal aorta and iliac arteries).
o = males, ● = females.

DISCUSSION

The increasing tortuosity of the abdominal aorta and iliac arteries is indicative of an aging process. It should be noted however that not all of the older patients had significant vessel tortuosity. It is known that longitudinal retraction of vessels decreases markedly with age (4) and the possible cause of vessel tortuosity is the loss of longitudinal stiffness. An age dependent loss of longitudinal stiffness may not be the sole causative factor leading to vessel tortuosity. This is indicated by the occurrence of tortuosity in some of the younger patients, suggesting that some individuals may have a greater inherited tendency for vessel tortuosity.

Previous work (5) on the effect of haemodynamic forces on atherogenesis have indicated that local changes in the flow shear stress patterns may lead to enhanced lipid uptake. The effect of the increased arterial curvature seen in a tortuous vessel would be expected to produce regions of both low and high shear stress. These haemodynamic changes would not be confined to a junction region and hence vessel tortuosity may provide an explanation for the more generalised appearance of the disease. That is not to state that vessel tortuosity has been established as having a definite causative relationship to atherogenesis. 35 of the 91 patients presented with moderate to severe atherosclerosis of the vessels as assessed radiographically. All of these patients were older than 40 years of age and had vessels which were to a greater or lesser extent tortuous. On the other hand, some patients with significant vessel tortuosity showed no radiographic evidence of the disease. The present results therefore, do not indicate that vessel tortuosity is a precursor to atherosclerosis. Without a knowledge of the other risk factors to which the patients are exposed it is clearly difficult to draw conclusions concerning the role of tortuosity in atherogenesis. However, in view of the changing haemodynamics invoked by vessel tortuosity it is unlikely that vessel tortuosity would not contribute to development and localisation of the disease. Furthermore, one could suppose that an individual with vessel tortuosity at an early age would be at greater geometrical risk of developing the disease.

Acknowledgment: The authors would like to thank the X-ray Departments of the Alfred Hospital and The Repatriation Hospital in providing access to radiographic archives.

REFERENCES

(1) Willis GC (1954) Canad Med Ass J   70:1
(2) Gessner FB (1973) Circ Res 33:259
(3) Nerem RM and Cornhill JF (1980) J Biomech Engng 102:181
(4) Learoyd BM and Taylor MG (1955) Circ Res 3:278
(5) Caro CG, Fitz-Gerald JM, Schroter RC (1971) Proc Roy Soc Lond 177:109

Chapter 4
Transport Phenomena and Underlying Mechanism of Atherogenesis

Wall Mass Transport and Other Mechanisms Underlying Atherogenesis

C.G. Caro

Physiological Flow Studies Unit, Imperial College, London, SW7 2AZ, England

This final session represents an important part of the Symposium, because much concerning atherogenesis remains to be considered and explained. Thus, although various observations lead to the conclusion that the development of atherosclerosis is associated with the local fluid dynamics, neither the flow pattern at sites of predilection nor the mechanisms which associate a particular flow pattern with predisposition to the disease is fully understood. Indeed, the distribution of the disease is not fully described by an association with a particular flow pattern. An additional characteristic is that it affects preferentially the intima (particularly the subendothelium) of thick-walled vessels, sparing thin-walled vessels.

The explanation for the preferential occurrence of atherosclerosis in the subendothelium of thicker-walled vessels is not known, but various studies suggest that a contributory factor is the accumulation of materials - including lipoproteins - within the subendothelial space, determined by the balance between their ease of ingress from the lumen across the endothelium and their ease of egress across the internal elastic lamella and media to the vasa vasorum and lymphatics in the adventitia and their interactions with the wall.

These remarks by no means imply that fluid dynamics plays no role in determining this distribution. The flow of solvent through the arterial wall can directly influence solute transport (via solvent drag effects) and can furthermore influence the transport properties of the poro-elastic interstitial matrix. There is, moreover, emerging evidence that the blood flow pattern can affect not only wall biology, but also wall mass transport and wall mechanics. These matters will be considered in several papers in this session.

It is of interest, in relation to these observations, that the underlying blood flow pattern varies widely in different parts of the arterial tree. There is, for example, prominent net flow reversal during the cardiac cycle in the femoral arteries and none in the carotids. It is, furthermore, of interest that the flow pattern in an artery is not given, but may be changed by various interventions. As shown by multi-channel Doppler ultrasound studies in healthy human subjects, a nitro-vasodilator can increase arterial compliance and flow pulsatility while cigarette smoking, which is an acknowledged 'risk factor' for atherosclerosis, can cause the opposite effects.

These and other observations reveal that the circulation is considerably more complicated than has often been supposed, both in terms of its mechanics and its biology. Thus, it would seem difficult in this elastic system with poro-elastic walls to uncouple pressure and flow and transport phenomena, and unwise to suppose that any haemodynamic change can occur without triggering a range of biological responses in, for example, the structure and metabolism of cells. Whether, therefore, a study is undertaken in vivo or with cells in culture, a precise description is needed of the mechanics (in the broadest sense) and the biology and biochemistry. Such a description will allow, inter alia, assessment of the appropriateness of the experimental conditions to those which obtain in vivo.

An exciting stage may be approaching in the study of atherosclerosis. Some of the underlying mechanisms are becoming clearer and the possibility is no longer unimaginable that the course of the disease may be altered by influencing not just the blood lipoproteins but also the factors which affect its localized occurrence in blood vessels. Such advancing understanding encourages the formulation of schemes to account for the disease. These should be subjected to testing against the full body of knowledge of the condition, including the effects of 'risk factors'.

There is evidently no single formula for the way ahead. One which has proved fruitful, and seems likely to continue to be so, is close collaboration between biomedical and physical scientists, but perhaps the extent of mechano-biological interaction, now apparent, should also encourage those inclined towards mechanics to extend their knowledge of biology and biochemistry and vice versa. The complexity of the problems in biology and physical science and the likelihood of the emergence of new fundamental findings implies, however, that the need is undiminished for talented specialists from both these fields.

Not everything in the complex cascade of events that comprises atherosclerosis necessarily involves mechano-biological interaction as a first stage. The challenge of clarifying the disease has led to important new insights into the mechanisms of cell migration and growth. These findings too will be discussed.

The Effect of Centrifugal Force on Glycosaminoglycans Synthesis and Cell Proliferation of Vascular Smooth Muscle Cells in Culture

M. Hamada, I. Nishio, Y. Kusuyama, M. Ura, H. Yoshikawa, and Y. Masuyama

Division of Cardiology, Department of Medicine, Wakayama Medical College, Wakayama, 640 Japan

ABSTRACT

To evaluate the role of hypertension independent of humoral factors on atherogenesis, synthesis of glycosaminoglycans(GAGs), protein and DNA were tested in the cultured vascular smooth muscle cells(NSMCs) from aortae of spontaneously hypertensive rats(SHR) and Wistar-Kyoto rats(WKY) under centrifugal force. Basal levels of GAGs and DNA were greater in SHR compared with WKY. Under the centrifugal force, cultured VSMCs synthesized more GAGs in both strains. DNA and protein syntheses were more suppressed by centrifugal force in WKY than in SHR. These results suggest that high blood pressure per se might promote atherosclerosis via metabolic changes in VSMCs, especially in genetic hypertensive animals.

INTRODUCTION

Hypertension, as well as hyperlipidemia, is believed to be a strong initiating or aggravating factor in atherogenesis. Our previous data revealed the close relationship between blood pressure levels and aortic GAGs levels in rats with experimental hypertension including SHR. GAGs levels were decreased in accordance with blood pressure fall in the hypertensive rats given anti-hypertensive agents[1]. Because of the coexistence of hypertension and some humoral factors related with hypertension, in these in vivo experiments, we could not elucidate the precise mechanism regulating aortic GAGs levels.

In this study, to evaluate the role of hypertension apart from humoral factors on GAGs synthesis in VSMCs, cultured aortic VSMCs from rats were loaded by centrifugal force as a simulation of blood pressure. Protein and DNA syntheses were also determined.

MATERIAL AND METHODS

(1)Stock culture

Smooth muscle cells were prepared by explant method[2]. In brief, the thoracic aorta was excised under sterile conditions from 12 weeks old male SHR and WKY. After careful removal of the adventitia and the intima, the aortic media was cleared of blood twice by Dulbecco-Vogt modified Eagle's medium(DMEM), cut into pieces and disposed onto flasks. After four weeks of culture in DMEM supplemented with 10% fetal calf serum(FCS), cells in

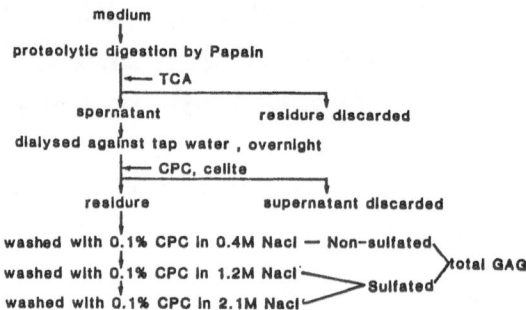

Fig.1 Method of analysis of glycosaminoglycans.

primary culture were trypsinized and dispersed into flasks approximately at a density of $4 \times 10^5/27$ cm^2 ,for subculture. The smooth muscle cells were identified by monoclonal antibody which recognizes actin filaments of VSMCs specifically(Fig.1).

Subculture 5 was used in these experiments. VSMCs were trypsinized and seeded at a density of $4 \times 10^5/28$cm^2 into screw capped flasks in DMEM containing 10% FCS. After incubation at 37C with 95% air and 5% CO_2 for four days, medium was exchanged to FCS-free DMEM. These flasks were centrifuged with a specially designed slow speed centrifuge at 0, 0.2, 2.0, 8.0G maintained at 37C, for 12 hours, twice, for a total spin time of 24 hours over a period of 48 hours.

(2)Glycosaminoglycans synthesis(Fig.1).

After the preincubation at each gravity level, the medium was changed to FCS-free DMEM containing 20 uCi of [^{3}H]-glucosamine for each flask. After 24 hours centrifugation, the medium was collected.   0.5ml of the medium was used to analyze GAGs by the method of Saani et al[3].   Subfractions of GAGs were measured using the method of Meir et al[4] .

(3)DNA synthesis.

To evaluate the effect of centrifugal force on the cell proliferation, [^{3}H]-thymidine incorporation into DNA was measured. After preincubation , these flasks were finally incubated for 6 hours with FCS-free DMEM containing 2.0 uCi of [^{3}H]-thymidine for each flask. VSMCs were sonicated and [^{3}H]-thymidine incorporation into PCA-insoluble fraction was counted using liquid scintillation counter.

(4)Protein synthesis.

To determine protein synthesis, 0.5 uCi of [^{14}C]-leucine was added to each flask and incubated for 2 hours at each gravity level.   [^{14}C]-leucine incorporated into TCA-insoluble fraction was also counted.

RESULTS

(1)Effect of centrifugal force on GAGs synthesis.

Basal level of incorporation of [^{3}H]-glucosasmine into total GAGs was 2.6 times more in SHR compared with WKY(Fig.2). Incorporation of [^{3}H]-glucosasmine into GAGs was increased by centrifugal forces. In SHR, the increase of incorporation of [^{3}H]-glucosasmine to total GAGs was greater at lower gravities

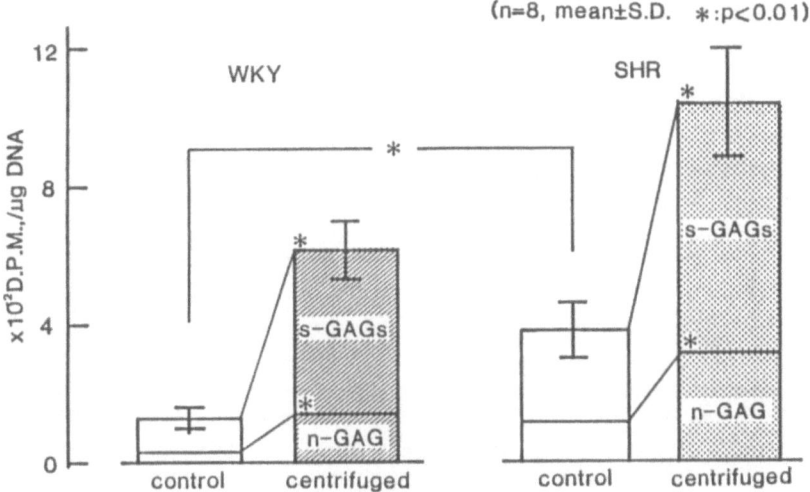

Fig.2 Effects of centrifugal force at 8G on [³H]-glucosamine incorporation into glycosaminoglycans.

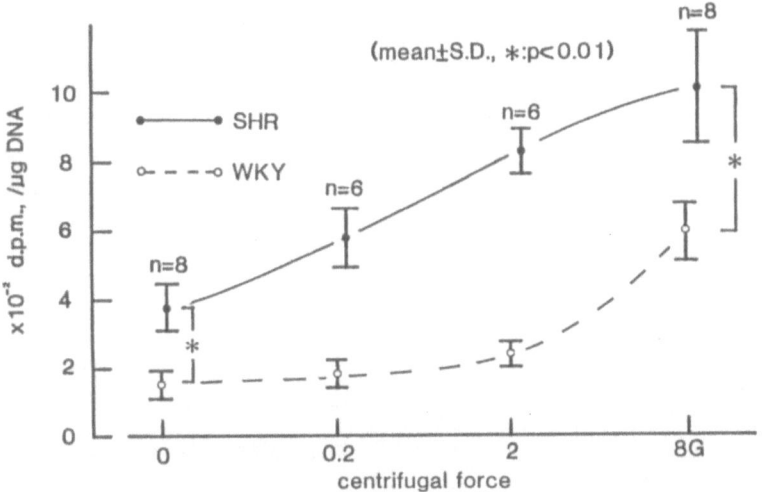

Fig.3 Effect of centrifugal force on glycosaminoglycans synthesis.

(Fig.3). These potentiations were equally observed in non-sulfated and sulfated GAGs in both strains(Fig.2).

(2)Effects of centrifugal force on DNA synthesis.

The basal level of [³H]-thymidine incorporation into DNA was significantly higher in SHR(Fig.4). Centrifugation of VSMCs resulted in decrease in proportion to the level of the gravities in both strains, especially in WKY at 8G(Fig.4,5).

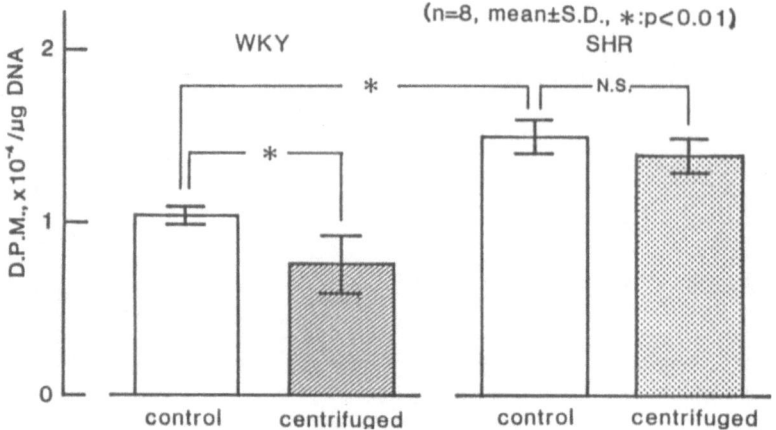

Fig.4 Effect of centrifugal force at 8G on
[³H]-thymidine incorporation into DNA

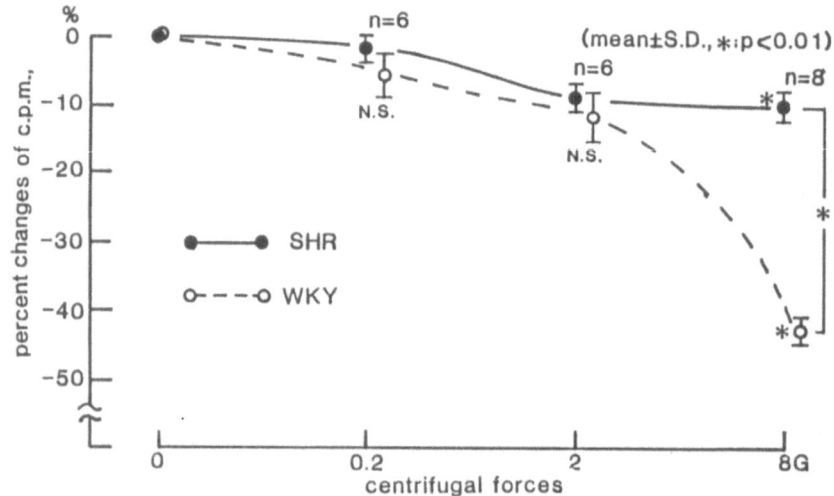

Fig.5 Percent changes of [³H]-thymidine incorporation
into DNA.

(3)Effects of centrifugal force on protein synthesis.

Actual protein contents measured by the method of Lowry showed no significant difference in these conditions. Total count of [¹⁴C]-leucine in TCA-insoluble protein was decreased by the centrifugal force. The suppression of protein synthesis by centrifugal force(0.2-8G) was less remarkable in SHR than in WKY. When the counts were corrected by DNA contents, no significant change was observed between centrifuged VSMCs and non-centrifuged controls(Fig.6).

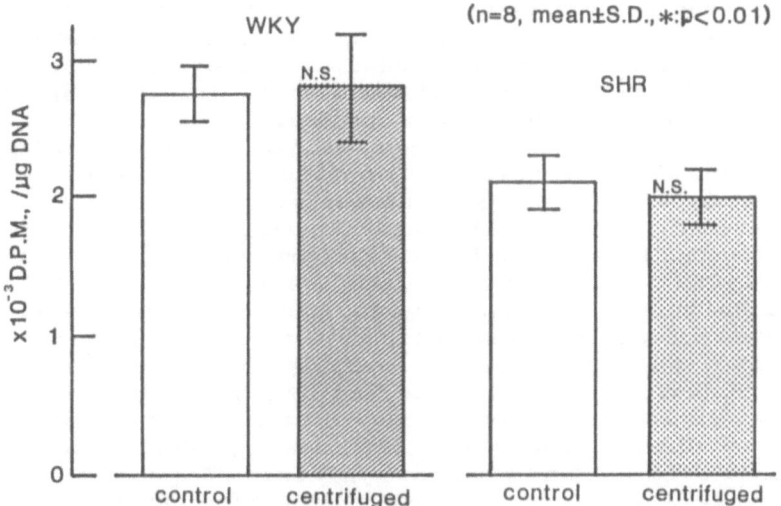

Fig.6 Effect of centrifugal force at 8G on [^{14}C]-leucine
incorporation into TCA-insoluble protein.

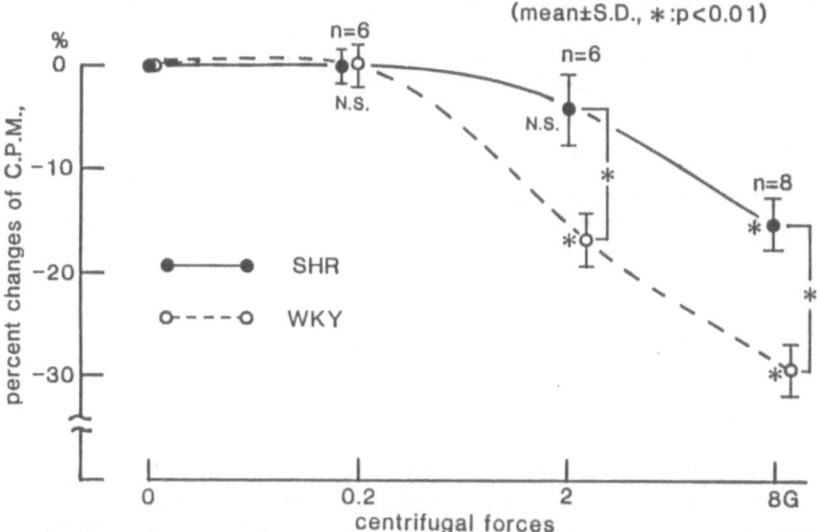

Fig.7 Percent changes of [^{14}C]-leucine incorporation
into TCA-insoluble protein.

DISCUSSION

In atherogenesis, glycosaminoglycans are one of the
important components of atherosclerotic plaques. GAGs are
excreted by the modified smooth muscle cells originating from the
medial layer and bind with low density lipoproteins in the
presence of calcium ion to constitute insoluble products in the
intima.

Among the several mechanisms regulating GAGs levels in the
arterial intima, hypertension is one of the most important
factors. Humoral factors, such as adrenergic neurotransmitters,

related to the pathogenesis of hypertension, might influence the GAGs synthesis by direct actions on VSMCs. In the present study, cultured VSMCs from rats were used, in order to eliminate the effects of humoral factors, and centrifugal force was applied as a mechanical stress of high blood pressure.

VSMCs from SHR showed a higher ability for GAGs synthesis in the non-centrifuged condition. Centrifugal force enhanced GAGs synthesis, in a gravity-dependent manner in both strains. Other investigators[5] reported that centrifugal force at 45G enhanced GAGs synthesis, especially in sulfated components in cultured pig aortic VSMCs. Our preliminary study revealed that 45G was too high for cultured VSMCs to survive, and that centrifugal force potentiated non-sulfated and sulfated GAGs almost equally.

As for DNA synthesis, the basal synthetic level of DNA was higher and that of protein corrected by DNA was lower in SHR in the basal condition, probably due to high frequency of diploids and tetraploids in the cells from SHR[6]. Centrifugal force suppressed both DNA and protein syntheses. This suppression is not due to cell viability, because tripan-blue staining showed no difference between the centrifuged and the non-centrifuged VSMCs. DNA- and protein-synthetic capacity under centrifugal force was more resistant in VSMCs from SHR compared with that from WKY. These characteristic changes in SHR might partly explain the vicious circle between hypertension and morphological changes of arterial wall in hypertensive animals.

CONCLUSION

In conclusion, independent of humoral factors, mechanical stress, as well as genetic factors, induces augmented GAGs and might induce atherosclerotic lesions via increased GAGs.

Acknowledgement: This study was supported by Grant-in-Aids for Scientific Research(61480211) from the Ministry of the Education, Science and Culture of Japan.

REFFERENCES

[1]Nishio I, Jimbo s, et al (1985): Acid Mucopolysaccharides in Rat's Aorta. J. Jap. Coll. Angiol., 25(4):259-262.
[2]Chamly-Chambell, J., Chambell, G.R. et al (1979):The smooth muscle cell in culture. Physiol. Rev., 59(1):1-61.
[3]Saani, H. and Tammi, M. (1977):A rapid method for separation and assay of radiolabeled mucopoly saccharides from cell culture medium. Analy. Biochem., 81(1):40-46
[4]Meir, P.D. and Wood, M. (1986):A simplified technique for the analysis of tissue acid mucopoly saccharides. Clin. Acta., 24(1):105-110.
[5]Merrilees, M.J. and Flint, M. (1977):The effect of centrifugal force on glycosaminoglycan production by aortic smooth muscle cells in culture. Atherosclerosis, 27:259-264.
[6]Gray K.Owens et al (1981):Smooth muscle cell hypertrophy versus hyperplasia in hypertension. Pro. Natl. Aad. Sci. USA, 788(12):7759-7763.

An *in vitro* Assay System for Measuring Both Vascular Permeability and Endothelial Cell Damage

S. Murota[1], I. Morita[1], and K. Kato[1,2]

[1] Section of Physiological Chemistry, Faculty of Dentistry, Tokyo Medical and Dental University, Tokyo, 113 Japan
[2] Research Center, Mitsubishi Chemical Industry, Yokohama, 227 Japan

ABSTRACTS

An assay system capable of measuring endothelial cell injury was established. The leakage of FITC-labeled bovine serum albumin through endothelial cell barrier was found to reflect the magnitude of endothelial cell injury. In the presence of complement, anti-ox red blood cell anti-serum caused severe injury to cultured endothelial cells derived from bovine carotid artery, followed by enormous increase in the albumin leakage. Exposure of endothelial cell monolayer to 15-HPETE (15-hydroperoxyeicosatetraenoic acid), one of the lipoxygenase metabolites of arachidonic acid, caused dose dependent injury to the endothelial cells. MCI-186 (3-methyl-1-phenyl-2-pyrazolin-5-one), a radical scavenger, had a remarkable protective effect on such endothelial cell injury.

INTRODUCTION

Endothelial cell injury has been recognized to be an initiation step toward the development of atherosclerosis. Therefore, it is very important to know what causes this endothelial cell injury, to know what the mechanism of this endothelial cell injury is, and to know how to protect the endothelial cells from the injury. The chromium-labeled technic has so far been used for detecting cytolysis. However, this technic has a defect in causing a high non-specific chromium release even from healthy normal cells. (1). Therefore, we tried to establish a more reliable method for examining endothelial cell injury.

EXPERIMENTAL METHODS

Endothelial cells were isolated from bovine carotid arteries and cultured with an Eagle's minimum essential medium containing 10% fetal calf serum (2). For assaying barrier activity of endothelial cell monolayers, the Boyden's chamber, a kind of chemotaxis chamber, was used (3). After setting up collagen coated (5μ g/ml gelatin, 100℃, for 1h) nucleopore filters (pore size: 5μ m) in Boyden's chambers, endothelial cells were cultured on the surface of the filters for 3 days when endothelial cell monolayers were obtained. After exposure of the monolayer to each one of the test drugs for 1h, bovine serum albumin (BSA) or FITC-labeled BSA was added only to the upper chamber. After 1h, the amount of leaked BSA or FITC-labeled BSA into the lower chamber across the endothelial cell monolayer was measured.

For assaying cell injury, dye exclusion test was performed for parallel cultures which were obtained by culturing the cells under the same conditions as indicated above except that the cells were grown in Petri dishes instead of in Boyden's chambers. The mono-layers of the parallel cultures were stained with erythrosine B. Only the dead cells were stained brown by the staining. The number of the dead cells was visually counted in micrographs.

RESULTS & DISCUSSION

BSA leakage from the upper chamber to the lower chamber across the nucleopore filter between them decreased sharply with increasing number of endothelial cells on the filter, and reached a constant low level after a monolayer of endothelial cells was completed on the surface of the filter (Fig.1). The permeability of BSA was found not to depend on the temperature during the experiments suggesting that this model refers to junctional transport.

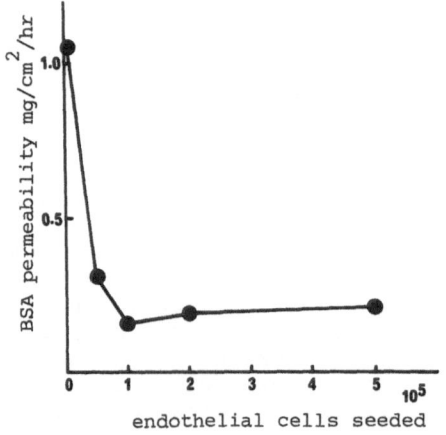

Fig.1. Effect of endothelial cell number seeded on BSA permeability across the mono-layer of endothelial cells. The experiments were carried out 3 day after the seeding.

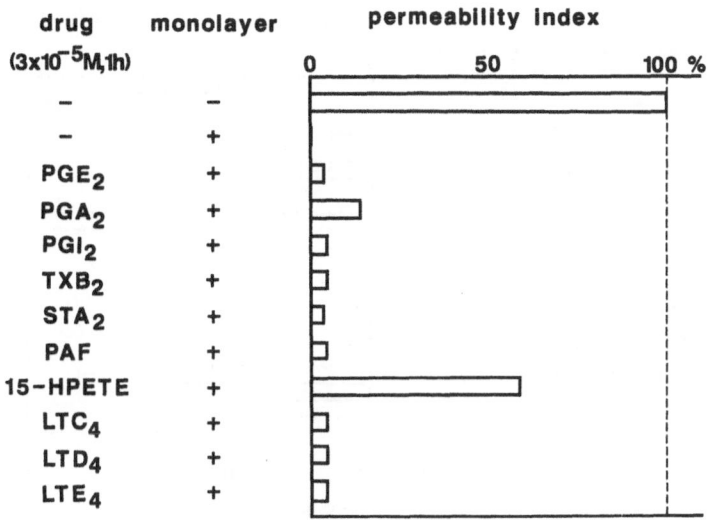

Fig.2. Effects of arachidonic acid metabolites on FITC-BSA permeability across endothelial cell monolayer

The above results indicate that the endothelial monolayer is keeping well its intrinsic barrier function during the experiments.
By using this model, we examined the effects of various arachidonic acid metabolites on endothelial cell permeability (Fig.2). Except PGA2 and 15-HPETE, most substances we tested have been known to cause vascular permeability increase in vivo and PGA2 and 15-HPETE have been known to be cytolitic. As shown in Fig.2, it is true that all the former substances caused some increase in the permeability of the fluorescent-BSA, but the values were very small. On the other hand, the cytolitic substances like PGA2 and 15-HPETE caused much larger permeability increases than the former substances. These results suggest that this in vitro model can be used for examining the change in both vascular permeability and endothelial cell injury, and that this model is much more sensitive to the change in cell injury than that in junctional transport system. To confirm this, next we examined the effects of cytochalasine B and anti-serum on the BSA permeability in the system.
Endothelial cell monolayers exposed to cytochalasin B were reported to show gaps between adjacent cells owing to retraction of cell cytoplasm and disruption of microfilaments (4). As shown in Fig.3, the cytochalasin B treatment resulted in an increase in the BSA leakage across the endothelial monolayers. By this experiment it was confirmed that such substances by opening gaps could increase BSA permeability in this assay system.
On the other hand, in the presence of complement, anti-ox red blood cell anti-serum caused severer injury to endothelial cells. This is perhaps because bovine endothelial cells have common anti-

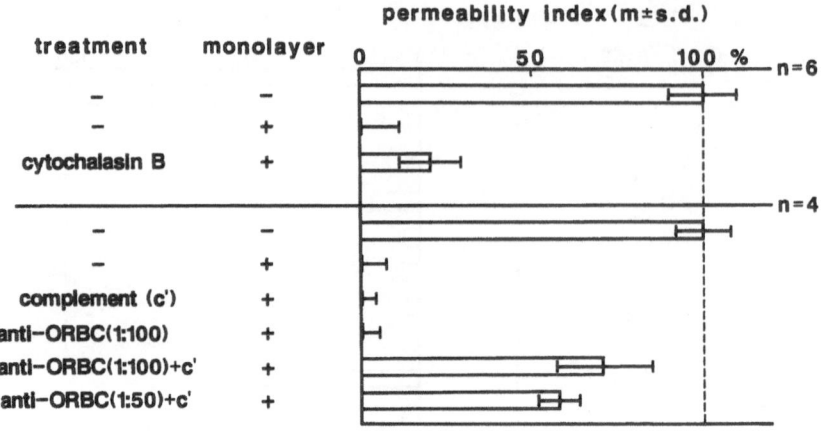

Fig.3. Effects of gap opening treatment and cytolitic treatment on BSA permeability across endothelial monolayer.

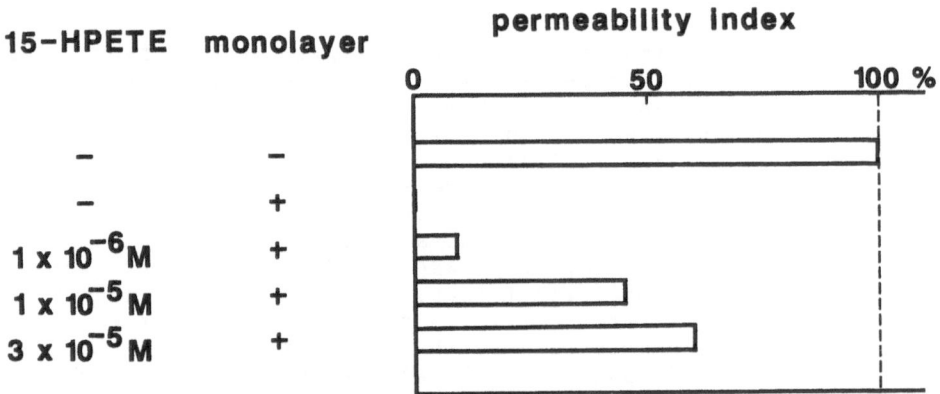

Fig.4. Effect of 15-HPETE on the leakage of FITC-BSA through the endothelial cell barrier

genicity to bovine red blood cells. As shown in Fig.3, anti-serum with complement caused prominent increase in the BSA permeability in a dose dependent manner. These results again indicate that this in vitro model is much more sensitive to endothelial cell injury than gap opening.

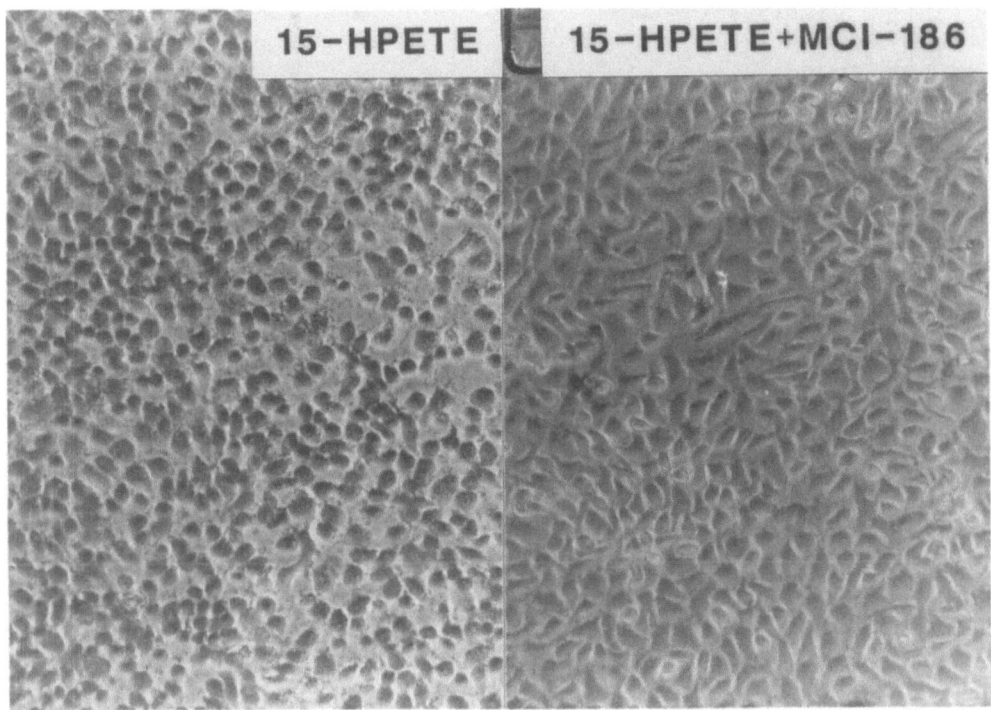

Fig.5. Injurious effect of 15-HPETE on endothelial cells, and
protective effect of MCI-186 on that. Each culture was stained
with erythrosine B. Only dead cells were stained brown. The left
micrograph shows the cells treated with 15-HPETE (3×10^{-5}M). The
right micrograph shows the cells treated with both 15-HPETE
(3×10^{-5}M) and MCI-186 (10^{-4}M)

        The effect of 15-HPETE on the permeability increase was also
dose dependent (Fig.4). To distinguish the BSA permeability increase due to cytolysis from that due to gap opening, the endothelial
monolayers in the paralel cultures were subjected to the dye exclusion test. By this test, cytolitic substances were easily distinguished from other types of substances. As shown in Fig.5 (left),
about 60% of the 15-HPETE treated cells were stained brown with
erythrosine B showing that these stained cells had been dead at the
test.

        Next we examined some drugs for their protective effect on the
endothelial cell injury. AVS, an anti-oxidant, dexamethasone, a
potent glucocorticoid and mepacrine, an inhibitor of phospholipase
A_2 failed to protect the endothelial cells against the injury caused
by 15-HPETE. In the case of mepacrine, it rather enhanced the cell
injury caused by 15-HPETE. Since mepacrine inhibits arachidonic
acid liberation from membrane phospholipids, this result suggests
that some of the arachidonic acid metabolites produced by the

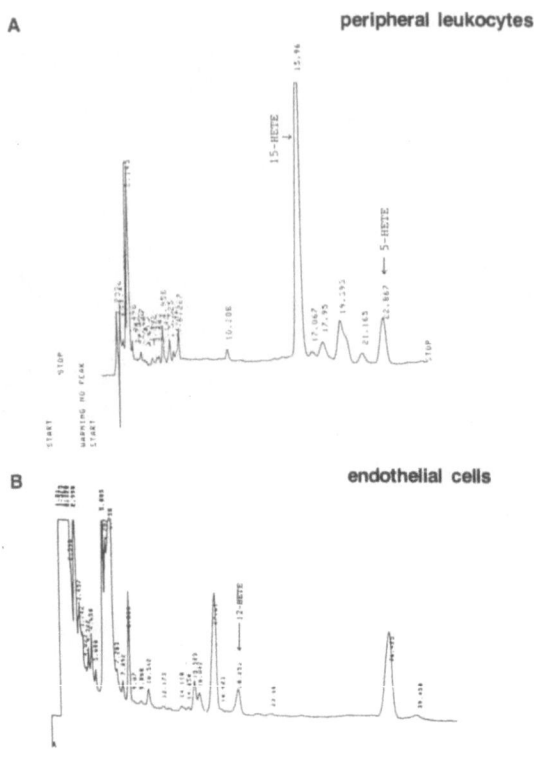

A: peripheral leukocytes

B: endothelial cells

Fig.6. HPLC profiles showing arachidonic acid metabolism by
leukocytes and endothelial cells.
 A: Homogenates of human peripheral leukocytes were incubated with
    arachidonic acid.
 B: Extract of the culture medium of bovine endothelial cells.

endothelial cells, perhaps prostacyclin, may have some beneficial
effect on the cell injury. MCI-186, a kind of radical scavenger,
showed a remarkable protective effect on the endothelial cell injury
due to 15-HPETE (Fig.5, right). MCI-186 was effective in both cases
when it was added to the cultures at the same time with 15-HPETE and
when it was added to the cultures 1h prior to the addition of
15-HPETE. MCI-186 at 3×10^{-5}M and at 3×10^{-4}M almost completely
abolished the endothelial cell injury caused by 15-HPETE. The cytoprotective effect of MCI-186 on the endothelial cells was dose
dependent (5).

    In our experiments, it was found that human peripheral leuko-
cytes were able to produce 15-HETE as well as 5-HETE, and that endothelial cells themselves were able to produce 12-HETE (Fig.6).
Therefore, it is suggested that such cytolytic lipid peroxides as
15-HPETE, 5-HPETE and 12-HPETE may actually be produced locally in
the lesion of atherosclerosis, and they injure endothelial cells
nereby.

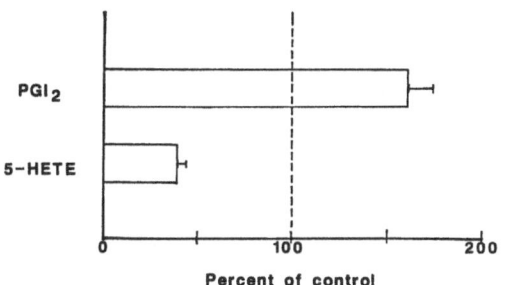

Fig.7. Effects of MCI-186 (10^{-5}M) on PGI_2 release by bovine endothelial cells in culture and on 5-HETE biosynthesis by the homogenates of RBL-1 cells.

It seems that MCI-186 shows such a remarkable cytoprotective effect partly because it can enhance PGI_2 production partly because it can inhibit 5-HETE production (Fig.7). However, it is also true that these activities of MCI-186 on arachidonic acid metabolism are not suficient to account for the prominent cytoprotective effect of MCI-186 in all. Most of the mechanism by which MCI-186 shows such a remarkable cytoprotection against the endothelial cells exposed to the lipid peroxide still remains unknown. In any case there is a possibility that MCI-186 may be developed to a unique anti-athero-sclerotic drug.

ACKNOWLEDGMENT

The authors wish to thank Mitsubishi Chemical Industries, Ltd., for the generous gift of MCI-186. We also wish to thank Mr.T. Watanabe and Mr.K.Noguchi for their technical assistance. This work was supported in part by a Grant-in-aid for Scientific Research from the Japanese Ministry of Education (No.62122004) and in part by a Research Grant for Cardiovascular Diseases (60C-2) from the Ministry of the Health and Welfare, Japan.

REFERENCES

1) Henriksen T et al (1979) Scand J Clin Lab Invest 39:369
2) Morita I et al (1984) Biochim Biophys Acta 792:304
3) Boyden SV (1962) J Exp Med 453:115
4) Shasby DM et al (1982) Circ Res 51:657
5) Watanabe T et al Prostagr. Leukotr. Med. in press

Endothelial Injury and Accumulation of Cholesterol Ester Derived from Circulating Lipoproteins

T. Takano, C. Mineo, R. Hashida, Y. Yagyu-Mizuno, K. Nakagami, and S. Ohkuma

Department of Microbiology and Molecular Pathology, Faculty of Pharmaceutical Sciences, Teikyo University, Sagamiko, 199-01 Japan

ABSTRACT

To elucidate the mechanism how lipoproteins transport through the endothelial barrier, an in vitro model of transcellular transport of macromolecules was developed.
In this paper, the involvement of endothelial cells and accumulation of cholesterol ester in arterial wall will be discussed from the following aspects. 1. Transcellular transport of lipoproteins through cultured endothelial monolayer. 2. Junctional transport of fluorescein dextran through cultured endothelial monolayer. 3. Endothelial injury in vitro and platelet aggregation.
These aspects may be helpful for understanding the fluid mechanism of blood flow atherogenesis.

INTRODUCTION

Vascular endothelial cells have an important function as a selective barrier and also have physiological mechanisms to prevent thrombosis on them to maintain smooth blood flow. There are so many indicators that endothelial injury and platelet aggregation are involved in the initial event of atherogenesis [1].
Studies of the transport of low density lipoprotein (LDL) are important for determining the mechanism of cholesterol ester accumulation in the arterial wall. Extensive studies of the internalization of LDL through receptors have been made on cultured endothelial cells. Recent cytochemical studies have shown that LDL passes through the endothelium in transcytotic vesicles in situ [2]. However, very little is known about the mechanism, kinetics and requirements of the transcellular transport of LDL across the endothelium, mainly because no simple, relevant in vitro model that uses cultured endothelial monolayers has been available.
To elucidate the mechanisms of transport of lipoproteins through the endothelial barrier such as vesicular transport, junctional transport and transport through endothelial injury, an in vitro model of transcellular transport of macromolecules was developed.

RESULTS

1. Transcellular transport of lipoproteins through cultured endothelial monolayer.

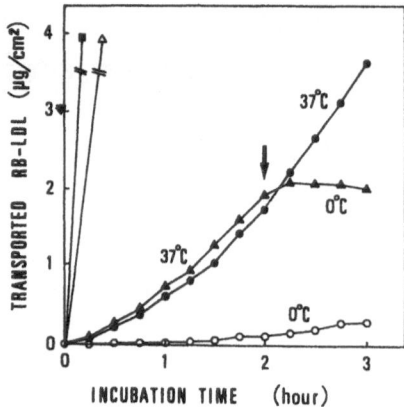

Fig.1 Time course of RB-LDL transport. RB-LDL (0.2 mg protein/ml) was introduced into upper compartment, and the RB-LDL transported through the membrane to the lower compartment was monitored: dacron sheet alone (■); dacron sheet with gelated collagen (△); endothelial monolayer on the dacron sheet with gelated collagen at 37°C (●), at 0°C (O), and at 37°C for 2 h then at 0°C (▲). The temperature was reduced at the time indicated by the arrow.

From in situ morphological studies, Simionescu et al. proposed that various tracers, such as ferritin and horseradish peroxidase, pass through the endothelium via transcytotic vesicles and/or through intercellular junctions [2]. Low molecular weight macromolecules tend to pass through intercellular junctions, and the transport seems to be regulated to some extent by the surface charge of the macromolecules and the charge of the cell surface in the microvascular endothelium.

To study the mechanism of lipoprotein transport through arterial cells, porcine endothelial cells were cultured on gelated type I collagen supported by a dacron sheet, and the transport of low density lipoprotein (LDL) labeled with Rhodamine-B isothiocyanate (RB-LDL) through the cells was measured [3].

Light microscopy showed that porcine endothelial cells became confluent 2-3 days after seeding. The surface and cellular arrangement of this endothelial monolayer appeared very similar to those of arterial endothelial cells in vivo. Transmission electron microscopy also showed that tight junctions are sometimes formed between cells like those formed between arterial endothelial cells in vivo.

A considerable amount of RB-LDL was transported at 37°C, but not at 0°C (Fig.1) [3], although it passed through the membrane freely in the absence of endothelial cells. There was no detachment of cells during incubation for 3 h at 37°C, because transport of RB-LDL decreased greatly when the temperature was reduced to 0°C after incubation at 37°C for 2 h.

RB-LDL transport in our study also was energy-dependent because it was inhibited by a combination of 2-deoxyglucose and NaN_3, inhibitors of ATP generation. Another important feature was the dose-response curve of RB-LDL transport; transport increased with increasing concentrations of RB-LDL up to 0.4 mg protein/ml, but was saturated at higher concentrations at 37°C. The maximum value in this condition was approximately 1.3 µg protein/cm^2/h. RB-^{125}I-LDL was not metabolized during transport because after transport at 37°C, no degradation products of apoprotein B were detected by SDS-polyacrylamide gel electrophoresis followed by autoradiography.

This present results suggest that RB-LDL is transported in transcytotic vesicles by a temperature- and energy-dependent process, but not through cellular junctions nor by endocytosis and exocytosis via a lysosomal system. This kind of study should be helpful in clarifying the physiological functions of lipoprotein transport, especially in pathological conditions such as atherosclerosis connected with the shear stress associated with blood flow.

2. Junctional transport of fluorescein dextran through cultured endothelial monolayer.

Transport via intercellular junctions also is well known. Dextrans labeled with fluorescein isothiocyanate (FDs) appear to be good tracers for the study of the vascular permeability of various tissues in situ [4], because FDs with a wide range of molecular weights can be obtained and can be measured quantitatively.

The transport of 4K-70K FDs did not depend on temperature, and the dose-respose curves showed that the transport of FDs of various sizes was non-saturable up to 100 μM FDs. In contrast, RB-LDL transport was temperature-dependent and saturable at approximately 200 μg/ml (about 0.2 μM).

The rate of transport of FDs through the endothelial monolayer depended on the molecular weight of FDs used in this in vitro system (Fig.2). Results were consistent with histological findings in situ. Measurements of transport rates of FDs in vivo compared with those found in our in vitro system may help widen our understanding of the construction and integrity of the cellular junctions of the endothelial monolayer, which seem to vary with the organ from which the cells are derived.

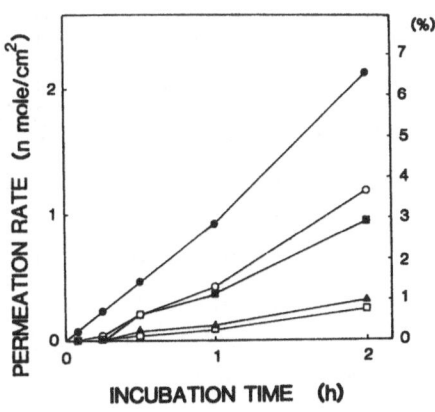

Fig.2 Time courses of FD transport. FD samples (50 μM) with molecular weights of 4K (●), 10K (○), 20K (■), 70K (▲) and 150K (□) were introduced into the upper compartment, and their passage through the membrane was studied for 2 h at 37°C. The transport of FD is shown in nmole per cm^2 membrane per h (left) and as the % of recovery per h of the amount of FD applied (right).

Table 1

	FD			RB-LDL		
	Molecular weight	0°C	37°C	Molecular weight	0°C	37°C
Transport rate (%/h)	4K	3.3	3.3			
	10K		1.8			
	20K		1.5	1,000K-1,500K	0.0	0.5-0.7
	70K	0.6	0.6			
	150K		0.4			
Temperature-dependence	Temperature-independent			Temperature-dependent		
Dose-response	Unsaturable			Saturable		

We now have examined the transport of FD, which differs from that of RB-LDL as shown in Table 1. The transport of 4K and 70K FD does not depend on temperature, and the dose-response curves show that the transport of FDs of various sizes is non-saturable up to 100 μM FD. In contrast, RB-LDL transport is temperature-dependent and saturable at approximately 200 μg/ml (about 0.2 μM).

We concluded from the results of our previous study that RB-LDL is transported in transcytotic vesicles (not through cellular junctions or by endocytosis and exocytosis via a lysosomal system) because its transport was temperature- and energy-dependent and saturable. In contrast, FD probably passes through the intercellular junctions of the endothelial monolayer.

3. Effect of PGI_2 on transcellular transport of fluorescein dextran.

Vascular integrity and function are mediated by the endothelial cell monolayer lining and the vascular wall. These endothelial cells are thought to act as a barrier to various macromolecules. Once endothelial cells are injured, the accumulations of lipoproteins such as LDL increase. This appears to be a primary event in atherogenesis. The surface of the endothelial cells also acts to protect against thrombosis, which stimulates permeability of the vascular wall. PGI_2, mainly produced in the endothelial cells, is one of the most potent known inhibitors of platelet aggregation.

In this work, we found PGI_2 at 3 x 10^{-9} M caused 20 % inhibition of transport of FD through an endothelial cell monolayer (Fig.3) [5]. The inhibitory effect of the stable PGI_2 deriv. (isocarbacyclin) persisted for at least 4 hr and that of native PGI_2 persisted for 2 hr. Our finding that although the half-life of native PGI_2 is only a few minutes, the inhibitory effect of PGI_2 was observed for at least 2 hr, suggested that a secondary mediator was involved in the inhibition. That the inhibitory effect lasted for at least 1 hr after removal of PGI_2 supports this interpretation.

One possible explanation of the inhibitory effects of prostaglandins is that the inhibition is due to their effects in increasing cAMP production as a secondary mediator. To confirm the involvement of cAMP in this system, we tested the effects of some reagents that modulate production of cAMP. In the presence of IBMX, which is an inhibitor of cAMP phosphodiesterase, PGI_2 deriv. increased the cAMP content from 3.3 pmol/10^6 cells to 17.1, in parallel with increase of its inhibition of FD transport from 42 % in the absence of, to 60.2 % in the presence of IBMX (Table 2). Addition of DDA, an inhibitor of adenylate cyclase, with PGI_2 deriv. reduced the amount of

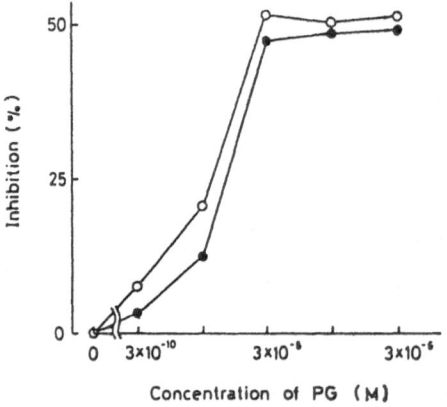

Fig.3   Dose-response curves of prostaglandins. The inhibitory effects (%) on FD transport in 2 hr of various concentrations of PGI_2 (—○—), PGI_2 deriv. (—●—).

Table 2   FD transport in the presence of reagents that affect the cAMP content of cells.

	FD (% inhibition)			FD (% inhibition)			FD (% inhibition)
None	76.3±10.7		PGI$_2$ deriv.	44.1±5.9 (42.2)		PGI$_2$	42.5± 7.5 (44.3)
dbcAMP	49.8± 7.4 (34.7)		+IBMX	30.4±6.0 (60.2)		+IBMX	23.2± 3.2 (69.6)
IBMX	56.5± 9.6 (26.0)		+DDA	70.9±6.5 (7.1)		+DDA	64.3±11.2 (15.7)
DDA	73.3±13.3 (3.9)		+IBMX DDA	61.2±9.3 (10.6)		+IBMX DDA	78.1± 8.6 (0)

FD transport (pmol/cm^2) in 1 hr in the presence of test reagents (PG; 3 µM, dbcAMP; 0.1 mM, IBMX; 0.5 mM, DDA; 0.1 mM) was measured. Data are the means ± SD. Inhibitory effects (%) are shown in parentheses.

cAMP from 17.1 pmol/10^6 cells to 3.0 and decreased the inhibitory effect of this prostaglandin derivative on FD transport from 60.2 % to 10.6.

The inhibitory effects of PGI$_2$ on FD transport may be explained by increase of tight junctional connections between endothelial cells, because PGI$_2$ increased the electrical resistance between the apical and basal layer from 18.4 $\Omega \cdot$ cm^2 to 26.6.   This interpretation is supported by evidence for a correlation between electrical resistance and the cAMP content of epithelial cells. Cyclic AMP, which increases on PGI$_2$ treatment probably acts as a secondary mediator in stimulating production of tight junctions.

4.   Endothelial injury in vitro and platelet aggregation.

Injury to endothelial cell layer and platelets adhesion and aggregation to these area are involved in the initiation of atherosclerosis. For the first step to reconstitute the injury of endothelium and to analyze the role of platelets, we made mechanical injury to the cultured endothelial cell layer, and investigated the binding of platelets. Platelets labeled with ^{51}Cr were added to the culture of endothelial cells injured by the teflon ring. Both fibronectin and fibrinogen were required for platelets binding to the cell layer (Fig.4).

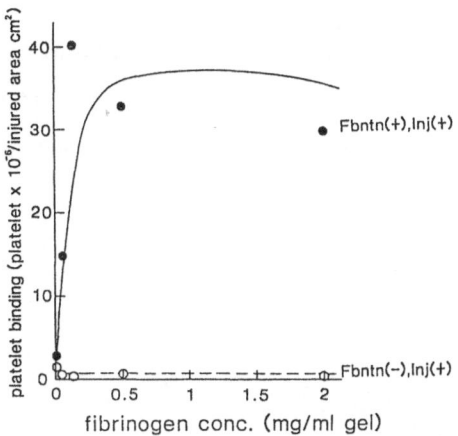

Fig.4   Effect of fibrinogen on platelet binding in injured area endothelial monolayer. Collagen solution (type I, 4 mg/ml, 1 ml) containing various amounts of fibrinogen with 20 µg/ml fibronectin (Fbntn) was gelated, and endothelial cells (EC) were cultured on the gel. ^{51}Cr-labeled platelets (1 x 10^8 cells/ml) were introduced and incubated for 20 h.

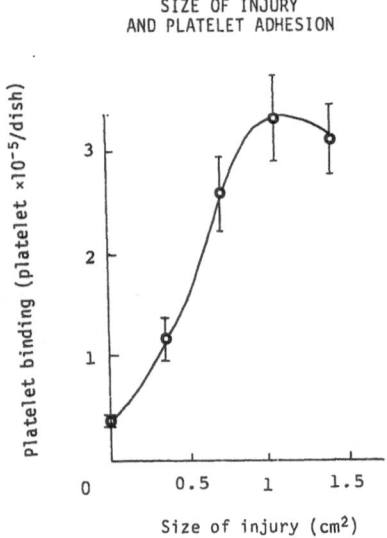

SIZE OF INJURY
AND PLATELET ADHESION

Platelet binding (platelet ×10⁻⁵/dish)

Size of injury (cm²)

Fig.5   Size of injury and platelet binding. With various sizes of injury of the endothelial cells on collagen gel containing 20 µg/ml fibronectin and 500 µg/ml fibrinogen, platelets (1 x 10^8 cells/ml) binding was assayed after 20 h incubation. The abscissa indicates arbitrary unit of detachment of the endothelial cells.

The amount of platelets adhered increased according to the size of injury (Fig.5) and the concentration of platelets added to the culture. The denuded area was repaired in time dependent manner by proliferation and migration of endothelium. The quantity of platelets bound decreased as endothelial cells repaired the injury. This in vitro model should be useful to investigate how modulators, such as protacyclin and PDGF produced by the platelets and cells, affect the binding of platelets, the repair of endothelium and the transport of macromolecules.

In this paper, the involvement of transcellular transport of macromolecules through endothelial cells and accumulation of cholesterol ester in arterial wall is discussed.

REFERENCES

[1] Ross R, (1986) New England J Med pp 314-500
[2] Simionescu N, (1983) Physiol Rev 63:1536-1579
[3] Hashida R, Anamizu C, Kimura J, Ohkuma S, Yoshida Y, Takano T, (1986) Cell Struct Funct 11:31-42
[4] Hashida R, Anamizu C, Yagyu-Mizuno Y, Ohkuma S, Takano T, (1986) Cell Struct Funct 11:343-349
[5] Mizuno-Yagyu Y, Hashida R, Mineo C, Ikegami S, Ohkuma S, Takano T, (1987) Biochem Pharmacol in press

The Modulation of Transport Through the Arterial Wall

M.J. LEVER

Physiological Flow Studies Unit, Imperial College, London, SW7 2AZ, England

ABSTRACT

The transport processes that occur within the arterial wall influence
wall biology and the development of arterial disease.Such processes are
influenced by the properties of the individual layers of the wall and
by interactions between them. Atherosclerosis is characterized by the
accumulation of material in the intima, a process which could result
from hindrance to transport across the media.The transport properties
of the media are influenced by those of the endothelium, local blood
flow, transmural pressure and vasoactive agents.The susceptibility of
different vessels to atherosclerosis may depend in part on their medial
properties.

INTRODUCTION

The accumulation of lipids and plasma proteins within the intima
of the arterial wall is one important feature of atherosclerosis. The
net rate of accumulation of materials within this layer depends on
various factors such as their metabolic turnover, the extent to which
they interact with tissue components and their ease of transport in and
out of the wall. Transport rates are determined by the properties of
all the wall structures: the endothelium, the intima, the media and the
adventitia as well as the vasa vasorum and adventitial lymphatics.
Modification of any of these can alter the extent and sites of
accumulation. Much attention has been focussed on the role of the
endothelium and, in particular, on how its high resistance to the
transport of fluid and solutes is modified by haemodynamic forces. Less
consideration has been given to the role of the deeper layers,
including the media, despite interdependence between the properties of
the layers. Hindrance of transport across the media may underly the
finding that marked accumulation of material normally occurs in the
intima of thick-walled arteries and not in thinner-walled vessels such
as veins (1). Indeed, the observations that the low density lipoprotein
concentration in the interstitial fluid of the intima can exceed that
of the plasma (2), and that lipid accumulates in the deeper layers of
the intima,could both be explained by a mechanism of ultrafiltration of
these materials by the deeper layers of the wall (3, 4).

TRANSPORT THROUGH THE MEDIA

The extracellular space of the media offers a route by which
plasma constituents and wall metabolites can pass across the whole

thickness of the wall. Transport can occur by convection, driven by the transmural pressure gradient and also by diffusion. Under normal in vivo conditions (in contrast to those pertaining in tracer uptake studies) diffusion will only be an important transport mechanism for metabolites and for larger solutes. For the latter, a concentration gradient exists between luminal plasma and adventitial lymph because of the partial reflection or ultrafiltration of these materials by the various layers of the wall. Diffusion of these large solutes including the plasma proteins will, however, be hindered by the exclusion properties of the various interstitial components such as the fibrous proteins, glycoproteins and glycosaminoglycans. The degree of exclusion of a solute can be assessed from measurement of its distribution volume, which is the ratio of the solute concentration in tissue to that in the bathing solution after incubation until equilibrium is reached. In such a series of experiments on fresh human mesenteric artery, the average distribution volume for albumin in the media was 0.13 which is 0.26 of the value for EDTA, a material whose distribution volume is a measure of the total extracellular space. Thus even a relatively small plasma protein is excluded from about 75% of the interstitial space. There was less exclusion by the intimal and adventitial tissues for which the mean distribution volumes for albumin were 0.22 and 0.45 respectively and for which the albumin/EDTA distribution volume ratios were 0.40 and 0.75 (5). Another study on the media of human aorta indicated that the distribution volume for LDL was negligibly small (2). Although a high degree of exclusion implies a considerable resistance to diffusive transport and the possibility of ultrafiltration by the excluding structures, drag-induced convective flux could transport material across the media through less restricted pathways in the interstitium in a similar manner to that by which larger solutes are transported through a gel fractionation column. The Peclet number has been estimated to be approximately 4 for albumin transport in the media of rabbit aorta, indicating an appreciable convective component to its transport within that tissue (6, 7). Larger plasma proteins will experience greater drag forces than albumin but there is also a greater probability that they will be ultrafiltered.

MODIFICATION OF MEDIAL TRANSPORT PROPERTIES

(a) Effects of endothelial properties on the media

Damage to the endothelium has often been observed to cause a marked increase in the rate of transport of macromolecules into the artery wall. This has commonly been attributed to removal of the high transport resistance of the endothelial layer. However, significant changes also occur in the transport properties of the underlying structures because of the role of the endothelium in modulating fluid flux across the wall (4). Destruction of the endothelium causes a pressure dependent increase in transmural fluid flux and this is associated with a slight swelling of the media as indicated by an increase in its water content (Fig. 1). Conversely, if the transmural fluid flux is abolished, a situation which is obtained experimentally by pressurizing arteries with air, the tissue compacts, with loss of interstitial fluid. While complete cessation of transmural fluid flux is unlikely in vivo, it will be low in thick-walled arteries because of the limited hydraulic conductivity of vessel wall tissue and may be particularly low in arteries with extensive plaque formation. Altered hydration produces marked changes in the exclusion properties of the media, these being very sensitive to

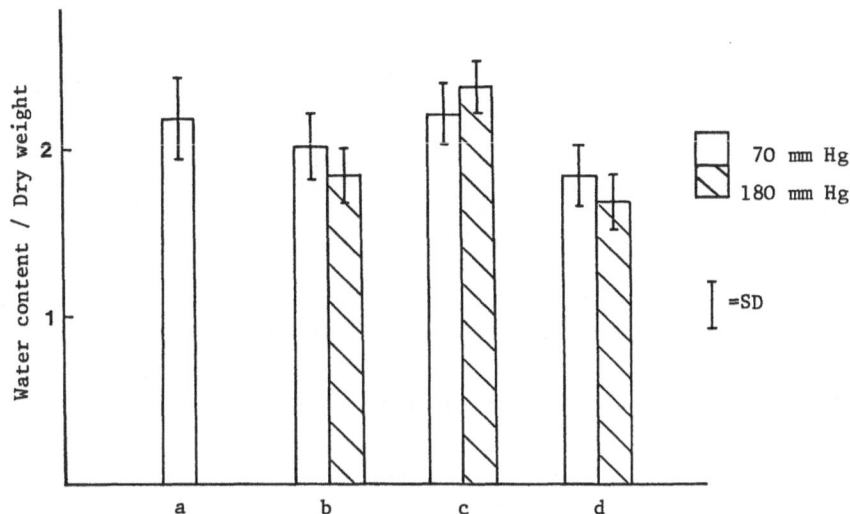

FIG. 1 The mean water contents of the media of rabbit aorta (a) zero transmural pressure and untethered (b) Liquid pressurized, intact, in vivo length (c) liquid pressurized, endothelium damaged, in vivo length (d) air pressurized, in vivo length.

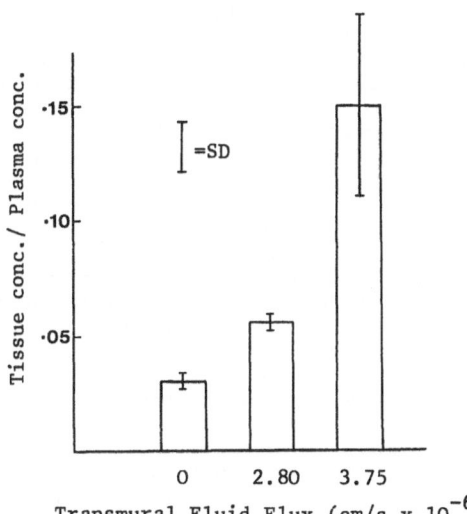

FIG. 2 The apparent mean medial distribution volumes for albumin in the rabbit aorta pressurized to 70 mmHg with air or with liquid while the endothelium is intact or damaged.

very small changes in the interstitial space. Fig. 2 shows that on changing the transmural fluid flux between 0 and 3.75×10^{-6} cm s^{-1}, the apparent medial albumin distribution volume can be varied by a factor of 7. Since the dependence of exclusion on hydration increases with solute size, much larger changes will occur in the transport properties for LDL than for albumin.

On damaging the endothelium therefore, the combined alteration of interstitial hydration and transmural fluid flow will enhance both the diffusive and convective transport of solutes across the wall. Under these conditions, the Peclet number for albumin increases by a factor of 2-3 (6, 7). It may be significant in this context that in experiments involving damage to the endothelium in experimental animals, intimal lipid accumulation tends to occur not immediately after damage but after regeneration of the endothelial layer.

(b) Effects of pressure on the media

Fig. 1 shows that an increase in wall strain of intact arteries by pressurization causes a fall in water content. When similar strains are produced in the absence of fluid convection, by pressurization with air, the water content is reduced further. Conversely, production of similar strains in de-endothelialized vessels causes an increase in water content which rises with increasing pressure and transmural flux. Thus, there appears to be an interaction between the circumferential hoop stresses caused by pressurization which tend to compress the tissue, and the drag forces associated with transmural flux which tend to expand the tissue. Alteration of the pressure not only changes the hoop stresses but also the driving force for transmural flux. The net changes in hydration will change the porosity of the wall tissue to solutes and may influence fluid transport itself. Thus, there is a decrease in the hydraulic conductivity of the intact rabbit aorta from 4.00×10^{-8} to 2.44×10^{-8}cm/s/mmHg on increasing the pressure from 70 to 180 mmHg (8). This fall in conductivity occurs despite the decrease in the thickness of the wall (indicating a much larger fall in specific conductivity) and may be associated with the observed decrease in wall hydration on increasing the pressure and perhaps also with increased tortuosity of the fluid pathways in the wall.

Solute transport into the artery wall is generally enhanced by increasing the transmural pressure and this is generally attributed to changes at the endothelium. The effects of pressure on solute transport across the media have been studied less, but the net effect of enhanced convection and a decrease in porosity could lead to greater ultrafiltration at the intima-media boundary.

(c) Effects of vasoactive agents on the media

An important mechanism involving the interaction of the endothelium and the media is the production of vasoactive agents by endothelial cells, a process which for EDRF and PGI$_2$, at least, is influenced by luminal wall shear. The altered wall strain caused by contraction or relaxation of vascular smooth muscle can also change the porosity of the tissue. For albumin, the distribution volume is 2.5 times lower in the fully contracted rabbit carotid artery than in the fully dilated vessel (9). Table 1 shows that the transmedial flux of albumin (measured by the rate of entry of Evans-blue labelled albumin into the wall) and fluid (measured volumetrically) both decrease on contraction of the vessel. How much of these falls is due to altered porosity, and how much to an increase in wall thickness caused by muscle contraction, is not clear.

Table 1. Effects on transport properties of de-endothelialized rabbit aorta at 70 mmHg following contraction with noradrenaline (10^{-5} M) or dilatation with ISDN (10^{-4} M).

	Noradrenaline	ISDN
Mean diameter (mm)	3.88 + 0.63	5.25 + 0.65
Apparent distribution volume for albumin	0.11 + 0.04	0.15 + 0.04
Albumin flux (cm s^{-1}x 10^{-6})	1.52 + 0.39	2.40 + 0.42
Water flux (cm s^{-1}x 10^{-6})	1.77 + 0.25	2.73 + 0.15

Changes in smooth muscle tone alter wall compliance which in turn can modify local blood flow and the fluid shear forces at the luminal surface.   Fluid and solute plasma-wall exchange processes which are sensitive to wall shear can therefore be modulated indirectly by medial properties.

HETEROGENEITY OF WALL TRANSPORT PROPERTIES

It is well-known that there is wide range of rates at which certain plasma-borne solutes are taken up by different blood vessels. Uptake of plasma proteins by the proximal part of the aorta, for example, occurs more rapidly than by the distal part and uptake by the pulmonary trunk is more rapid still (10).

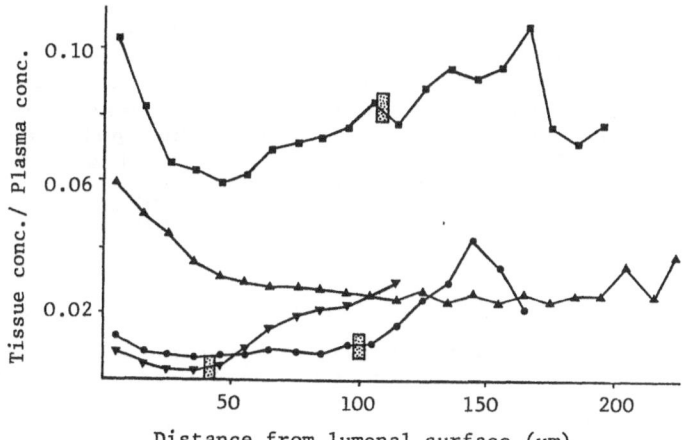

FIG. 3 In vivo steady state distribution of labelled albumin across the walls of various rabbit arteries, obtained by en face serial sectioning. ▼ carotid   ● dorsal thoracic aorta   ▲ ascending aorta   ■ pulmonary   trunk.   ▨ indicates   the   position   of   the medial-adventitial boundary.

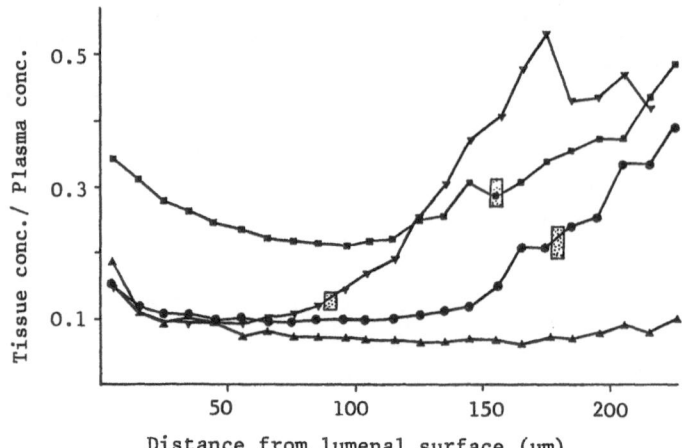

FIG. 4 In vitro measurements of the distribution volume of labelled
albumin across the walls of various rabbit arteries, obtained by en
face serial sectioning, ▼ carotid ● dorsal thoracic aorta
▲ ascending aorta ■ pulmonary trunk. ▨ indicates the
position of the medial-adventitial boundary.

Figure 3 shows the in vivo distribution of albumin across the walls of
four different arteries of the rabbit. In these vessels, the intima is
negligibly thin and the distribution curves are comprised of data from
the media and adventitia, the concentration of tracer generally being
lower in the former (for the ascending aorta,only medial data is
given). In vivo the arteries experience different amplitudes and
patterns of shear stress and also exhibit differences in some features
of their endothelial structure such as glycocalyx thickness and cell
shape.Such factors may contribute to the different patterns of label
uptake, but in vitro measurements of the albumin distribution volume in
the different vessel layers(Fig.4) suggest that the much greater medial
porosity of the pulmonary trunk compared with that of the other vessels
may be an additional factor in determining its greater in vivo uptake.
Measurements of flux across the wall of these vessels are required to
test whether the low predilection of the pulmonary artery to
atherosclerosis is due to the readier passage of material across the
media resulting from its greater porosity.

CONCLUSION

Blood flow and the associated wall shear stresses can have effects
on the transport properties of the surface layers of the vessel and can
also affect the properties of the deeper layers in a number of indirect
ways. These include the release of vasoactive agents and the modulation
of transmural water flux by changes in the degree of protein
ultrafiltration at the surface or by changes in the glycocalyx or
intercellular clefts.The resulting changes in the media may influence
the ultimate fate of materials transiently in the sub-endothelial or
intimal spaces.

Acknowledgements: I should like to acknowledge the contributions of various colleagues with whom I have collaborated, including Colin Caro, Alain Tedgui, John Tarbell, Nat Cary, Mark Jay and Nasrin Sharifi. The work has been supported by the MRC, National Heart Research Fund and Pharma Schwarz GmbH.

REFERENCES

(1) Caro C G, Lever MJ, Laver-Rudich Z, Meyer F, Liron N, Ebel W, Parker KH, Winlove CP (1980) Atherosclerosis 37:497-511
(2) Smith EB, Staples EM (1982) Atherosclerosis 41: 295-308
(3) Fry DL, Cornhill JF, Sharma H, Pap JM, Mitschelen J (1986) Arteriosclerosis 6:475-490
(4) Tedgui A, Lever MJ (1987) Am J Physiol 253 (in press)
(5) Cary N, Jay MT, Lever MJ (1987) J Physiol (Lond) 388:26P
(6) Truskey GA, Colton CK, Smith KA (1981) Quantitative analysis of protein transport in the arterial wall. In: Schwartz CJ, Werthessen NT, Wolf S (eds) Structure and function of the Circulation Vol 3 Plenum Press New York 287-355
(7) Tedgui A, Lever MJ (1985) Circ Res 57: 856-863
(8) Tedgui A, Lever MJ (1984) Am J Physiol 247: H784-791
(9) Caro CG, Lever MJ (1983) Atherosclerosis 46: 137-146
(10) Christensen S, Stender S, Nyvad O, Bagger H (1982) Atherosclerosis 41: 309-319

Effect of Tissue Hypoxia on the Development of Atherosclerosis

Y. Ishikawa, J. Mukodani, R. Okamoto, M. Hatani, M. Tsukitani, N. Watanabe, T. Taniguchi, N. Miyazaki, M. Tsunemitsu, S. Takano, and H. Fukuzaki

First Department of Internal Medicine, Kobe University School of Medicine, Kobe, 650 Japan

ABSTRACT

It has been suggested that hypoxia enhances the development of atherosclerosis. The aim of this study was to clarify the mechanisms. Experiments were designed to observe the effects of hypoxic and hyperoxic inhalation in WHHL rabbits and have revealed that atherosclerotic lesions in the hypoxia group were larger than those in the hyperoxia group. Since there was no fluctuation in plasma cholesterol level, the effect of hypoxia was probably a direct one. Cell culture studies were carried out, using rabbit aortic smooth muscle cells and fibroblasts, and the cells were incubated in the medium supplemented with hyperlipidemic serum. The esterified cholesterol contents in the cells under the hypoxic condition were 2-3 times higher than those under control conditions. Analysis of cholesterol metabolism revealed that hypoxia increased ACAT activity and suppressed cholesterol efflux.

From these results, we conclude that under the hyperlipidemic condition, cell hypoxia plays an important role in atherogenesis. The hypothetical mechanisms of hypoxia on the development of atherosclerosis are proposed.

INTRODUCTION

The inner layers of the artery are avascular. The supply of oxygen and nutrients to this area depends upon direct diffusion from the vascular lumen and vasa vasorum. The avascular zone is always jeopardized because it is located a critical diffusion distance from the lumen [1]. Arterial tissue hypoxia could be induced easily by a deterioration in the diffusion and an interruption of blood flow through the vasa vasorum.

Since Heuper [2] introduced the anoxemia theory of atherogenesis, much interest has centered around the possible mechanisms. We investigated the effect of systemic hypoxia and hyperoxia on the development of atherosclerosis in Watanabe Heritable Hyperlipidemic (WHHL) rabbits. These rabbits lack low density lipoprotein (LDL) receptors and therefore provide us with a unique model for human familial hypercholesterolemia. In addition, we studied the effect of hypoxia on the lipid metabolism in cultured cells.

METHOD

In vitro study

Twelve WHHL rabbits were exposed to either 40% oxygen (hyperoxia group) or 10% oxygen (hypoxia group) for 5 hours a day, 5 days a week for 8 weeks. Four control rabbits inhaled ordinary room air. Fasting blood was collected every two weeks for the determination of plasma cholesterol and triglyceride. At the end of 8 weeks, the animals were sacrificed, using excess intravenous pentobarbital. The aortas were then isolated from their origin down to the bifurcation, incised longitudinally and stained with Sudan III for evaluation of lesion areas.

To evaluate the effect of hypoxia and hyperoxia on the collagen metabolism, hydroxyproline was measured in an intima-media preparation of WHHL rabbits by the method of Prodkop.

Cell culture study

Serum

Normolipemic rabbit serum (NRS) was obtained from male Japanese White rabbits fed a normal rabbit chow diet (ORC-4 Oriental Yeast Co. Japan). Hyperlipemic rabbit serum (HRS) was obtained from white rabbits fed a rabbit chow diet supplemented with 1% cholesterol for at least 1 month. Blood was collected from the unanesthetized rabbits by puncture of the marginal ear vein, after the rabbits were fasted overnight. Serum was obtained by centrifugation and sterilized by filtration through 0.45 µm filters (Millipore Japan, Tokyo). Serum cholesterol, triglyceride and phospholipid were measured by enzymatic methods, using Determinec TC 5 (Kyowa Hakko Kogyo, Tokyo), Triglyceride CII-Test (Wako Pure Chemical Industries, Osaka), and PL Kit-K (Nihon Shoji, Tokyo), respectively.

Preparation of lipoprotein-deficient serum (LPDS)

LPDS (d>1.21 g/ml) from NRS was isolated by ultracentifugation, as described by Havel et al. The fraction was dialysed against 0.15M NaCl-containing 0.01% ethylenediamine tetraacetic acid (EDTA), pH 7.4, and sterilized by passage through 0.45 µm filters.

Cells

The method of isolation of aortic smooth muscle cells has been described previously [3]. In brief, the thoracic aorta was removed from anesthetized 3 month-old rabbits. Then ten 2mm x 2mm intima-media segments were placed in a 25cm² Corning flask and grown in Dulbecco's modified Eagle's medium (Nissui, Tokyo) supplemented with 10% newborn calf serum (GIBCO) and $NaHCO_3$ at pH 7.4. Penicillin (100 IU/ml) and streptomycin (100 µg/ml) were routinely added to the culture media. The flasks were maintained in an incubator with humidified air and 5% CO_2 at 37°C.

LDL receptor-positive skin fibroblasts were obtained from normal Japanese White rabbits. LDL receptor-negative fibroblasts were obtained from WHHL rabbits. Cells were incubated in the same conditions and medium.

For the experiments, aortic smooth muscle cells were seeded in 35-mm plastic petri dishes at a density of 2×10^5 cells/dish. Skin fibroblasts were seeded in 60-mm plastic petri dishes at a density of 4.5×10^5 cells/dish. Cells were incubated for 2-3 days until subconfluency. After the growth medium was removed, the cells were washed once with PBS and incubated with 3 ml of medium containing LPDS (2.5 mg of protein/ml)for 24h in order to activate LDL receptors.

Then the medium was removed and 3 ml of medium containing 20% NRS or
HRS were added to each dish. The cells were transferred either to the
incubator conditioned with $20\%O_2$, $75\%N_2$, and $5\%CO_2$ (control cells) or
to the incubator with 2% or 5% O_2, 93 or $90\%N_2$, and $5\%CO_2$ (hypoxic
cells). After 48h incubation, the culture medium was removed, the
cells were rinsed twice with PBS, and harvested with 0.05%
trypsin-0.02% EDTA solution. Cells from these dishes were collected
in a conical centrifuge tube and washed three times with PBS by
repeated centrifugation. Cell counts were carried out using a
Burker-Turk hemocytometer. Cell viability was estimated by the trypan
blue exclusion test.

Cellular lipid analysis
    Lipids were extracted from the washed cell pellet using the
method of Folch et al. Namely, 1 ml of methanol was added to each
tube containing a washed cell pellet. After sonication of the cell
pellet for 1 min using the microtip of the sonifier (Sonifier B-12,
Branson Sonic Power, USA), 2 ml of chloroform were added. After
mixing and centrifugation, the clear supernatant was transferred to a
glass tube and the sediment was washed twice with 1 ml of
chloroform-methanol (2:1) mixture by repeated centrifugation (3000 rpm
for 10 min). The dry sediment was dissolved in 0.5N NaOH and an
aliquot was taken for protein determination by the method of Lowry et
al. One ml of 0.5% NaCl was added to 5 ml of crude lipid extract, and
the two liquids were mixed vigorously. After centrifugation (3000 rpm
for 10 min), the lower phase was taken for lipid analysis and an
aliquot was evaporated under reduced pressure. Free and total
cholesterol was determined by the enzymatic fluorometric method of
Heider and Boyett. The esterified cholesterol content was determined
by subtraction of free cholesterol content from that of total content.
All results were expressed per mg of cell protein.

Analysis of cholesterol metabolism
    Cholesterol synthesis was determined by measuring the amount of
[^{14}C]acetate incorporated into cholesterol. ACAT activity was
determined by measuring the incorporation of [^{14}C] oleate into the
cholesteryl ester of cells. Cholesteryl ester efflux from cells was
measured by the change of cholesteryl ester content in cells.

Statistical analysis
    All the results were expressed as mean±SD, unless specified.
Statistical significance was calculated using Student's t-test.

Results

In vitro study

    At the beginning of the study, the plasma levels of cholesterol
in WHHL rabbits were as follows: 368±16 mg/dl (mean±SE) in the
hyperoxia group, 408±42 mg/dl in the hypoxia group, and 448±53 mg/dl
in the control group. These differences were not statistically
significant. No significant fluctuations in plasma cholesterol were
observed in any of the three groups throughout the 8 weeks.
    The percentage of lesion area was 6.9±1.9 % (mean±SE) in the
hyperoxia group, 8.8±2.8% in the control group, and 11.8±0.6% in the
hypoxia group (Fig.1). The average lesion area in the hypoxia group
was significantly larger than that in the hyperoxia group (p<0.05).
The severity of the lesions was not significantly correlated with
either plasma cholesterol or triglyceride (r=0.35 and 0.36,

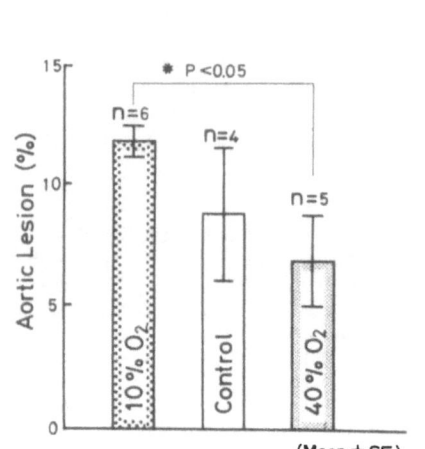

Fig.1

(Mean ± SE)

Effects of O₂ inhalation on aortic lesion.

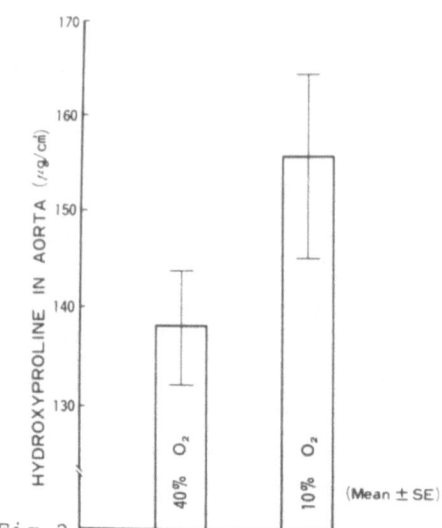

Fig.2

Effects of O₂ inhalation on aortic hydroxy-proline content in hyperlipidemic rabbits (WHHL-Rabbit).

respectively). The mean content of hydroxyproline in the aortic intima-media preparation was 155 μg/cm² for the hypoxia group and 138 μg/cm² for the hyperoxia group (Fig.2).
Lipid components of cultured normal and WHHL rabbit fibroblast.

The total cholesterol, triglyceride, and phospholipid contents of HRS were 2,200 mg/dl, 210 mg/dl, and 592 mg/dl, respectively. For NRS, the contents were 43 mg/dl, 22 mg/dl, and 57 mg/dl, respectively.
Table 1 shows the lipid contents of the control (20%O_2) and the hypoxic (2%O_2) cells after 48h incubation in the medium containing 20%NRS or 20%HRS. The esterified cholesterol levels of hypoxic cells incubated with 20%HRS were much higher than those of control cells: 2.3-fold in normal cells and 1.9-fold in WHHL cells. In NRS-containing medium, hypoxia did not promote the accumulation of either free or esterified cholesterol in the cells. The triglyceride levels of control cells in HRS-containing medium were much higher than those of cells incubated in NRS-containing medium. In the hypoxic cells, there was a much higher triglyceride accumulation.
Fig.3 shows the ratio of lipid content in hypoxic cells (2%O_2 or 5%O_2) to control cells (20%O_2). The ratios for esterified cholesterol and triglyceride increased markedly. Thus, the increased lipid contents were inversely correlated with O_2 concentrations.
In rabbit aortic smooth muscle cells incubated in NRS-containing medium, the free cholesterol content of hypoxic cells was higher than that of control cells (p<0.02). In HRS-containing medium, the free cholesterol level was 20% higher and the esterfied cholesterol 2.6-fold higher in the hypoxic cells compared to control cells (Fig.4).

Table 1   Lipid content of cultured normal and WHHL fibroblasts
           incubated with a medium containing 20% NRS or HRS under
           either control or hypoxic conditions for 48h.

	Normal fibroblasts		WHHL fibroblasts	
	$20\%O_2$	$2\%O_2$	$20\%O_2$	$2\%O_2$
Free fatty acid				
LPDS	27.7±1.3		30.5±1.8	
NRS	23.8±0.8	34.3±1.8***	27.4±0.7	39.4±1.2***
HRS	25.8±1.1	32.6±2.1**	27.4±2.3	32.9±1.2*
Triglyceride				
LPDS	9.4±1.7		9.1±0.8	
NRS	5.4±0.5	127.3±1.5***	6.6±0.2	
				113.0±5.3***
HRS	67.6±2.1	292.3±9.7***	86.0±1.0	250.3±5.7***
Free cholesterol				
LPDS	12.8±0.7		14.4±0.4	
NRS	10.7±0.1	11.2±0.4	11.5±0.4	9.5±0.3***
HRS	14.6±0.2	21.3±1.1***	15.4±1.0	19.8±1.5*
Esterified cholesterol				
LPDS	1.7±0.6		1.1±0.3	
NRS	0.6±0.2	0.7±0.7	0.4±0.4	0.9±0.2
HRS	14.4±0.8	32.5±2.3***	12.4±1.3	23.2±1.0***
Phospholipid				
LPDS	161±3		149±2	
NRS	168±4	166±2	168±4	166±3
HRS	183±5	184±7	176±3	175±2

(mean±SD)   * p<0.05, ** p<0.01, *** p<0.001

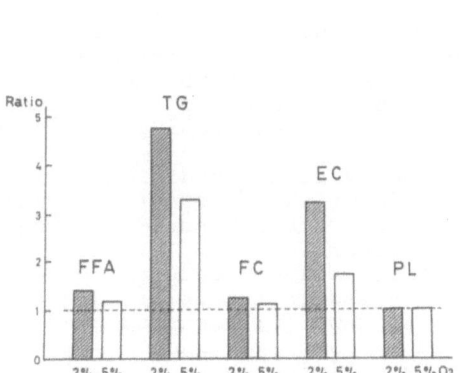

Fig.3   Lipid content ratio of Hypoxia/Normoxia in 20% hyperlipemic serum.

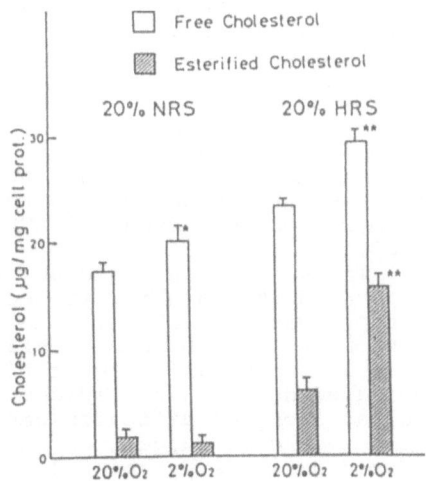

Fig.4

Cholesterol content of cultured rabbit aortic smooth muscle cells incubated with a medium containing 20% NRS or HRS under either control or hypoxic conditions for 24 h.

(* p<0.02, ** p<0.001)

Cholesterol metabolism

Hypoxia suppressed cholesterol synthesis in cells cultured in NRS-containing medium. In the HRS-containing medium, cholesterol synthesis was suppressed markedly in both control and hypoxic cells. ACAT activity was $12.1\pm2.0 \times 10^3$ cpm/mg cell protein under hypoxia and $6.1\pm0.3 \times 10^3$ cpm/mg cell protein under control conditions ($p<0.05$). These results suggest that ACAT activity is increased under hypoxic conditions.

In the preincubation period, the CE content was 59.7 ± 1.3 nmol/mg cell protein after cholesterol loading. After 24h incubation in the LPDS-containing medium, cholesterol ester decreased to 36.6 ± 6.3 nmol/mg cell protein under control conditions and 53.1 ± 3.0 nmol/mg cell protein under hypoxia ($p<0.05$). These results suggest that hypoxia suppresses the efflux of cholesteryl ester.

DISCUSSION

·Lipid accumulation in the arterial wall is one of the main features of atherosclerosis. In order to elucidate the process of atherogenesis, it is important to clarify the mechanism of lipid accumulation. Heughan et al [4] reported that in experimental atheromata oxygen tension was as low as 10 and 12 mmHg. We therefore investigated the effect of hypoxia on the development of atherosclerosis.

Kjeldsen et al[5] reported that systemic hypoxia aggravated atheroma formation, and caused an increase in lipid levels, relative to the control. In our study of WHHL rabbits, plasma cholesterol level was not differentially influenced under hypoxic vs. hyperoxic conditions. These results suggest that hypoxia has a direct effect on lipid accumulation in aortic intima. To test this hypothesis, we investigated the effect of hypoxia on lipid accumulation in cultured cells. Under these conditions, cells were free from humoral and neural regulations. The levels of lipid in the medium were the same in both hypoxic and control cells. Hypoxia accelerated cholesterol accumulation in cultured rabbit aortic smooth muscle cells incubated in HRS-containing medium. Futhermore, hypoxia enhanced the accumulations of cholesterol, triglyceride, and free fatty acid in fibroblasts. Thus hypoxia associated with hyperlipidemia appears to play an important role in atherogenesis. By cholesterol metabolism analysis, it was determined that hypoxia enhanced cholesteryl ester accumulation by increasing ACAT activity and by decreasing the efflux of CE.

Tissue hypoxia could be induced under various conditions. It is well known that smoking is one of the major risk factors for coronary atherosclerosis. The stimulatory effect of carbon monoxide on the development of atherosclerosis has been reported [6].

Talbott et al[7] reported that arterial oxygen saturation decreased during hyperlipidemia and suggested that this was due to the decreased oxygen diffusion capacity. Ishikawa [8] reported that intramyocardial oxygen tension measured by mass spectrometer was reduced during experimental exogenous hyperlipidemia and speculated that during postalimentary lipemia oxygen diffusion capacity might be reduced, thereby inducing arterial tissue hypoxia. Heistad et al [9] showed that the vasa vasorum failed to increase blood flow to the aortic wall during acute hypertension. In diabetes mellitis, polyol metabolism is accelerated and cells are exposed to hypoxic state because of the accumulation of sorbitol. It also has been suggested that the platelet mass formation on the surface of damaged vessel

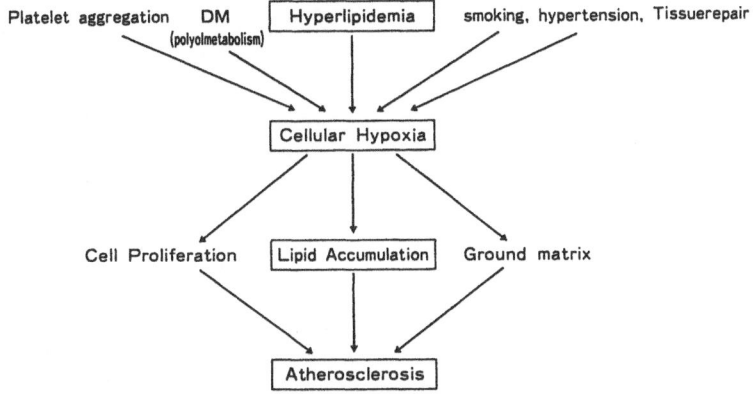

Fig.5   Hypothetical Mechanisms of Hypoxia
in Development of Atherosclerosis

walls causes local hypoxia which affects the cells beneath the thrombus.

In addition to the deleterious effects on lipid metabolism, hypoxia has other potentially atherogenic effects. Pietila et al [10] reported that the synthesis of sulphated glycosaminoglycans and hyaluronic acid was stimulated and collagen synthesis decreased by hypoxia. Kuehl et al [11] showed that at lowered oxygen tension, cell proliferation was increased in its early stages.

We conclude that tissue hypoxia enhances cholesteryl ester accumulation and promotes atherosclerosis. A proposed mechanism for hypoxia-induced atherogenesis is shown in Fig.5.

ACKNOWLEDGEMENTS

We greatly acknowledge Dr. Yoshio Watanabe for providing WHHL rabbits. We also thank Ms. Kayoko Nokihara for her secretarial assistance.

REFERENCES

[1] Geiringer E (1951) J Pathol Bacteriol 63:201.
[2] Heuper WC (1944) Arch Path 38:245.
[3] Tsukitani M, Okamoto R, Suehiro A, Hatani M, Fujino M, Imai N, Takano S, Watanabe Y,Fukuzaki H (1982) Kobe J Med Sci 28:171.
[4] Heughah C, Niinikoski J, Hunt TK (1973) Atherosclerosis 17:361.
[5] Kjeldsen K, Wanstrup J, Astrup P (1968) J Atheroscler Res 8:835.
[6] Astrup P, Kjeldsen K, Wanstrup J (1967) J Atheroscler Res 7:343.
[7] Talbott GD, Frayser R (1963) Nature 200:684.
[8] Ishikawa Y (1979) Kobe J Med Sci 25:19.
[9] Heistad DD, Marcus ML, Law EG, et al. (1978) J Clin Invest 62:133.
[10] Pietila K, Jaakkola O (1984) Atherosclerosis 50:183.
[11] Kuehl KS, Brutting SP, Singer EV, Rubio R, Bern RM (1980) Cell Tissue Res 216:591.

An Hypothesis for the Localization of Atherogenesis and Its Relationship to Endothelial Regulation and Transport

S. Weinbaum[1], R. Pfeffer[2], and S. Chien[3]

[1]Department of Mechanical Engineering, The City College of the City University of New York, New York, NY 10031, USA
[2]Department of Chemical Engineering, The City College of the City University of New York, New York, NY 10031, USA
[3]Department of Physiology, Columbia University Medical School, New York, NY 10032, USA

ABSTRACT

A new hypothesis is advanced for the localization of atherogenesis in which the initial event in the formation of a foam cell lesion is a localized increase in endothelial permeability to LDL due to transient open junctions in regions of elevated cell turnover. The new hypothesis attempts to relate this initial event to a complex sequence of reactions involving a new model for the mediation of LDL receptors on the basal side of the endothelial cell, the subsequent recruitment of monocytes and their conversion to macrophages subject to endothelial mediation and finally the migration and proliferation of smooth muscle cells in the intima.

INTRODUCTION

The two fundamental questions that have attracted the most interest in the development of an hypothesis for atherogenesis are (i) what determines the blood serum LDL-cholesterol levels in "normal" adults and (ii) why does the disease process appear to have a predilection for certain specific sites near bifurcations and other regions where flow reversal and separation is anticipated in the major arteries. The pioneering research of Brown and Goldstein [1] has provided considerable insight into the first question over the past decade. These investigators through an ingenious series of experiments with cultured human fibroblasts were able to identify and determine the genetic structure of a high affinity receptor protein for LDL and demonstrate the competing intracellular regulatory mechanisms that determined the population of the receptors and the intracellular metabolism of the LDL.

While the studies of Brown and Goldstein summarized in [1] directly explain the very early development of atherosclerosis in the small fraction (less than one percent) of the adult human population with greatly elevated blood serum LDL levels (in excess of 300 mg/dl) that result from receptor defects associated with the genetic disease, familial hypercholesterolemia, it has long been a puzzling issue why only a 25 percent change in blood LDL levels from 150 to 200 mg/dl can cause a more than five fold increase in risk for the development of the disease in the population at large and a 14 fold increase at 250 mg/dl. The new hypothesis proposed herein shall attempt to explain how the regulation of the subendothelial lipid environment by the endothelial layer might provide a sensitive detection system via which relatively small changes in blood LDL levels cited above can lead to such a large increase in incidence of the disease and also provide an explanation to the second question concerning the localization of atherogenesis.

It is generally recognized that there are three principal events in the early formation of lesions; the accumulation of intimal lipid, the proliferation of smooth muscle cells (SMC) and the appearance of macrophages in the subendothelial space. These events are associated with a complicated sequence of mechanisms involving the transendothelial transport of LDL, the lipid metabolism of the various cellular components of the intima, the release of various chemotactic agents and growth factors and the possible modification of LDL in the subendothelial space. While individual processes have been examined in depth the relationship between the events and the various mechanisms has remained a mystery and in some cases the experimental observations have been contrary to one's intuition. A classic example is the well known experiment by Minick et al. [2] to study dietary induced lesions following endothelial denudation. The endothelium has commonly been viewed as the principal barrier to the entry of lipid yet in these diet fed animals the lesions formed under the leading edge of the reendothelialized regions and in the central areas where the endothelium was still denuded there was SMC proliferation but no lipid accumulation.

The most commonly accepted causitive mechanism for the focal nature of the disease is the "response to injury" hypothesis formulated by Ross and coworkers [3]. This hypothesis initially placed a strong emphasis on local denuding injury to the endothelium as the initial event, since the attachment of platelets at the site of the injury and the release of platelet derived growth factor (PDGF) were the primary mechanisms in the initial lesion formation and it is well recognized that platelets will not attach to an intact endothelium. The hypothesis has recently undergone a major modification [4] in light of extensive experiments that have conclusively shown that overt endothelial denudation is seldom seen in early lesion formation [5] and platelets do not normally attach to an intact endothelium. Ross [4] now suggests that a more subtle form of endothelial injury must be present and that growth factors released by other cellular components, as opposed to PDGF, may play a primary role.

The new hypothesis described herein shall attempt to build on the modified model in [4] by establishing the relationship between four main areas of research: (i) the new model proposed by Weinbaum and coworkers [6] for the ultrastructural correlate of the large pore and the relationship of endothelial cell turnover to local variations in macromolecular permeability, (ii) the Brown and Goldstein model [1] for fibroblasts as applied to the lipid metabolism of the intimal cells, (iii) the work of Steinberg and coworkers [7] on the localization of LDL degradation and (iv) the role of the macrophage in early lesion formation.

THE LOCALIZATION MECHANISM

A new hypothesis for the ultrastructural correlate of the large pore has been proposed by the authors that has important implications for the focal origin of atherogenesis [6]. It was suggested that the regional variations in macromolecular permeability might be associated with normal cell turnover and transient openings in the intercellular junctions of either dying or newly replicated endothelial cells. This idea was motivated by a number of experiments summarized in [6] which have shown that there is a close spatial correlation between regions of enhanced cell turnover and increases in endothelial permeability to Evans blue labeled albumin and a variety of radioactively labeled tracer molecules including LDL. Since at any given time less than one percent of all endothelial cells are involved in turnover and the cross plane area of the clefts of these cells occupies less than 1 in 10^5 of the endothelial surface, the quantitative feasibility of this hypothesis required careful examination. A series of mathematical models of increasing sophistication were developed to predict the steady state and time dependent permeability and uptake behavior that should be anticipated according to this hypothesis. Specially designed experiments were then performed to test these predictions in the laboratory of Dr. S. Chien. The latest version of the model [8] is shown schematically in fig. 1. The artery wall is broken into a periodic array of units in which each unit contains one cell with a transient open junction, shown shaded, at its center. In the initial version of the model in [6] the finite resistance of the open cleft was neglected, the large non-isotropy in the diffusional resistance

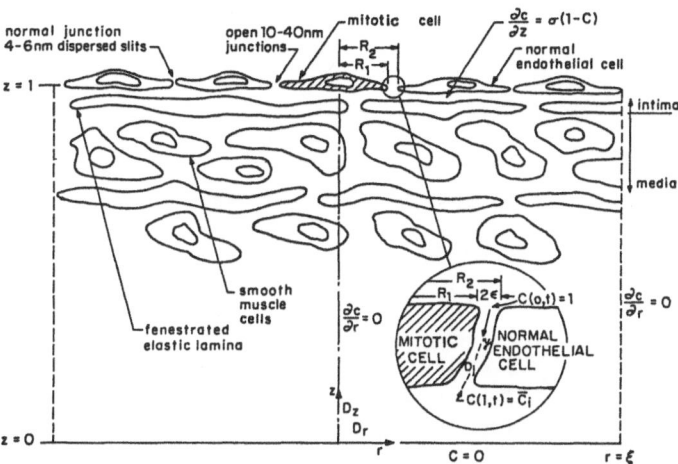

Fig. 1 Schematic of periodic unit in model for the artery wall where shaded endothelial cell at origin has transient open junction.

in the r and z directions due to the presence of the elastic lamina was not considered and the background flux through the remaining endothelium was ascribed to vesicular transport. Recent serial section electron microscopic reconstructions and transport studies with cationized ferritin strongly indicate that the plasmalemma vesicles do not shuttle across the cell's cytoplasm and serve this transport function. These deficiencies are accounted for in the new model [8] by introducing a separate diffusion coefficient for the open cleft D_j, different diffusion coefficients D_r and D_z for each medial direction and, replacing vesicular transport by an intermediate size pore that is formed by small breaks (4-6 nm dispersed slits) in the intramembraneous protein strands of the normal junctional complexes. This pore allows for the restricted passage of albumin and other small proteins.

Fig. 2 shows the predictions of the model in [8] for the subendothelial concentration distribution in the intima at different nondimensional times (t = .001 corresponds to roughly one minute for an artery wall of 0.2 mm thickness), when one cell in 200 has a fully open 20 nm cleft and labeled albumin is used as the tracer molecule. One observes that for short enough times t < .01 (10 minutes) there is a clearly definable elevation in concentration that is confined to a relatively small region beneath and surrounding the cell in question. One should easily be able to observe these isolated leakage sites optically if they existed. (The spikes at the cleft exit are beyond the resolution of light microscopy). The theory also predicts that for larger times the much more rapid diffusion in the r as opposed to the z direction due to the presence of the first elastic lamina (this is particularly evident for D_r/D_z = 100) would quickly lead to a filling of the entire subendothelial space and thus make it difficult to distinguish the localized leaks from the background labeling. Localized hot spots suggestive of this behavior have recently been reported in [9] where 200 μm brown reaction foci were observed for short duration (1 min.) uptake studies using HRP as the tracer molecule. They are not observable in traditional uptake studies using light microscopy where the labeling period is typically 15 minutes or longer.

The reaction foci observed in [9] are obviously much larger than a single cell, but the new theory has been instrumental in defining a time window and probe molecule size for the design of a prototype experiment in which the time dependent growth of such localized leakage sites could systematically be studied if they existed. A typical enface micrograph after one minute labeling

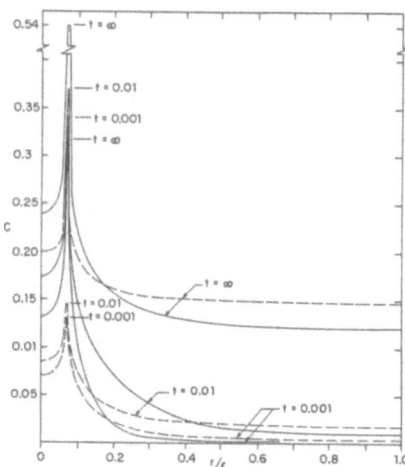

Fig. 2 Time dependent subendothelial concentration distribution for albumin. $D_j/D_z = 87.5$.
Dashed curves $D_r/D_z = 100$; solid curves $D_r/D_z = 10$.

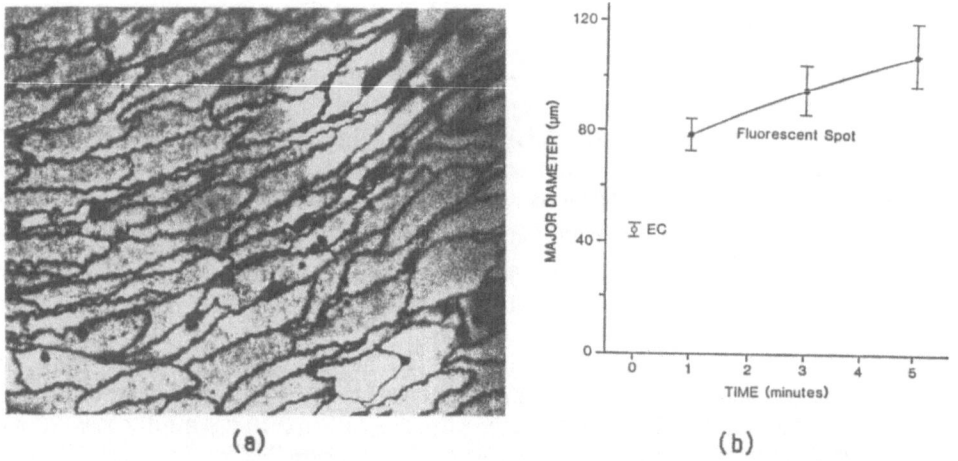

        (a)   (b)

FIGS. 3 (a,b) (a) Enface micrograph of rat thoracic aorta one minute after the introduction of
FITC albumin. Cell borders are stained with silver nitrate. (b) Time dependent growth of average
fluorescent spot diameter. The major diameter of the endothelial cell is shown for comparison.
(courtesy Dr. K. M. Jan).

using FITC albumin is shown in Fig. 3a where the cell borders are delineated using silver nitrate
stain. Two leakage sites are noted, each slightly larger than two cells. The time dependent growth
of the leakage sites has been monitored using both enface and cross-sectional micrographs. These
results are shown in fig. 3b.
      When the new hypothesis for the large pore was first introduced in [6] little was known
about the state of the endothelial junctions during cell turnover. This is important in
understanding the basic leakage mechanism. If the leakage occured during the process of cell death
when the cell was in the process of being sloughed off by its neighbors one should be able to detect

this by performing a painstaking labeling experiment in which one simultaneously identifies a dead or dying cell in the endothelial population (the plasmalemma of these cells are permeable to small probe molecules) and determines the integrity of its junctions. These experiments, which have been performed by Dr. M. Lee and are reported in [8], have shown that the junctions of these cells do not readily permit the passage of HRP in short time labeling studies of the order of a minute. Equivalent direct evidence is not yet available for the state of the junctions in newly replicated cells; however, the results in fig. 3(b) provide a valuable indirect clue. If the curve is extrapolated back to zero time one finds that the fluorescent spot has an initial area which is very close to that of two cells. This indicates that the leakage occurs shortly after cell division when the two daughter cells are contiguous and suggests that the junctional strands of these newly replicated cells may be incomplete. A reasonable conjecture is that that the two daughter cells must initially share the complement of junctional proteins provided by the parent cell until their own protein synthesizing apparatus has provided sufficient new proteins to form a mature junction. Based on the time scale for the synthesis of other membrane proteins, e.g. the LDL receptor [1], this formation process could last from 8 to 24 hours. These questions are currently under further study.

Another important prediction of the theoretical model is the change in steady state local endothelial permeability to macromolecules due to regional variations in cell turnover. In [6] it was first shown that 50 to 100 percent increases in permeability could result when the cell turnover rate doubled in the physiologically meaningful range .001 to .01. The revised non-isotropic model in [8] predicts results which are of the same order, but with somewhat higher increases in permeability due to the enhanced lateral diffusion in the r direction. These predictions are in close correspondence with experimental observations. While the possibility that regional variations in cell turnover account for focal regions of enhanced macromolecular permeability is a very attractive hypothesis, it does not explain the localization of diet induced lesions and the apparent distribution of permeability observed in the healing wound experiments of Minick et al. [2] mentioned earlier. This apparent paradox will be explained in the new hypothesis by examing the cellular LDL degradation pattern in the artery wall and other possible roles the endothelium may play in the formation of the early lesion.

THE DISTRIBUTION OF LDL DEGRADATION IN THE ARTERY WALL

The research of Steinberg, Carew and Pittman described in [7] has been instrumental in distinguishing the degraded intracellular lipid pool from the total lipid uptake (both intracellular and extracellular) and determining the spatial distribution of the degradation within arterial wall tissue. In the early studies of these investigators an LDL molecule tagged with ^{14}C-sucrose was developed to quantify the irreversible lysosomal degradation of LDL in various body organs, such as the liver, spleen and adrenals. This same principle was then applied to the artery wall except that the specific activity of artery wall catabolism is two orders of magnitude smaller than organs like the liver and adrenals where large amounts of LDL need to be degraded since these organs need free cholesterol for the production of hormones. To this end a much more sensitive tagged LDL molecule was developed, radioionidated tyramine cellobiose LDL.

In a series of studies using TC LDL these researchers were able to show the relative and absolute amounts of the lysosomal degradation in the intima and media of a rabbit aorta and also the fraction of the total LDL flux into the aortic wall that was catabolized by its cellular components. The results indicated that (i) the total amount of receptor mediated degradation was comparable in the intima and media but that on a per unit volume basis the activity of the intima was nearly 50 fold larger, (ii) the rate of influx of LDL across the endothelium was much larger than the total rate of degradation and hence most of the LDL that entered the intima was transported by diffusion and convection across the artery wall and exited at the adventitial surface. Carew also observed that in cholesterol fed rabbits the surface pattern of fatty lesion formation around the ostia of the intercostal arteries as they branch from the aorta as indicated by a non-specific Sudan IV stain for lipid was virtually identical to the pattern observed for the degradation of TC LDL after only 24 hours of labeling. One thus concludes that the slow long time gradual accumulation of lipid in the intracellular pool clearly overshadows the interstitial extracellular lipid concentration. However, it would seem reasonable based on the Brown and Goldstein model [1] for the native LDL receptor that the interstitial LDL concentration plays a critical role in determining at any given moment how much LDL will be entering the cellular components of the arterial intima and media.

The experiments just described do not identify just which cells in the intima are performing the degradation. More recent studies using autoradiographic grain counts indicate that in these cholesterol fed rabbits most of the degradation was occuring in a layer of macrophage type foam cells, one to two cells deep, that completely underlies the endothelial cell layer [10]. Furthermore, Carew had also performed preliminary experiments following the protocol of Minick [2] using the balloon catheter injury. These experiments showed that the pattern of fatty lesions which had formed under the leading edge of reendothelialized regions following the partial healing closely corresponded to the surface pattern observed for the localization of the degradation of the TC LDL and that significant degradation did not occur in areas which were still denuded although there was significant SMC proliferation.

THE NEW HYPOTHESIS FOR THE LOCALIZATION OF ATHEROGENESIS

The combined evidence summarized herein has been used to formulate an overall hypothesis for the formation of the intial lesion. This is outlined below.

(1) Regional variations in endothelial permeability to macromolecules are associated with local enhancement in cell turnover in regions of low blood shear where flow reversal is encountered. The large pore through which the LDL molecule is assumed to enter are transient open junctions around newly formed daughter cells where the junctional strands are hypothesized to be incomplete following mitosis. This arises from the initial sharing of junctional proteins of the parent cell and the finite time it takes to synthesize the missing proteins.

(2) The sensitivity of the endothelial cell as a detector of small changes in its subendothelial environment is due to the large asymmetry in the loading of the LDL receptors on the blood and tissue sides. The theoretical model in Fig.1 predicts that for normal cell turnover the subendothelial LDL concentration on the tissue side is approximately 1 µg/dl and thus less than the saturation level of 2 µg/dl observed for the optimal functioning of the receptor pathway in human fibroblasts and also significantly less than the level at the adventitial surface due to the effects of convection. Since all receptor sites on the luminal plasmalemma are occupied at normal blood serum levels, the endothelial cell responds primarily to changes in its subendothelial LDL concentration. In regions of high cell turnover increases in LDL permeability are, therefore, readily detected by the endothelial cell. The studies of Reckless et al. [11] have shown that the endothelial cell expresses a high affinity receptor for LDL but the rates of uptake followed by degradation are very low. We thus conjecture that the importance of the endothelium in the lipid metabolism of the intima is not to catabolize LDL but to serve as the detection system for evaluating and responding to the subendothelial LDL concentration.

(3) Local increases in LDL permeability have two important consequences. First, once the LDL pathway is fully downregulated due to the saturation of abluminal LDL receptors the endothelial cell is unable to respond on its own to further increases in its subendothelial lipid environment. Second, the endothelial cell sends out a distress signal to circulating monocytes which causes them to adhere in these localized regions. Faggiotto et al. [5] have observed the adhesion of monocytes within a period of 12 days after the primates were put on a high cholesterol diet. These monocytes are recruited to restore normal subendothelial LDL levels in regions of high LDL permeability since the endothelial cells are incapable of doing this themselves. The fact that macrophages are

present only where the endothelium has regrown in Minick's experiments strongly suggests that the endothelium is the origin of the chemotactic signals for the recruitment of monocytes. The release of the chemoattractant could be associated with endothelial cell replication or an unwanted increase in the cellular free cholesterol content.

(4) Monocytes are able to penetrate the endothelial cell layer in junctional regions through pseudopod motion and thereafter enter the intima. Monocytes do not possess the apoprotein B 100 receptor for LDL and thus the LDL must first be modified before it can be internalized by the monocytes if they are to function as a macrophage for the LDL. Henriksen et al [12] has observed that macrophages when incubated with endothelial cells in culture are able to modify LDL in a manner which enables the macrophages to degrade the LDL 4 to 5 times faster than native LDL. This scavenger receptor for EC modified LDL does not appear to be regulated like the native LDL receptor and thus the macrophage should be capable of consuming vast amounts of modified LDL and storing it in esterified form. It has recently been found that LDL when exposed to macrophages in culture is oxidized and that this oxidized LDL can be noxious to skin cells. Such behavior in vivo could be a further mechanism for increasing the turnover rate of the endothelium.

(5) There are two lipid pools, an extracellular pool of primarily native LDL and an intracellular pool of degraded LDL that is stored in the cell primarily as cholesterol oleate. The lipid level of extracellular LDL is very low compared to the latter, even in regions of high cell turnover or overt denudation. The principal intracellular depository for degraded lipid is the macrophage since this cell, in contrast to the endothelial cell and SMC, is not able to regulate its LDL receptor number.

(6) The migration of SMC into the intima and their proliferation, is not due to platelet derived growth factor PDGF, but to growth factors and chemoattractants that are released by either the endothelial cells or the macrophages. Both these cells have been demonstrated in tissue culture to release growth factors that closely resemble PDGF. The entrainment of SMC and their replication is a normal reparative response. Their presence in the growing lesion may therefore be only a secondary passive response to the primary injury sequence summarized in (1) to (5) above.

This research is supported by an NSF "Creativity Award" ENG 85-00301 and NIH grant HL-19454.

REFERENCES

1. Brown MS, Goldstein JL (1984) Scientific. Am. **251**, 58-66
2. Minick CR, Stemerman MB, Insull Jr. W (1977) Proc. Natl. Acad. Sci. **74**, 1724-1728
3. Ross R, Glomset JA (1976) N. Engl. J. Med. **295**, 369-377
4. Ross R (1986) N. Engl. J. Med. **314**, 488-500
5. Faggiatto A, Ross R, Harker L (1984) Arteriosclerosis, **4**, 323-340
6. Weinbaum S, Tzeghai G, Ganatos P, Pfeffer R, Chien S (1985) Am J. Physiol. **248**, H945-H960.
7. Steinberg D (1983) Arteriosclerosis **3**, 283-301
8. Weinbaum S, Wen GB, Ganatos P, Pfeffer R, Lee M, Chien S (1987) "On Transient Diffusion of Macromolecules Through Leaky Junctions and their Subendothelial Spread" J. Theor. Biol., in review.
9. Stemerman MB, Morrel EM, Burke KR, Colton CK, Smith KA, Lees RS (1986) Arteriosclerosis, **6**, 64-70
10. Steinberg D, Pittman RC, Carew TE (1985) Annals New York Acad. Sci., Atherosclerosis, ed. K. T. Lee, **454**, 195-206
11. Reckless JPD, Weinstein DB, Steinberg D (1978) Biochim. Biophys. Acta, **529**, 475-487
12. Henriksen T, Mahoney EM, Steinberg D (1983) Arteriosclerosis **3**, 149-159

Models of Endothelial Cell Junctions

R. Skalak

Bioengineering Institute, Department of Civil Engineering and Engineering Mechanics,
Columbia University, New York, NY 10027, USA

ABSTRACT

This paper reviews some recent theoretical models of endothelial cell
junctions and transport of fluid through the clefts. The classical
system of small and large pores is replaced by a system of slits. It
is postulated that the uniform spacing of 200 Å is maintained by
macromolecules which bridge between two cell membranes. Such
bridging molecules could maintain the observed cell spacing without
causing a major increase in flow resistance. The molecular forces at
tight junctions account for the bending of cell membranes and
discontinuities in the tight junctions leave tortuous pathways
allowing passage of solutes up to the size of albumin.

INTRODUCTION

Endothelial cell junctions provide a mechanical function of
keeping the endothelial cell layer intact, and on a finer scale, form
a selective barrier to the movement of fluid and macromolecules thru
the clefts. The latter function of providing a selective
permeability has been extensively explored experimentally and can be
described as a system of small pores through which fluid can pass and
larger pores which allow selective passage of macromolecules.
Several excellent reviews summarize data and theory [1,2,3].
However, the ultrastructural details of the endothelial cell layer
which correspond to the various sizes of pores is still undergoing
clarification. One aspect of these developments is the role of
transendothelial transport by vesicles. It has been shown that most
vesicles are attached directly, or through a chain of vesicles, to
the surfaces of endothelial cells so that there are few free vesicles
available for transport [4,5]. Consequently, the role of vesicles in
transendothelial transport is probably small and more attention has
been focused again on the structure and function of the endothelial
cell junctions [6,7]. In particular, more structural detail and
theoretical modeling of the role of tight junctions in the
endothelial cell clefts have suggested that non-uniformity in space
and time may be important to observed permeabilities.

The basic geometry of the endothelial cleft in cross-section is
a remarkably uniform spacing of about 200 Å for most of its length
with short regions of closer apposition of the adjacent cell
membranes at the tight junctions. The strands of intramembranous
proteins which form the connections at tight juctions have been shown
to be discontinuous, leaving tortuous paths through the endothelial
cell junctions, winding between the tight junction segments. This
spatial inhomogeneity provides possible paths corresponding to small
pores allowing passage of fluid and small molecules only, through the

spatial inhomogeneity provides possible paths corresponding to small pores allowing passage of fluid and small molecules only, through the tight junctions, and larger molecules up to size of albumin through the tortuous paths which circumvent the tight junctions. For the largest pores, allowing passage of larger macromolecules, it has been suggested [8] that transient opening of the cell junctions during death and replacement of individual endothelial cells may be the principle pathway. This is an inhomogeneity in time and a comparatively rare event so it could be expected to be difficult to demonstrate directly in electron-microscopic sections.

In theoretical models of flow through the endothelial clefts, it is most often assumed that they may be represented as a slit with a two-dimensional Poiseuille flow at each cross-section [6,9], An alternative view is that the wider parts of the clefts are filled by a fibrous network which controls the selectivity of the endothelium with respect to molecular size [7]. Such a network is not seen in the usual electron-microscopic sections, but cytochemical methods have established that endothelial cells have a glycocalyx layer at least on the lumenal surface of the cell. Another reason to anticipate that there is some connection across the uniform (200 Å) gap that appears in electron-microscopic section of endothelial cell clefts is that this spacing must be maintained by some regular system of molecular forces.

The mechanical functions of the endothelial cell are less well explored than the permeability properties. To begin with, the normal spacing of 200 Å requires some explanation in terms of forces involved because this spacing is quite uniform even though the surfaces of two cells are wrinkled and convoluted (Fig. 1). Since the cells themselves are fairly stiff and the pressure in the cleft probably varies from arterial pressure to some lower value, the forces holding the cleft spacing uniform must be quite large and stiff.

A mathematical model of the uniform spacing of cell membranes as well as tight junctions can be based on the electrostatic repulsions,

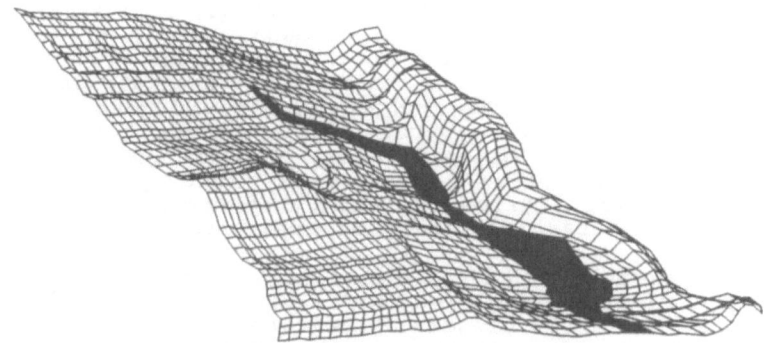

Fig. 1   A portion of the surface of an endothelial cell junction reconstructed from serial sections. The darkly shaded pportion is the area of tight junction formation which is discontinuous, as shown.   (Personal communication from Drs. Shu Chien and Nihat Ozkaya).

van der Waal forces and membrane bending stiffness [9]. The forces
due to the protein strands at tight junctions interacting with the
bending stiffness of the membrane can be shown to reproduce shapes
similar to those observed in electron micrograph sections. The
normal gap width of approximately 200 Å can also be shown as an
equilibrium between van der Waal forces and electrostatic repulsions
[9]. However such an equilibrium would be relatively easily upset
and a pressure range of the order of 50mmHg would produce a
noticeably wider gap width whereas the actual clefts appear to be
quite uniform in their spacing. It is therefore suggested [10] that
the normal spacing is maintained by a sparsely distributed system of
macromolecules which bridge from one cell to the other. It can be
shown that such a system is possible with little influence on the
pressure drop due to fluid flow through the cleft. These models are
still in an early stage of development and their predictions and
confirmation by experimental observation in different situations
needs further exploration.

Another aspect of the endothelial cell junctions which is not
very well explored is the mechanical strength and mechanisms by which
the endothelial cell layer maintains its mechanical integrity. The
stress required to separate two endothelial cells joining at a cleft
has not been measured directly. If bridging macromolecules are
present some rupture strength of their bonds must determine the
extent of the normal endothelial cleft. It may be anticipated that
the tight junctions provide an increased strength over that of the
normal gap width. No measurements or theory of such ultimate
strengths are available. These factors may enter into considerations
where the endothelial cell layer is injured or mechanically
removed. Mechanical considerations of the endothelial cell layer as
a whole will also involve the properties of the cytoplasm and the
cytoskeleton within the endothelial cell. There are some
measurements of the properties of individual endothelial cells, but
the range of such properties, their variation when the cells are
changing form or dividing and other conditions of interest are not
known at this time.

SLIT MODELS

In most theoretical models of the endothelial cell junctions,
the clefts are assumed to be slits containing only fluid. The tight
junctions are represented as narrowed portions as shown in Fig. 2A.
The exact geometry (shape) of the narrowed portion is not important,
but the resistance depends on the minimum width and its effective
length primarily. In any case, a variable width of slit can be
replaced by a slit of uniform width which has the same overall
resistance [6]. A complication arises when the tortuous paths around
the tight junctions are considered. These pathways have a different
(wider) effective width and must be considered as paths in parallel
to those passing directly through the tight junctions. Such multiple
path theories are not yet fully developed and may also help to
explain the selectivity observed with respect to molecular size
[2,3].

A further complication arises when considering the interaction
of the endothelial cell layer and the underlying tissue,
particularly, the arterial walls. The pressure drop across the
endothelial layer depends on the resistance offered by the arterial
wall which is in series with the endothelial cleft resistance.

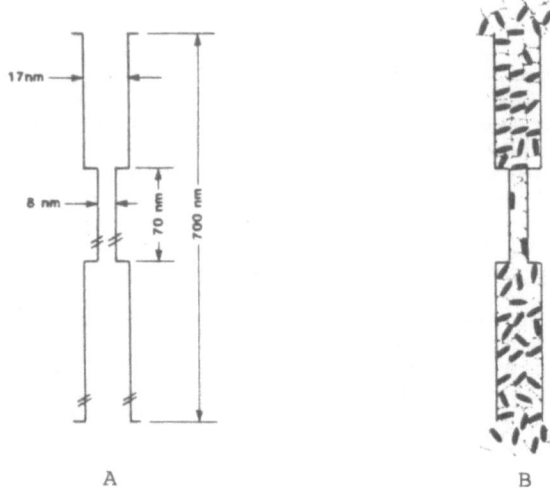

A   B

Fig. 2 Two models of the molecular ultrafilter at the capillary
wall. A. The molecular filter is assumed to be a narrow
constriction within the channel. The slit is drawn using mean values
of cleft geometry in the frog mesenteric capillary. Similar
structures have been proposed for the junctions in mammalian
continuous capillaries. The slit is 17 nm wide except for the
constriction (7-8 nm wide), which occupies 10% of the cleft depth.
B. The molecular filter is assumed to be a network of fibrous
molecules. The fiber matrix is contained within the wide part of the
channel and consists of fibers 0.6 nm in radius to which albumin
molecules are absorbed. (From Curry [7] by permission)

However, at the abluminal side of the endothelial cell layer, the
fluid flow is concentrated at the cell junctions and hence cannot be
a uniform flow in the arterial wall. A transition zone just below
the endothelium results through which the flow is more evenly
distributed. This transition zone is of the order of the endothelial
cell dimensions in thickness [6]. In this analysis the arterial wall
is assumed to behave as a porous medium. The arterial wall
permeability is probably larger in the lateral directions, compared
to the radial direction. This distorts the flow pattern, but the
qualitative behavior will remain the same. Slit theories are
amenable to extensive and precise analysis, but the critical
questions remaining are of experimental nature, namely, what is the
effective minimum width that properly represents a tight junction and
whether or not a fiber matrix exists in the endothelial cleft which
obstructs flow more than Poiseuille flow predicts.

THE FIBER MATRIX MODEL

Consideration of various capillary beds and the variation of
solute permeability for various size solutes, has led to the
suggestion that the wide part of the endothelial cleft is filled with
a fiber matrix [7]. Figure 2B shows a schematic diagram of the
endothelial cleft with the fiber matrix as a opposed to an open slit
with a tight junction narrowed portion in Figure 2A. One reason for
suggesting this model is that an equivalent pore radius which
describes the selectivity of the capillary wall to intermediate size
solutes is smaller than the equivalent pore radius described by

hydraulic conductivity. Another reason is that when different beds are considered (e.g. frog mesentery and muscle) the hydraulic conductivity may vary by a factor of ten while the selectivity or reflection coefficient for various size of solutes remains relatively constant. The fiber matrix theory allows independent control of the hydraulic permeability and the selectivity to various size solutes. The permeability is dependent upon the area available in the cross section of the endothelial clefts which are open. The implication is that the presence of tight junctions reduces the available area. The selectivity to various size molecules is assumed to be controlled by the size and distribution of a network of fibrous molecules within the wide part of the junction. This provides a system in which transport may be modulated by charge and specific chemical interactions also [7]. The primary manner in which the fiber matrix provides selectivity is by steric hindrance. The measured permeability in frog mesenteric capillaries have been interpreted in terms of a matrix consisting of fibers of 0.6 nm radius and occupying 5% of the endothelial cleft volume. Computations show that such a matrix would restrict the movement of albumin to the same extent as a cylindrical pore 5.5 nm in radius and at the same time provide a hydraulic resistance equivalent to a cylindrical pore 8 nm in radius. Moreover it is shown that the theoretical values of the reflection coefficient for molecules varying from 0.5 nm to 3.5 nm is more realistically predicted by the fiber matrix model particularly in the range of 2 nm or more solute radius. The fiber matrix theory has thus been shown to be consistent with a wide variety of experimental data. However it remains to demonstrate the structural details and chemical composition of the hypothesized fiber matrix.

STRUCTURAL MODELS OF THE ENDOTHELIAL CLEFT

A model which can maintain the uniform spacing of membranes in an endothelial cleft has been developed assuming bridging molecules which connect the membranes in an array of posts [10]. Each macromolecular link is assumed to have a single chain core which can develop a tensile force τ_p in a partially coiled position. Further, it is assumed there are fixed negative charges on side chains of the core chain. These fixed charges result in a cylindrical region around the core in which an increased pressure Δp results due to the Donnan effect. This pressure tends to separate the membranes and this tendency is resisted by the tensile force τ_p. The numerical estimates of these forces are important to the concept of how such a system will behave. For single molecule posts spaced at 200 Å , the net stiffness of the system is high, yielding a stiffness of the order of 10 mmHg per 1 Å of displacement (increase in cell spacing). Thus, the electrostatic, van der Waal and pressure forces due to fluids and intracellular pressures would have small effects on the membranes spacing. This could account for the very uniform spacing observed. It can be shown that at a 200 Å spacing, the bending of the cell membrane between posts should also be small. Another aspect of concern is the increase in pressure drop due to the presence of the posts when there is fluid flow in the clefts.

The pressure drop due to a distributed system of macromolecules connecting the membranes of an endothelial cell cleft can be estimated from an idealized model. Consider an array of circular posts of radius "a" spanning between two membranes spaced 2h apart as shown in Fig. 3A. The mean pressure drop ($\partial p / \partial x$) due to slow flow of a viscous fluid at mean velocity U in the x direction has been

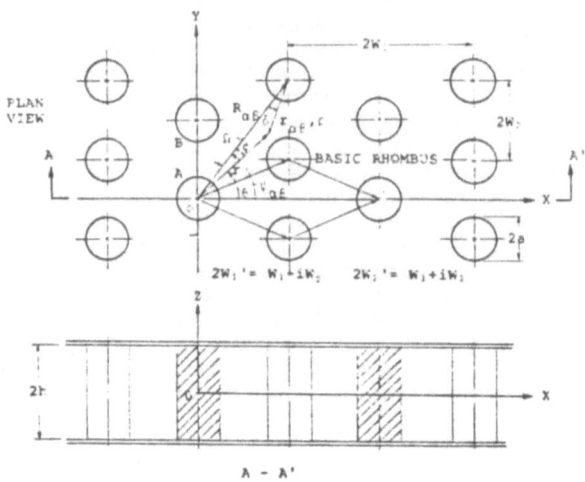

A

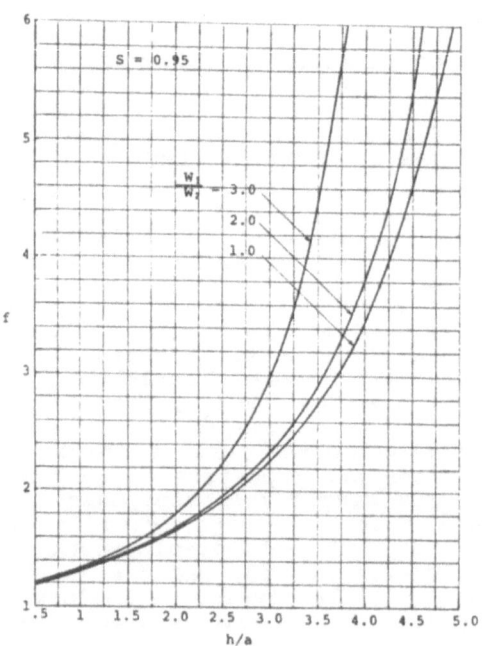

B

Fig. 3 A. Regular array of circular solid posts between parallel plates. B. Pressure drop factor f (Eq. 1) for fluid flow through arrays arranged as shown in (A). (From "Mechanics of Endothelial Cell Junctions" C.C. Hsuing, Doctoral Dissertation, Columbia University, New York, 1983, by permission).

derived from solutions of the Stokes flow equations. The results can be expressed in the form

$$\frac{\partial p}{\partial x} = \frac{3 \mu U}{h^2} f \qquad (1)$$

where U is the mean velocity of the flow, μ is the viscosity of the fluid and f is a dimensionless factor which depends on the solidity ratio S, and on the ratios (h/a) and (W_1/W_2), (see Fig. 3). The solidity ratio is the fraction of the total area in plan that is occupied by fluid:

$$S = 1 - \frac{\pi a^2}{2W_1 W_2} \qquad (2)$$

The factor f is the ratio of the pressure drop with the posts present to the pressure drop at the same mean velocity in the absence of posts (Poiseuille flow). The variation of f with (h/a) for S=0.95 and various values of (W_1/W_2) is shown in Fig. 3B. It can be seen that if the post width to membrane spacing ratio is unity (h/a = 1), then the increase in pressure drop over that due to an unobstructed Poiseuille flow is about 30% (f=1.3). If the cell spacing is large (h/a >> 1), then the percentage of the pressure drop due to the posts increases because the pressure drop due to Poiseuille decreases as h increases. In the endothelial cell junctions, it is anticipated that h/a would be of order unity so that the increase in pressure due to 5% (by volume) of posts would be less than a factor of two.

REFERENCES

[1]Curry FE (1984) Mechanics and thermodynamics of transcapillary exchange. In: Renkin EM, Michel CC (eds) Handbook of Physiology Vol. IV, The Microcirculation, Sec. 2: The Cardiovascular System. Amer. Physiol. Soc., Bethesda, pp 375-409
[2]Michel CC (1984) Fluid movements through capillary walls. In: Renkin EM, Michel CC (eds) Handbook of Physiology Vol. IV, The Microcirculation, Sec. 2: The Cardiovascular System. Amer. Physiol. Soc., Bethesda, pp 375-409
[3]Taylor AE, Granger DN (1984) Exchange of macro-molecules across the microcirculation. In: Renkin EM, Michel CC (eds) Handbook of Physiology Vol.IV, The Microcirculation, Sec. 2: The Cardiovascular System. Amer. Physiol. Soc., Bethesda, pp 467-520
[4]Bundgaard M, Frokjaer - Jensen J (1982) Microvasc. Res. 23: 1-30
[5]Chien S, Laufer L, Handley DA (1982) J. Ultrastruc. Res. 79: 198-206
[6]Tzeghai G, Weinbaum S, Pfeffer R (1985) J. Biomech. Engrg. 107: 123-130
[7]Curry FE (1986) Circ. Res. 59: 367-380
[8]Weinbaum S, Tzeghai G, Ganatos P, Pfeffer R, Chien S (1985) Am. J. Physiol. 248: H945-H960
[9]Hsuing CC, Skalak R (1984) Biorheology 21: 207-221
[10]Silberberg A, Skalak R (1987) Passage of macromolecules and solvent through clefts between endothelial cells: Conditions controlling cleft patency. Fourth World Congress for Microcirculation, Tokyo, Abstracts, p 340.

Subject Index